METHODS IN MOLECULAR BIOLOGY

Series Editor
John M. Walker
School of Life and Medical Sciences
University of Hertfordshire
Hatfield, Hertfordshire, AL10 9AB, UK

For further volumes:
http://www.springer.com/series/7651

Malaria Vaccines

Methods and Protocols

Edited by

Ashley M. Vaughan

Center for Infectious Disease Research, Seattle, WA, USA

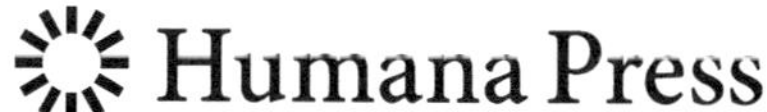

Editor
Ashley M. Vaughan
Center for Infectious Disease Research
Seattle, WA, USA

ISSN 1064-3745 ISSN 1940-6029 (electronic)
Methods in Molecular Biology
ISBN 978-1-4939-2814-9 ISBN 978-1-4939-2815-6 (eBook)
DOI 10.1007/978-1-4939-2815-6

Library of Congress Control Number: 2015945589

Springer New York Heidelberg Dordrecht London

Printed on acid-free paper

Humana Press is a brand of Springer
Springer Science+Business Media LLC New York is part of Springer Science+Business Media (www.springer.com)

Preface

The most effective way to control and ultimately eliminate an infectious disease is through vaccination. Man has successfully eliminated small pox with this ingenious strategy but other diseases are proving harder to eradicate, even when highly effective vaccines do exist. Malaria is caused by the eukaryotic pathogen parasite *Plasmodium*, and to date no efficacious vaccine against any eukaryotic pathogen is widely available. Nevertheless seminal studies in the 1960s showed the power of immunity in controlling malaria disease. In 1961 Sydney Cohen and colleagues showed that the passive transfer of gamma immunoglobulin from adults living in areas of high malaria endemicity to young children with severe malaria disease could help eliminate parasites from the blood. This study clearly demonstrated the ability of humoral immunity to control severe disease. In 1967, Ruth Nussensweig and colleagues demonstrated that the immunization of mice with irradiated *Plasmodium berghei* sporozoites led to the generation of an immune response that completely protected the immunized mice from a sporozoite challenge. Subsequently, in 1973, David Clyde and colleagues repeated these studies in man using irradiated *Plasmodium falciparum* parasites and again showed that complete protection could be achieved. These pivotal breakthroughs have fueled decades of research into malaria vaccine efforts focusing on both blood stage vaccines and preerythrocytic vaccines. It is now known that both humoral and cellular immunity are important partners in effective vaccine design, and large bodies of work have shown that antibodies can prevent both merozoite and sporozoite invasion while $CD4^+$ T cells and $CD8^+$ T cells play critical roles in the destruction of infected erythrocytes and hepatocytes respectively.

The goal of this volume, which focuses exclusively on malaria vaccinology, is to introduce researchers to a subset of the many methods regularly being used in this field. This volume complements a recent "Methods in Molecular Biology" volume that is devoted exclusively to malaria and provides a complete overview of the protocols and tools used by the molecular and cellular malariologist. Working with the human malaria parasite both in vitro and in vivo is challenging due to its unique tissue tropism, and research efforts on malaria vaccine design have required the creation of novel methodologies for determining vaccination efficacy as well as pinpointing correlates of protection. These methodologies have been fine-tuned over the years, and this volume brings together a large number of nuanced chapters from leading experts in the field that will help any aspiring malaria vaccinologist determine the effectiveness of vaccine regimens. Thus, the volume provides a unique resource and exquisitely detailed methodologies that are not typically found in published literature.

The chapters contained within talk to interventions concerning all aspects of life cycle progression—measuring antibody responses to blood stage parasite survival, the T cell responses engendered by attenuated sporozoite vaccination, and the unique effect on transmission of antibodies that target the mosquito stage of the life cycle. Additionally, methods concerning the ability to generate targeted gene deletions and replacements in the genome of *Plasmodium* parasites convey how *Plasmodium* parasite phenotypes can be created to precise specifications. More recently, the potential power of humanized mouse models of disease progression has been demonstrated and these are discussed herein.

We thank all authors for their dedication in creating step-by-step methodologies that will undoubtedly lead to further discoveries and further improvements. Hopefully these findings will ultimately lead to the creation of an effective vaccine regimen for the elimination and ultimately the eradication of malaria.

Seattle, WA, USA *Ashley M. Vaughan*

Contents

Contributors

MARION AVRIL • *Center for Infectious Disease Research formerly known as Seattle Biomedical research Institute, Seattle, WA, USA*

AMY KRISTINE BEI • *Harvard T. H. Chan School of Public Health, Boston, MA, USA*

ELKE S. BERGMANN-LEITNER • *Malaria Vaccine Branch, Walter Reed Army Institute of Research, Silver Spring, MD, USA*

PHILIPPE BOEUF • *Centre for Biomedical Research, Macfarlane Burnet Institute of Medical Research, Melbourne, VIC, Australia*

HASNAA BOUHAROUN-TAYOUN • *Faculty of Public Health, Lebanese University, Fanar El Metn, Lebanon*

TEUN BOUSEMA • *Department of Medical Microbiology, Radboud University Medical Center, Nijmegen, The Netherlands; Department of Immunology and Infection, London School of Hygiene and Tropical Medicine, London, UK*

KATHERINE J. BREMPELIS • *Department of Global Health, University of Washington, Seattle, WA, USA*

PETER C. BULL • *KEMRI-Wellcome Trust Research Programme, Kilifi, Kenya; Centre for Tropical Medicine, Nuffield Department of Medicine, Oxford University, Oxford, UK*

NOAH S. BUTLER • *Department of Microbiology and Immunology, University of Oklahoma Health Sciences Center, Oklahoma City, OK, USA*

I. NICHOLAS CRISPE • *Department of Pathology, University of Washington, Seattle, WA, USA*

ALYSE N. DOUGLASS • *Center for Infectious Disease Research, Seattle, WA, USA*

PIERRE DRUILHE • *VAC4ALL, Paris, France*

PATRICK E. DUFFY • *Laboratory of Malaria Immunology and Vaccinology, NIAID, NIH, Rockville, MD, USA*

ELIZABETH H. DUNCAN • *Malaria Vaccine Branch, Walter Reed Army Institute of Research, Silver Spring, MD, USA*

MANOJ T. DURAISINGH • *Harvard T. H. Chan School of Public Health, Boston, MA, USA*

MOHAMMAD R. EBRAHIMKHANI • *Department of Biological Engineering, Massachusetts Institute of Technology, Cambridge, MA, USA*

LANDER FOQUET • *Center for Vaccinology, Ghent University and University Hospital, Ghent, Belgium*

MICHAL FRIED • *Laboratory of Malaria Immunology and Vaccinology, NIAID, NIH, Rockville, MD, USA*

JENNA J. GUTHMILLER • *Department of Microbiology and Immunology, University of Oklahoma Health Sciences Center, Oklahoma City, OK, USA*

WINA HASANG • *Department of Medicine, The University of Melbourne, The Doherty Institute Level 5, Parkville, VIC, Australia; Victoria Infectious Diseases Service, The Doherty Institute, Parkville, VIC, Australia*

CORNELUS C. HERMSEN • *Medical Centre, Radboud University Nijmegen, Nijmegen, The Netherlands*

CHRIS J. JANSE • *Leiden Malaria Research Group, Department of Parasitology, LUMC, Leiden, The Netherlands*
STEFAN H.I. KAPPE • *Center for Infectious Disease Research, Seattle, WA, USA*
ALEXIS KAUSHANSKY • *Center for Infectious Disease Research, Seattle, WA, USA*
SHAHID M. KHAN • *Leiden Malaria Research Group, Department of Parasitology, LUMC, Leiden, The Netherlands*
KIRAKORN KIATTIBUTR • *Faculty of Tropical Medicine, Mahidol Vivax Research Unit, Mahidol University, Bangkok, Thailand*
URSZULA KRZYCH • *Department of Cellular Immunology, Malaria Vaccine Branch, Walter Reed Army Institute of Research, Silver Spring, MD, USA*
CHALERMPON KUMPITAK • *Faculty of Tropical Medicine, Mahidol Vivax Research Unit, Mahidol University, Bangkok, Thailand*
WOLFGANG W. LEITNER • *National Institute of Allergy and Infectious Diseases, National Institutes of Health (NIH), Bethesda, MD, USA*
GEERT LEROUX-ROELS • *Center for Vaccinology, Ghent University and University Hospital, Ghent, Belgium*
JING-WEN LIN • *Leiden Malaria Research Group, Department of Parasitology, LUMC, Leiden, The Netherlands; Division of Parasitology, MRC National Institute for Medical Research, London, UK*
PETER G. METZGER • *Center for Infectious Disease Research, Seattle, WA, USA*
PHILIP MEULEMAN • *Center for Vaccinology, Ghent University and University Hospital, Ghent, Belgium*
JESSICA L. MILLER • *Center for Infectious Disease Research, Seattle, WA, USA*
CATHERIN MARIN MOGOLLON • *Leiden Malaria Research Group, Department of Parasitology, LUMC, Leiden, The Netherlands*
ISAAC MOHAR • *Gradient, Seattle, WA, USA*
SARA A. MURRAY • *Systems Immunology, Benaroya Research Institute, Seattle, WA, USA*
MORTEN A. NIELSEN • *Centre for Medical Parasitology, Department of International Health, Immunology and Microbiology, Faculty of Health and Medical Sciences, University of Copenhagen, Copenhagen, Denmark*
ALEXANDER PICHUGIN • *Department of Cellular Immunology, Malaria Vaccine Branch, Military Malaria Research Program, Walter Reed Army Institute of Research, Silver Spring, MD, USA*
FIONA J.A. VAN PUL • *Leiden Malaria Research Group, Department of Parasitology, LUMC, Leiden, The Netherlands*
STEPHEN ROGERSON • *Department of Medicine, The University of Melbourne, The Doherty Institute Level 5, Parkville, VIC, Australia; Victorian Infectious Diseases Service, The Doherty Institute, Parkville, VIC, Australia*
WANLAPA ROOBSOONG • *Faculty of Tropical Medicine, Mahidol Vivax Research Unit, Mahidol University, Bangkok, Thailand*
BRANDON K. SACK • *Center for Infectious Disease Research, Seattle, WA, USA*
ALI SALANTI • *Centre for Medical Parasitology, Department of International Health, Immunology and Microbiology, Faculty of Health and Medical Sciences, University of Copenhagen, Copenhagen, Denmark*
AHMED M. SALMAN • *Leiden Malaria Research Group, Department of Parasitology, LUMC, Leiden, The Netherlands; The Jenner Institute, University of Oxford, Oxford, UK*

JETSUMON SATTABONGKOT • *Faculty of Tropical Medicine, Mahidol Vivax Research Unit, Mahidol University, Bangkok, Thailand*
ROBERT SAUERWEIN • *Medical Centre, Radboud University Nijmegen, Nijmegen, The Netherlands*
TRACY SAVERIA • *Center for Infectious Disease Research, Seattle, WA, USA*
MARTHA SEDEGAH • *Naval Medical Research Center, Silver Spring, MD, USA*
WILL J.R. STONE • *Department of Medical Microbiology, Radboud University Medical Center, Nijmegen, The Netherlands*
JOSHUA TAN • *KEMRI-Wellcome Trust Research Programme, Kilifi, Kenya; Centre for Tropical Medicine, Nuffield Department of Medicine, Oxford University, Oxford, UK*
ANDREW TEO • *Department of Medicine, The University of Melbourne, The Doherty Institute Level 5, Parkville, VIC, Australia*
ASHLEY M. VAUGHAN • *Center for Infectious Disease Research, Seattle, WA, USA*
RYAN A. ZANDER • *Department of Microbiology and Immunology, University of Oklahoma Health Sciences Center, Oklahoma City, OK, USA*
STASYA ZARLING • *Department of Cellular Immunology, Malaria Vaccine Branch, Walter Reed Army Institute of Research, Silver Spring, MD, USA*

Part I

Pre-erythrocytic Stages

Chapter 1

Isolation of Non-parenchymal Cells from the Mouse Liver

Isaac Mohar, Katherine J. Brempelis, Sara A. Murray, Mohammad R. Ebrahimkhani, and I. Nicholas Crispe

Abstract

Hepatocytes comprise the majority of liver mass and cell number. However, in order to understand liver biology, the non-parenchymal cells (NPCs) must be considered. Herein, a relatively rapid and efficient method for isolating liver NPCs from a mouse is described. Using this method, liver sinusoidal endothelial cells, Kupffer cells, natural killer (NK) and NK-T cells, dendritic cells, CD4+ and CD8+ T cells, and quiescent hepatic stellate cells can be purified. This protocol permits the collection of peripheral blood, intact liver tissue, and hepatocytes, in addition to NPCs. In situ perfusion via the portal vein leads to efficient liver digestion. NPCs are enriched from the resulting single-cell suspension by differential and gradient centrifugation. The NPCs can by analyzed or sorted into highly enriched populations using flow cytometry. The isolated cells are suitable for flow cytometry, protein, and mRNA analyses as well as primary culture.

Key words Liver, Perfusion, Cell isolation, Sinusoidal endothelial cells, Kupffer cells, Hepatic stellate cells

1 Introduction

The principle cell types in a healthy liver are hepatocytes, liver sinusoidal endothelial cells (LSEC), Kupffer cells, and hepatic stellate cells (HSC) [1–3]. Fewer in number are bile duct cells, venous and arterial endothelial cell, hepatic progenitor cells, and dendritic cells. Furthermore, the number and proportion of leukocytes can increase tremendously in an infected or damaged liver [4, 5]. As a result, granulocytes, monocytes, natural killer (NK) and NK-T cells, dendritic cells, CD4+ and CD8+ lymphocytes, and B cells are important determinants of the liver biology. Thus, the dissected dynamics of each cell type can provide powerful information to understand the pathology and immunology of the tissue. This information, in combination with serological, histological and tissue-level observations, allows for a comprehensive assessment of each experimental mouse, thus reducing the number of experimental mice while increasing the likelihood of discovery.

Isaac Mohar and Katherine J. Brempelis are co-first authors of this chapter.

Ashley M. Vaughan (ed.), *Malaria Vaccines: Methods and Protocols*, Methods in Molecular Biology, vol. 1325, DOI 10.1007/978-1-4939-2815-6_1, © Springer Science+Business Media New York 2015

The purpose of this protocol is to provide a detailed description of materials and methods by which liver cell populations can be isolated from the mouse liver and studied, while also permitting the collection of blood and intact liver tissue. The liver dissociation protocol is derived from the method published by Seglen [6] for isolating rat liver cells. Dr. Seglen provides an extensive description of the theory behind rat liver dissociation that extends to the mouse. We have evolved the method of Seglen to allow rapid, yet effective, isolation of mouse liver cells, permitting the dissociation of up to five livers per hour by two skilled technicians—one conducting perfusions and dissections, the other processing cell suspensions.

The basic protocol relies upon in situ perfusion of the liver via the portal vein. Peripheral blood and cells are flushed from the liver in a Ca^{2+}-free buffer, prior to perfusion with the collagenase digestion solution. Following liver digestion, the liver is removed and mechanically dissociated. Hepatocytes are separated by low-speed centrifugation, and then non-parenchymal cells (NPCs) are enriched by gradient separation. The enriched NPCs allow for relatively efficient cell type-specific analysis and/or further purification by flow cytometry [7]. For purification, magnetic bead-based methods can be applied and in certain circumstances are preferred [8], however, cell sorting allows for multi-way separation from each preparation.

Although liver NPCs are the focus of this protocol, hepatocytes are readily purified and cultured with good success. In addition, it is not yet clear if this protocol is able to isolate the population of sessile Kupffer cells, which are radioresistant and appear somewhat distinct in function from their non-sessile counterparts [2]. This caveat in mind, this protocol establishes a reproducible method to isolate and enable the study of many cell types from the mouse liver. Indeed, a parallel understanding of cell-specific responses associated with tissue immune and pathological responses offers promise of new insights into treatment and prevention of infection and disease.

2 Materials

All solutions and consumables should be purchased as "tissue culture tested" from a trusted commercial source in order to assure minimal contamination with endotoxin and sterility. All surgical instruments should be thoroughly washed, rinsed and autoclaved for sterility, especially if primary culture is the end goal. As with any protocol involving animals, institutional guidelines for handling, anesthesia, and waste disposal should be followed.

2.1 Anesthesia

1. Anesthesia approved for terminal procedures such as Avertin; 1.25 % (w/v) 2,2,2-tribromomethanol, 2.5 % (v/v) 2-methyl-2-butanol, sterile water. Filter-sterilize and then store at 4 °C protected from light (*see* **Note 1**).

2. 28G ½ inch needle, suitable for intraperitoneal injections.
3. 1-cc syringe.

2.2 Perfusion/Liver Dissociation Hardware Components

1. Peristaltic pump; such as Gilson MINIPULS 3 with medium flow-rate pump head.
2. Pump tubing and connectors; such as F1825113 and F1179951.
3. Tubing extension with slip-tip end; such as Hospira 1265528.
4. Catheter; 24G, IV, such as BD 381412 (*see* **Note 2**).
5. Scissors, straight fine-tipped dissection.
6. Forceps, 2 blunt tip.
7. 50-ml conical tubes.
8. 15-ml conical tubes.
9. 5-cm sterile petri dish (optional).
10. 10-cm sterile petri dish.
11. Stainless steel mesh "tea strainer."
12. 10-cc syringe.
13. 100-μm filter.
14. 70-μm filter (optional).
15. Gauze pads, large-size.
16. Surgical tape, such as 3 M Transpore.
17. Disposable absorbent underpads.
18. 37 °C water bath with 50-ml conical rack.

2.3 Perfusion/Liver Dissociation Solution Components

1. Hank's Balance Salt Solution (HBSS); no Ca^{2+}, no Mg^{2+}, no phenol red.
2. HBSS with phenol red.
3. Phosphate buffered saline (PBS), pH 7.4.
4. Distilled water, TC-grade.
5. PBS, 10×.
6. HEPES; 1 M (Stock).
7. EDTA; 0.5 M (Stock).
8. $CaCl_2$; 0.5 M (Stock).
9. Fetal bovine serum (FBS).
10. Collagenase; *Clostridium histolyticum*, Sigma-Aldrich C5138 (*see* **Note 3**).
11. OptiPrep; 60 % iodixanol solution in water.
12. Tissue fixative; 4 % formaldehyde in PBS.
13. 70 % ethanol.

Table 1
Antibodies for FACS-based purification of some of the major liver NPC and leukocytes

Epitope	Fluorophore	Clone	Dilution
CD8a	Pacific Blue	53-6-7	1:250
CD4	PerCP-Cy5.5	RM4-5	1:250
CD11b	FITC	M1/70	1:200
NK1.1	Per-Cy7	PK136	1:200
Tie2	PE	TEK4	1:250
F4/80	APC	BM8	1:200
GR1	APC-Cy7	RB6-8C5	1:200
N/A	Live/Dead Violet	N/A	1:1000

The antibodies listed here will allow for selection or analysis of some of the most numerous liver NPC as well as some leukocytes

These solutions can be prepared in advance and stored at 4 °C.

1. Perfusion Buffer, 5–10 ml per mouse; HBSS, 5 mM HEPES, 0.5 mM EDTA.
2. Wash Buffer, 50 ml per mouse; PBS, 4 % FBS, 0.5 mM EDTA.
3. PBS Flow Buffer (PFB), 20 ml per mouse; PBS, 1 mM EDTA, 2 % FBS.

These solutions should be prepared on the day of isolation.

1. Collagenase solution, 5–10 ml per mouse; HBSS (w/phenol red), 5 mM HEPES, 0.5 mM $CaCl_2$, 0.5 mg/ml collagenase.
2. 40 % iodixanol in PBS, 2.5 ml per mouse; 1.67 ml OptiPrep + 0.25 ml 10× PBS + 0.58 ml TC-grade water.

2.4 Cell Analysis and Purification Components

1. Flow cytometer; such as BD Biosciences, LSRII or Aria.
2. Flow cytometry tubes (*see* **Note 4**).
3. Antibodies for sorting cell type and/or analysis (Table 1) (*see* **Note 5**).

3 Methods

3.1 Prepare for Perfusion(s)

1. Warm perfusion and collagenase solutions to 37 °C for approximately 15 min prior to beginning the perfusion.
2. Prepare tubing for perfusion (*see* **Note 6**).
3. Prepare perfusion area with absorbent pad, dissection tools, gauze, 10-cm petri dish, tea strainer, and 10-cc syringe (Fig. 1).
4. Fill perfusion line with perfusion solution.

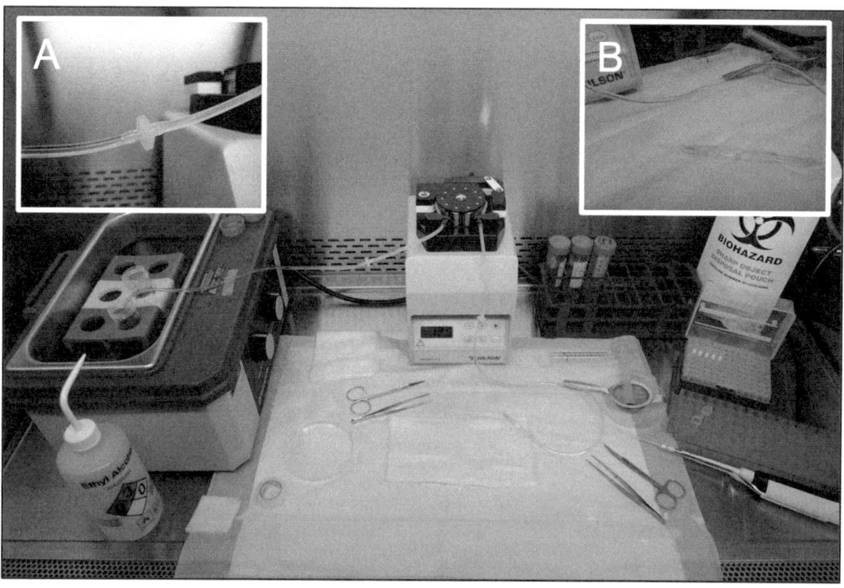

Fig. 1 Suggested workspace set-up. Position the water bath and pump to allow the perfusion tubing to reach the bottom of the 50-ml conical tubes. The water bath should be to the *left*, in order to allow switching of the perfusion line while holding the catheter with the *right hand.* Place absorbent pad on the work surface; this pad will both absorb perfusion solutions and act as the foundation to adhere the mouse. Place large gauze pad in the center of the work area; this small pad will absorb most of the perfusion solutions as well as blood and should be changed after every other if not every mouse. Place tea strainer in a 10-cm petri dish. Place the lid of the dish to the left of the smaller gauze pad. Place one pair of sharp scissors and forceps above the gauze. Place the other scissors and forceps to the right of the gauze. Position the surgical tape, small gauze pads, and 70 % ethanol within easy reach. *Inset* (**a**) illustrates the connection between extension tubing and silicon peristaltic pump tubing. *Inset* (**b**) illustrates the catheter connected to the male end of the extension tubing

3.2 Anesthetize Mouse

1. Inject mouse with appropriate amount of anesthesia.
2. Once adequate level anesthesia is obtained, proceed to Subheading 3.3 (*see* **Note 7**).

3.3 Surgical Preparation

1. Place mouse belly-up on large gauze pad.
2. Secure mouse by footpads using surgical tape in an X orientation (Fig. 2a).
3. Disinfect and wet mouse fur using 70 % ethanol. Wipe off excess.
4. Open skin to expose the peritoneal membrane (Fig. 2b).
5. Open peritoneal membrane (Fig. 2c), gently move intestines and stomach to the right and very gently "stick" the liver to the diaphragm. This should expose the portal vein and descending vena cava (*see* **Note 8**) (Fig. 2d).
6. Use sharp scissors to nick the portal vein; blood will flow (*see* **Note 9**).

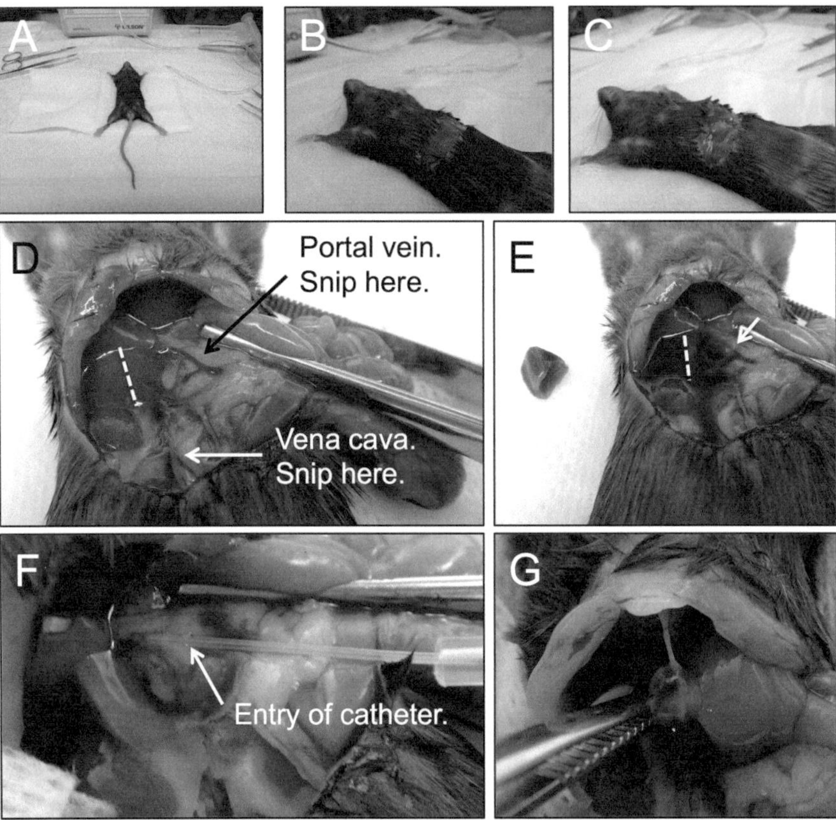

Fig. 2 General perfusion anatomy and procedure. (**a**) Adhere anesthetized mouse overtop of the gauze in an X-configuration. (**b**) Make a crosswise incision through the mouse skin to reveal the peritoneum. (**c**) Being careful to avoid cutting internal organs, make a crosswise incision through the peritoneum. (**d**) Move the gastrointestinal organs to the *left*, revealing the portal vein. Place forceps to hold tissue off of the vein. (**e**) Snip the portal vein (collect blood if desired), then remove a portion of the intact *right* posterior lobe. Catheterize the portal vein, then immediately cut the descending vena cava. (**f**) The liver will blanch once the portal vein is catheterized, and will fully perfuse once the vena cava is cut. Avoid pushing the catheter too far into the vein. The tip of the catheter should be easily observed within the vein. (**g**) Once digested, remove the liver by the falciform ligament, along the top of the medial lobe. The gall bladder is a good landmark for identifying the ligament

3.4 Blood and Tissue Collection (Optional)

1. Collect 0.2–0.5 ml of blood as it pools near the portal vein. Transfer to proper collection tube.
2. Locate and remove ~2/3 of the right posterior liver lobe (Fig. 2d, e). Transfer to 4 % formaldehyde for fixation or further divide for other assessments.

3.5 In Situ Liver Dissociation

1. Turn on pump to flow of ~2 ml/min.
2. Drip perfusion buffer onto the cut portal vein.
3. Use gauze sponge to draw perfusion solution to the left.
4. Identify the opening in the vein (*see* **Note 10**).

5. Gently catheterize the vein; the liver should blanch (*see* **Note 11**) (Fig. 2f).
6. Cut the descending vena cava; blood and buffer should visibly flow from the vena cava.
7. Relax your hand (*see* **Note 12**).
8. Perfuse liver with 5–10 ml of perfusion buffer. Most perfusion tubing setups hold about 5 ml of solution, thus once the descending vena cava is cut, proceed to **step 9**.
9. Stop pump.
10. Switch line to collagenase, using the left hand.
11. Resume pump flow (*see* **Note 13**).
12. Swell the liver using forceps to occlude buffer flow from the vena cava, every 45–60 s for 5–10 s. If part of the right posterior lobe was removed, use the forceps to occlude flow into this lobe (*see* **Note 14**).
13. Perfuse liver with 5–10 ml of collagenase buffer. After 3–4 min, the liver should soften and the left lobe will begin to fall over the portal vein. When this happens, use forceps to lift up the lobe to periodically check that the catheter is properly positioned. After 5 min, the internal structure of the liver cracks. This indicates a good digestion, and is most evident in the right anterior lobe.
14. Stop the pump.
15. Remove catheter from vein.
16. Reverse pump to return unused collagenase solution to the 50-ml conical tube.
17. Switch line back to perfusion solution and refill the line in preparation for the next mouse.

3.6 Single Cell Suspension

1. Using wide-tipped forceps, grasp the liver just to the left of the gall bladder along the falciform ligament (Fig. 2g).
2. Use scissors to separate the liver from the diaphragm and all other points of connection. Care should be taken to avoid cutting the gastrointestinal tract.
3. Transfer the digested liver into the tea strainer within a 10-cm petri dish.
4. Remove the gall bladder (*see* **Note 15**).
5. Add 30 ml of cold wash buffer to the dish.
6. Use the rubber plunger of 10-cc syringe to gently massage the liver through the tea strainer, shake the strainer to disperse the cells. The liver should easily disperse with only the capsule and ligament remaining in the strainer.

7. Use 10-cc syringe (or 10-ml pipet) to gently disperse any clumps.
8. Filter (100 μm) the cell suspension into a 50-ml conical tube.
9. Store on ice or at 4 °C for no longer than 15 min before proceeding to Subheading 3.8.

3.7 Isolate Splenocytes (Optional, See Note 16)

1. Locate and remove spleen.
2. Place spleen into 5-ml petri dish filled with 10 ml of PFB.
3. Place the spleen on the rough surface of a glass slide.
4. Use the rough surface of a second glass slide to dissociate the spleen by gentle pressure applied in a circular motion. Continue this gentle mashing until the tissue is clearly dispersed.
5. Scrape the cells into the buffer using the edge of the slide.
6. Disperse the cells by pipetting.
7. Filter (70 μm) into 50-ml conical tube.
8. Store on ice until the NPC isolation reaches Subheading 3.10, **step** 7, then process as NPC.

3.8 Crude Liver Cell Fractionation

1. Centrifuge the cell suspension at 50 × *g* for 3 min at room temperature. At this speed and duration, hepatocytes and debris will pellet while most NPCs will remain in suspension.
2. Transfer the supernatant, which contains the hepatocyte-depleted NPCs, to a new 50-ml conical tube.

3.9 Hepatocyte Enrichment (Optional)

1. Wash the hepatocyte pellet in 40 ml of wash buffer.
2. Pellet at 50 × *g* for 3 min.
3. Resuspend in 10 ml of media.
4. The resulting hepatocytes can be further enriched by magnetic bead depletion of contaminating cells and/or plated on collagen-coated tissue culture dishes. For the mouse, anti-CD45 and anti-CD146 microbeads will deplete most immune cells and endothelial cells, respectively.

3.10 Non-parenchymal Cell Enrichment

1. Pellet the NPC suspension at 500 × *g* for 5–7 min at 4 °C.
2. Gently resuspend in 2.5 ml of PFB.
3. Mix cell suspension with 2.5 ml of 30–40 % iodixanol solution in 15-ml conical. A final concentration of 20 % iodixanol will enrich for most if not all intact NPCs.
4. Gently overlay with 2 ml of PFB.
5. Centrifuge at 1500 × *g* for 25 min at room temperature. If available, turn the brake OFF on the centrifuge to minimize disturbance to the cell interface.

6. During the centrifugation add 10 ml of cold PFB to a 15 ml conical tube.
7. After centrifugation a well-defined interface of cells should be visible. Carefully transfer this cell layer from the iodixanol gradient to the 10 ml of PFB in order to wash away excess iodixanol.
8. Centrifuge at 500 × *g* for 5 min at 4 °C.
9. Resuspend the enriched NPC pellet in 0.5 ml of cold PFB or appropriate buffer for desired applications.

3.11 Staining NPCs for Flow Cytometry

1. Prepare the necessary number of flow cytometry tubes.
2. Add anti-CD16/anti-CD36 (Fc receptor blocking) antibody to each sample to a final concentration of 1:250 (*see* **Note 17**).
3. Incubate for 5 min at room temperature.
4. Add antibody cocktail (*see* Table 1).
5. Vortex briefly and gently.
6. Incubate for 20 min at 4 °C.
7. Wash the cells by adding 1 ml of PFB to each sample.
8. Centrifuge at 500 × *g* for 5 min at 4 °C.
9. Aspirate supernatant.
10. Resuspend cell pellet in 0.5 ml of PFB.
11. In order to minimize clogs during cell sorting, filter the cell suspension.

3.12 Identifying and Sorting Liver NPC by Flow Cytometry

Liver NPCs have yet to become absolute in their defining characteristics. However, many distinct cell populations can be sorted from a mouse liver. Those identified here represent a cross-section of major cell types, including endothelial cells, macrophage, quiescent hepatic stellate cells, lymphocytes, and natural killer cells. If a population of cells appears diffuse in characteristics, separation by an additional dimension may reveal multiple cell populations. The successful isolation of pure and viable cells is as much art as science and will be aided by the direction and advice of a skilled flow cytometrist with an appreciation for the complexity of sorting from dissociated tissue. The gating strategy depicted in Fig. 3 is one approach to sorting liver NPCs.

3.13 Quality Control Analysis of Enriched Liver Cell Populations

Quality control analysis of enriched and sorted liver cell populations can be conducted by in vitro culture of the cells to confirm morphology and/or function [7]. In addition, enriched cells can be analyzed for expression of genes known to be relatively specific to cell types. The basic protocol and representative results are presented below.

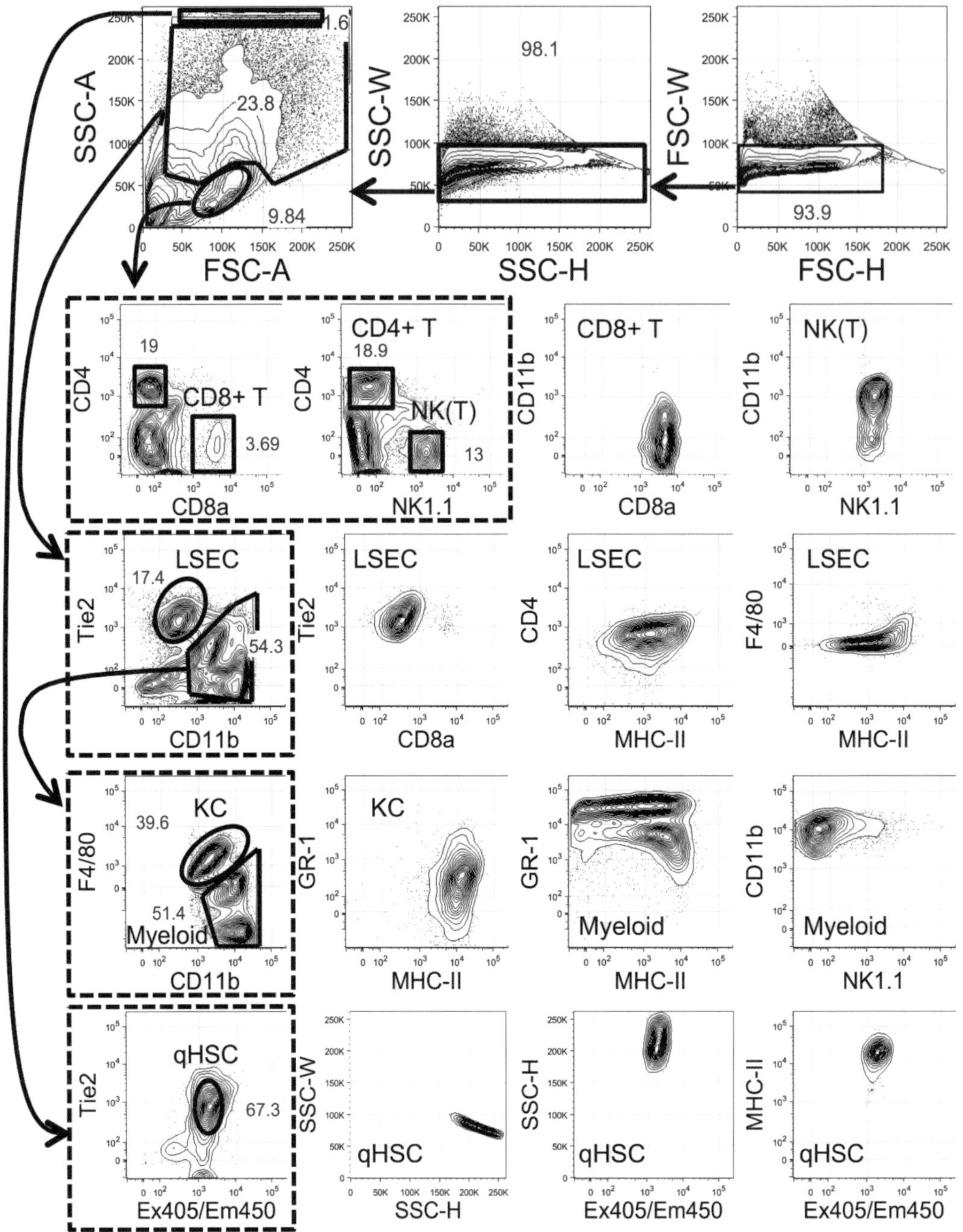

Fig. 3 NPC sort strategy. Representative NPC sorting strategy from a C57BL/6J mouse 68 h following injection of 50,000 *Plasmodium yoelii* sporozoites. Labeled gates are sorted populations. Exclude doublets by FSC-H vs. FSC-W and SSC-H vs. SSC-W, but if quiescent hepatic stellate (qHSC) are desired, be sure to include the SSC-H events. From a standard FSC-A vs. SSC-A scatter plot, separate lymphocyte-sized cells from cells with high granularity (SSC) and larger size (FSC). Hepatic stellate cells contain highly refractive retinol droplets and are autofluorescent when excited with 405 nm and emitting at 450 nm. Lymphocytes can be separated into many populations. Here, CD8+ T cells are collected against CD8a vs. CD4. CD4+ T cells and NK(T) cells are collected against NK1.1 vs. CD4. A significant population of NK-T cells are CD4+ in the mouse. The best identifier of NK-T cells is CD1d (stained by tetramer, not conducted here). NK(T) cells induce CD11b expression when activated. From the larger cells, LSEC, Kupffer cells (KC), and infiltrating myeloid cells (including monocytes and granulocytes) can be collected. LSEC are selected against CD11b vs. Tie2. From the CD11b$^{int/hi}$ Tie2$^{int/lo}$

The described liver cell isolation method was used to purify liver LSECs, Kupffer cells (KCs), qHSCs, and hepatocytes from five 9-week-old C57BL/6 J male mice purchased from The Jackson Laboratory (Bar Harbor, ME). Briefly, hepatocytes were processed through Subheading 3.9 and enriched using anti-CD45 and anti-CD146 microbeads. Liver NPCs were processed through Subheading 3.10 and then stained for cell sorting on a BD Aria III, as touched upon in Subheading 3.12. The antibodies used to discriminate cell populations during sorting were as follows: Live/Dead Violet (Pacific Blue), CD11b (BV605), IA/IE (FITC), Tie2 (PE), Ly6C (PerCP-Cy5.5), F4/80 (APC), and Ly6G (APC-Cy7). There were minimal differences in the concentration of antibodies used in sorting (*see* **Note 18**) and while the gating strategy was similar to that shown in Fig. 3, it was not identical (*see* **Note 19**).

Post-sort analyses of sorted LSECs, KCs, and qHSCs show average cell purities of 93.02 %, 93.82 %, and 87.02 % respectively (averaged value of $n=5$). To further assess the purity of these cell populations, RNA was isolated using TRIzol (Invitrogen) and then cDNA was synthesized (QIAGEN QuantiTect) and quantified using microfluidic PCR (Fluidigm Corp, South San Francisco CA, USA) with cell-type-specific TaqMan® assays (Invitrogen) (Fig. 4). The qRT-PCR analysis shows that isolated hepatocytes, LSECs, KCs, and qHSCs are enriched for their cell-type-specific genes. Genes commonly associated with each cell type—*Alb* for hepatocytes, *Tek* (Tie2) for LSECs, *Emr1* (F4/80) for KCs, and *Pdgfrb* for qHSCs—are enriched in the expected populations (*see* **Note 20**).

4 Notes

1. Avertin becomes toxic when exposed to light. Although concentrated stock solutions can be prepared, preparation of smaller volumes of working solution minimizes the likelihood of accumulating toxic by-products.
2. Some researchers use the needle to catheterize, others simply use a 24G needle. We prefer to use the Vialon™ catheter alone and reuse it on multiple mice.

Fig. 3 (continued) cells, KC and general myeloid cells can be distinguished by CD11b vs. F4/80 staining. Here we see that KC are MHC class-II high and GR-1 (Ly6G/Ly6C) intermediate. The myeloid infiltrate contains GR1^{hi} and GR1i^{nt} population with varying degree of MHC-II staining. Lastly, qHSC show very high SSC and autofluorescence (Ex 405 nm/Em 450 nm) and often show autofluorescence in many channels. Since many of these characteristics are that of dead cells or debris, the best validation of sorted qHSC is direct observation under a light microscope. In all cases, heterogeneity may exist in these populations, and further selection or validation of purity may be needed

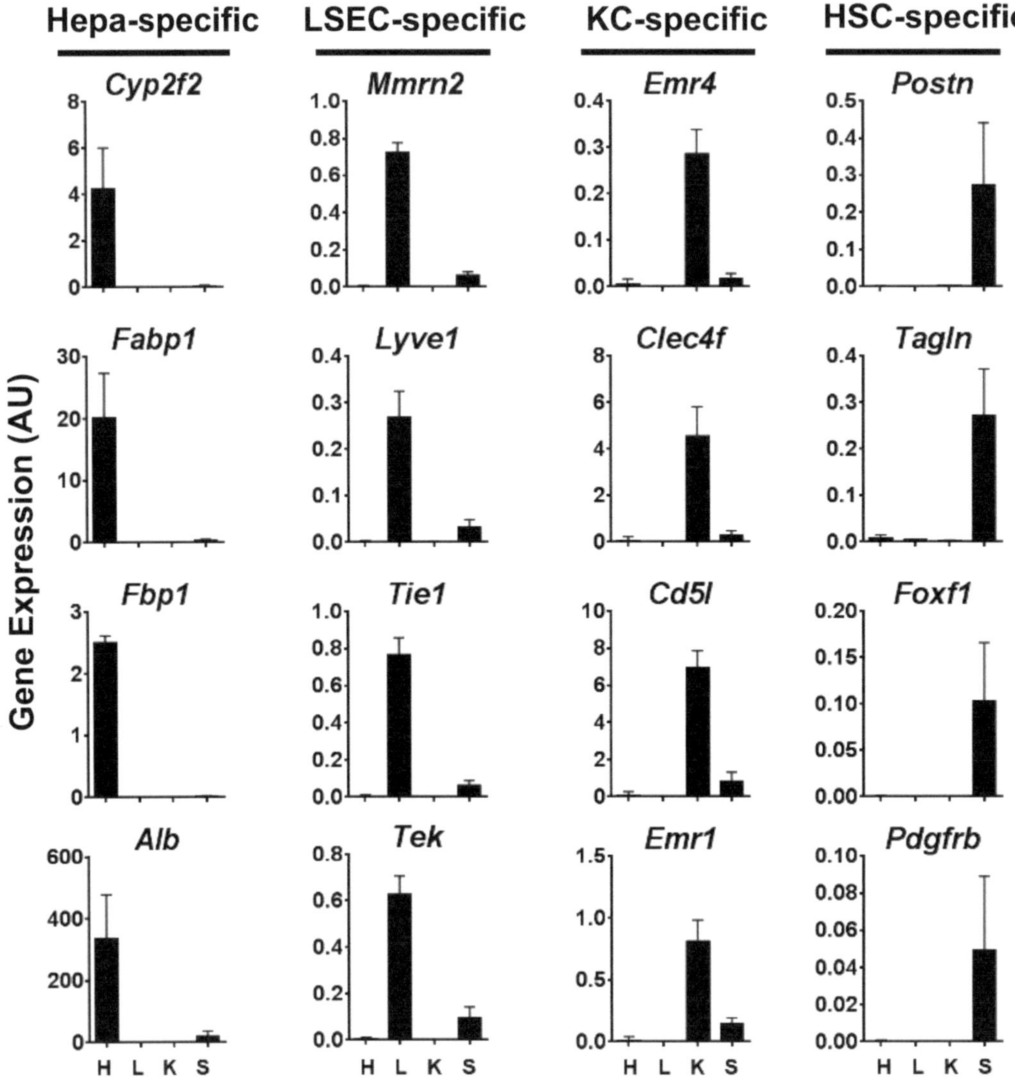

Fig. 4 Quality control by qRT-PCR of hepatocytes and sorted liver NPCs. The relative expression of genes in enriched liver cell types illustrates the efficacy of the method. Gene expression is normalized to the average of three house-keeping genes: *Gapdh*, *Actb*, and *Hprt*. Each bar is the mean (+SD) of n = 5 mice. H = Hepatocyte, L = LSEC, K = Kupffer cell, and S = Hepatic stellate cell. Graphed using Prism6 (GraphPad Software, San Diego CA, USA)

3. Collagenase is available in many fractions and sources. We have found that collagenase from *C. histolyticum*, Type IV, from Sigma-Aldrich dissociates the liver efficiently and maintains expected cell function.
4. Standard polystyrene tubes are suitable for most applications. However, prior to sorting samples, it is important to filter (40 μm) each sample in order to reduce the likelihood of clumps and clogs. Use sterile tubes when necessary.

5. The choice of antibodies and fluorophores is highly dependent upon the cell(s) of interest. Those listed in Table 1 allow for separation of relatively pure populations of LSEC, Kupffer cells, CD8+ T cells, CD4+ T cell, infiltrating myeloid cells, and quiescent HSC. During inflammation or pathology, the morphology and cell surface molecules of most cells change, resulting in heterogeneity. Thus, additional antibodies may be necessary to achieve homogenous cell populations.
6. Prepare a perfusion tubing set using two IV extensions, two adaptors, and one length of silicon peristaltic pump tubing. Cut and discard the male end from one extension set and the female from the other; remove the slide clamps from both and discard. Connect the cut ends of the extension tubes to the pump tubing using the connectors (Fig. 1a). Connect the catheter to the male end (Fig. 1b). Perfusion tubing may be reused for many months with proper cleaning and storage. Flush the tubing with 5 ml of 70 % ethanol followed by 15 ml of sterile distilled water. Allow the tubing to run dry then store in a plastic zip-lock bag, protected from light. Tubing will become brittle with prolonged exposure to ethanol. Upon reuse, flush the tubing with ethanol then distilled water, run dry, then fill with perfusion buffer.
7. Toe-pinch reflex is a standard method for assessing depth of anesthesia in mice. The mouse should not flinch. If flinching occurs, allow more time or administer additional Avertin.
8. Exercise care when moving the liver in order to avoid hemorrhage. Once the portal vein is exposed, place forceps in order to hold back other tissue. Excess fat (or pancreas) may partially hide the portal vein. This is more likely in older (>8 months of age) male mice.
9. It will be more difficult to catheterize the vein if it is cut clean through. A "nick" in the vein will allow an entry point for a catheter without a needle, while preserving structural support.
10. Blood will generally flow from the right—the opening towards the intestines. As perfusion buffer washes the blood away, the nick in the portal vein should be clear. Gently catheterize the vein towards the liver.
11. Do not cut the descending vena cava until the portal vein is catheterized. The liver should blanch as soon as the vein is catheterized, if it doesn't the vein is not catheterized, so try again. The most likely "miss" occurs in the smooth muscle layer surrounding the vein. This layer will puff up. If this occurs, remove the catheter and try for the vein opening again. The catheter is visible within the vein.
12. It is important to maintain a steady hand or else the catheter will slip, tear or puncture (if pushed too far toward the liver)

the vein. Mindful relaxation of the right hand will minimize shaking and fatigue, which is especially important for multiple mouse experiments. If with time and practice, shaking persists and is the cause of failed perfusions, consider the method of Seglen and secure the catheter with a noose. Alternatively, with practice, the catheter can be fully released from grip, once the mouse has expired.

13. When switching the line from perfusion buffer to collagenase, air bubbles are occasionally introduced. A small bubble (<3 mm) in the line is not an issue. Larger bubbles may occlude the perfusion of regions of the liver, but not always. If a very large bubble (>2 cm) is seen in the line, it is best to remove the catheter just before the bubble reaches the catheter, run the bubble out, then catheterize the vein again. With practice, this is easily done. When in doubt, let the bubble run its course.

14. The liver should swell. The left lobe, in particular, should clearly swell and fall over the portal vein. If the liver does not swell, inspect the catheter in the portal vein. Diseased livers (i.e., fibrotic) do not digest or swell very well.

15. The gall bladder contains bile acid salts, digestive enzymes, and fat-soluble compounds destine for excretion in the feces. Ideally, the gall bladder is removed intact. However, we have not observed a difference in NPC phenotype due to gall bladder rupture. If working with an assistant, pass the digested liver to the assistant to complete the processing, then continue with Subheading 3.7 or begin another mouse.

16. Although it is optional, removal and isolation of cells from the spleen is useful for preparing compensations for flow cytometry and providing additional (and validating) immunological information. The cell surface staining of lymphocytes isolated from the liver often shows a bias towards mixed activation and polarization states. By contrasting the immunophenotype of cells in the liver to those of the spleen, one is better able to assure: (1) an intact and "proper" immune system, (2) proper staining protocol, and (3) proper gating strategy in flow cytometry.

17. A concentration of 1:50 Fc block is generally adequate to identify populations of liver NPCs with proper compensation. Increasing the concentration of Fc block will reduce the amount of nonspecific antibody binding, and has the potential to further resolve cell populations. LSEC and KC are abundant liver NPC and show affinity for most flow cytometry antibodies.

18. Anti-CD16/anti-CD36 (Fc receptor blocking) was used at a final concentration of 1:50 to increase the resolution between cell populations. The Live/Dead Violet stain was used at a final concentration of 1:1000. All other antibodies were used at a final concentration of 1:200.

19. Cells were sorted in the manner illustrated in Fig. 3, with modification. In brief, following size gating on the FSC-A vs. SSC-A plot, Live/Dead was used to exclude dead cells. Cells staining $CD11b^{int}/^{hi}Tie2^{int/lo}$ CD11b vs. Tie2 plot were further gated on CD11b vs. Ly6G to gate out the $Ly6G^{hi}$ neutrophils then selecting Kupffer cells by CD11b vs. F4/80. Of note, since the size gate from the FSC-A vs. SSC-A plot is mostly sufficient to separate qHSC from LSEC and KC, this panel uses the Pacific Blue channel to sort qHSC as the highly autofluorescent population and to define dead cells as the Pacific Blue positive population. The qHSC are generally more Pacific Blue "positive" than dead cells.
20. The low-level expression of LSEC- and KC-specific genes in the qHSC population is likely due to a small contaminating fraction of dead LSECs and KCs, and resulting from the use of the Pacific Blue channel for both qHSC autofluorescence and the Live/Dead-violet stain. We suspect this issue to be solved if a different channel for Live/Dead discrimination is used. Autofluorescence from debris, however, renders many other channels frustratingly nonspecific for absolute exclusion of dead cells. As a result, exclusion of dead cells should be considered on a case-by-case basis.

Acknowledgements

This protocol was developed under support by the National Institutes of Health grants R21AI099872 and T32AI007411 and Seattle Biomedical Research Institute.

References

1. Baratta JL, Ngo A, Lopez B, Kasabwalla N, Longmuir KJ, Robertson RT (2009) Cellular organization of normal mouse liver: a histological, quantitative immunocytochemical, and fine structural analysis. Histochem Cell Biol 131:713–726.
2. Klein I, Cornejo J, Polakos N, John B, Wuensch S, Topham D, Pierce R, Crispe I (2007) Kupffer cell heterogeneity: functional properties of bone marrow derived and sessile hepatic macrophages. Blood 110:4077.
3. Winau F, Quack C, Darmoise A, Kaufmann SHE (2008) Starring stellate cells in liver immunology. Current opinion in immunology, 20:68–74.
4. Wynn TA, Ramalingam TR (2012) Mechanisms of fibrosis: therapeutic translation for fibrotic disease. Nature Medicine 18:1028–1040.
5. Crispe IN (2009) The liver as a lymphoid organ. Annu Rev Immunol 27:147–163.
6. Seglen PO (1976) Preparation of isolated rat liver cells. Methods in cell biology 13:29 -83.
7. Ebrahimkhani MR, Mohar I, Crispe IN (2011) Cross-presentation of antigen by diverse subsets of murine liver cells. Hepatology (Baltimore, Md), 54:1379–1387.
8. Brownell J, Wagoner J, Lovelace ES, Thirstrup D, Mohar I, Smith W, Giugliano S, Li K, Crispe IN, Rosen HR, Polyak SJ (2013) Independent, parallel pathways to CXCL10 induction in HCV-infected hepatocytes. Journal of hepatology, 59 (2013) 701–708.

Chapter 2

Measurement of the T Cell Response to Preerythrocytic Vaccination in Mice

Jenna J. Guthmiller, Ryan A. Zander, and Noah S. Butler

Abstract

Whole attenuated parasite vaccines designed to elicit immunity against the clinically silent preerythrocytic stage of *Plasmodium* infection represent the most efficacious experimental platforms currently in clinical trial. Studies in rodents and humans show that T cells mediate vaccine-induced protection. Thus, determining the quantitative and qualitative properties of these T cells remains a major research focus. Most rodent models of preerythrocytic anti-*Plasmodium* vaccination focus on circumsporozoite-specific CD8 T cell responses in BALB/c mice. However, CD4 T cells and non-circumsporozoite-specific CD8 T cells also significantly contribute to protection. Here we describe alternative approaches that enable detection and functional characterization of total CD8 and CD4 T cell responses induced by preerythrocytic vaccination in mice. These flow cytometry-based approaches rely on monitoring the modulation of expressed integrins and co-receptors on the surface of T cells in vaccinated mice. The approaches enable direct determination of the magnitude, kinetics, distribution, phenotype, and functional features of T cell responses induced by infection or whole-parasite vaccination using any mouse-parasite species combination.

Key words Radiation attenuated sporozoite, Genetically attenuated parasite, Vaccine, *Plasmodium*, Malaria, CD8 T cell, CD4 T cell, Integrins

1 Introduction

Malaria remains a global health crisis and it has been argued that eradication of the disease cannot be achieved without the development of efficacious vaccines against *Plasmodium* parasites [1]. Although there are several subunit and vectored antimalarial vaccines under clinical evaluation [2], current experimental vaccines that elicit the most potent and long-lasting protection in humans are those formulated using live attenuated sporozoites incapable of causing disease [3–6]. Radiation and genetically attenuated parasites, and the prophylactic use of antimalarial drugs targeting blood stage parasites, are promising strategies currently under evaluation in clinical trials as preerythrocytic vaccine platforms [7–10]. Notably, each of these leading preerythrocytic vaccine platforms

Ashley M. Vaughan (ed.), *Malaria Vaccines: Methods and Protocols*, Methods in Molecular Biology, vol. 1325, DOI 10.1007/978-1-4939-2815-6_2,

was first predicted and qualified using rodent models [11–13]. Thus, experimental mouse models continue to provide fundamentally important information regarding the mechanisms of immune resistance induced by preerythrocytic vaccination.

Studies in rodents have conclusively shown that a central component of protective preerythrocytic vaccination involves the induction of parasite-specific CD8 T cells targeting *Plasmodium-infected* hepatocytes [11, 14, 15]. Data from human studies also show strong correlations between the activity of CD8 T cells and protection against experimental mosquito bite challenge [5, 6, 10, 16]. CD8 T cells limit parasite survival by several pathways, including direct cytolysis of infected hepatocytes, and by expressing antiparasitic cytokines that act to limit parasite survival within infected hepatocytes [14, 17–19]. Although data supporting a role for CD4 T cells in limiting liver stage infections is less abundant, several studies demonstrate that CD4+ major histocompatibility (MHC) class II-restricted T cells can exert cytolytic activity against parasite-infected cells [20–23]. Moreover, MHC class I deficient mice, which lack CD8 T cells, are resistant to sporozoite challenge following multiple vaccinations with attenuated *Plasmodium* sporozoites [24]. Protection in the latter studies depended on CD4 T cells and correlated with neutralizing parasite-specific antibody responses. Finally, CD4 T cells also are important regulators of CD8 T cell responses, as *Plasmodium*-specific CD8 T cells fail to form sizable memory populations in the absence of CD4 T cells [25]. Thus, parasite-specific CD4 T cells are also important regulators of vaccine-induced anti-*Plasmodium* immunity via their provision of help for CD8 T cells and B cells, and perhaps through direct cytolysis of parasite-infected cells [20–22]. Collectively, these studies underscore the critical role for T cells in mediating preerythrocytic vaccine-induced protection against *Plasmodium*. Therefore, defining the numerical, phenotypic and functional features of parasite-specific CD8 and CD4 T cells activated by preerythrocytic vaccination remains an important goal.

High-resolution study of pathogen-specific T cells classically requires knowledge of defined T cell epitopes and MHC restriction elements, or access to immunologic tools such as MHC tetramers or T cell receptor transgenic (TCR Tg) mice. For both *Plasmodium yoelii* and *Plasmodium berghei* liver stage parasites several tools exist and at least one dominant CD8 T cell epitope from each parasite has been mapped in inbred BALB/c mice [26]. These CD8 T cell epitopes derive from the sporozoite- and liver stage-expressed circumsporozoite (CS) protein (*P. yoelii*, amino acids 280–288, $CS_{280-288}$; *P. berghei*, $CS_{252-260}$, e.g., Fig. 1) [26]. Notably, TCR Tg mice have been generated for the *P. yoelii* CD8 T cell determinant [27]. *Plasmodium*-specific TCR Tg CD4 T cells have also been generated, but the MHC class II-restricted TCR is specific for a blood stage antigen (MSP-1) and the epitope is only

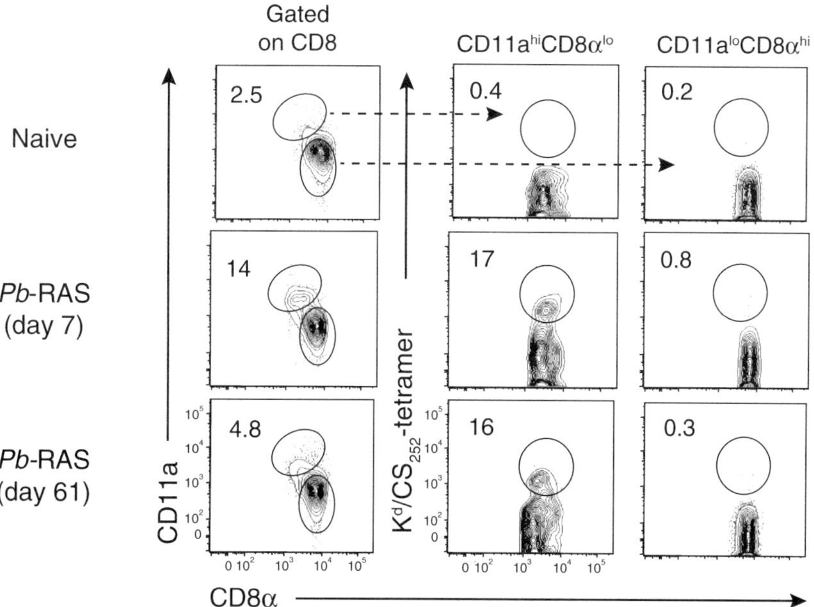

Fig. 1 Peripheral blood from BALB/c mice was collected before (naïve) and 7 and 61 days after vaccination with 20,000 *Plasmodium berghei* radiation attenuated sporozoites (*Pb*-RAS). Flow cytometric analyses were conducted to determine the fraction of vaccine-induced CD8 T cells (CD11a^{hi}CD8α^{lo}) that were specific for the dominant CD8 T cell epitope that derives from the parasite circumsporozoite (CS) protein (amino acids 252–260). Cells were processed and stained with MHC class I tetramer (K^{d}/CS$_{252}$) followed by anti-CD90.2, anti-CD8α, and anti-CD11a as described in the text. Numbers refer to the fraction of cells within each defined population gate. These examples highlight that MHC class I tetramer reagents can identify epitope-specific CD8 T cells induced by preerythrocytic vaccination, enabling subsequent examination of measures of phenotype or function. These data also show that the vast majority (>80 %) of the CD8 T cells induced by RAS are specific for undefined or unknown epitopes, further underscoring the utility of surrogate approaches to measure the quantity and quality of the total T cell response following preerythrocytic vaccination

expressed by *Plasmodium chabaudi* rodent parasites [28–30]. More recently, Heath and colleagues developed a new TCR Tg mouse line bearing CD8 T cells responsive to an antigen expressed during both blood and liver stage [31]. Strikingly, the epitope from this antigen is conserved in *P. berghei*, *P. yoelii*, and *P. chabaudi*, so future applications of this new research tool should reveal important information about cross-stage (blood and liver) specific CD8 T cell immunity. Because the experimental use of TCR Tg CD8 T cells in malaria models was recently reviewed [32], specific protocols are not described herein.

It is well known that CS-specific CD8 T cell populations can be sufficient to limit or stop the progression of liver stage *Plasmodium* parasites [17, 26, 27, 33, 34]. Thus, there are clear advantages to studying CS-specific endogenous (polyclonal) or TCR Tg (monoclonal) CD8 T cells. On the other hand, as noted above, CD4 T cells also contribute to resistance and several studies have shown that non-CS-specific CD8 T cells significantly limit *Plasmodium* liver stage infection [35, 36]. Indeed, more than 80 % of CD8 T cells induced by radiation attenuated sporozoite (RAS) vaccination of BALB/c mice are responding to non-CS antigens [15] (Fig. 1), so studying the biology and behavior of these cells is equally important. However, the lack of additional and validated non-CS-specific CD4 and CD8 T cell epitopes has hampered direct study of these T cell populations of unknown antigenic specificity. To overcome these limitations, cell surface markers of T cell activation have been widely used to monitor *Plasmodium* vaccination-induced T cell responses. For example, modulation of CD62L, CD44, CD122, and CD45RB expression has been used to identify RAS-induced, liver-resident CD8 T cells in mice [37–40]. However, several of these molecules are expressed on both naïve and memory T cells (e.g., CD62L and CD122 [41]) or they exhibit a continuum of expression (e.g., expression of CD44 is not bimodal). Moreover, the expression of several of these markers can be modulated by T cell homeostatic proliferation [42]. These variables add to the difficulty of distinguishing among bona fide naïve, effector and memory T cells through monitoring CD62L, CD44, and CD122.

In an effort to further enhance resolution and more clearly distinguish true naïve and effector and memory T cells, we developed alternative methods to track T cell responses following *Plasmodium* infection or vaccination in both inbred and outbred mice [15, 43]. Notably, these methods were first validated using models of virus and bacterial infection [44, 45]. We determined that antigen activated CD8 T cells could be distinguished from naïve CD8 T cells based on the coordinate modulation of the integrin CD11a (the alpha L chain of LFA-1) and downregulation of the CD8α chain of the co-receptor. Effector and memory CD8 T cells are CD11a^{hi}CD8α^{lo} and naïve CD8 T cells are CD11a^{lo}CD8α^{hi} (Fig. 2). Unlike CD8 T cells, antigen activated CD4 T cells do not appreciably downregulate the CD4 co-receptor, so monitoring the coordinate modulation of CD11a and an additional integrin, CD49d (the alpha 4 chain of VLA-4), is used to distinguish naïve CD4 T cells from antigen-activated CD4 T cells [43, 45]. Effector and memory CD4 T cells are CD11a^{hi}CD49d^{hi} and naïve CD4 T cells are CD11a^{lo}CD49d^{lo} (Fig. 2). There are three main advantages to using these approaches: (1) modulation of CD8α, CD11a and CD49d requires TCR cross-linking and does not occur following exposure of T cells to inflammation or homeostatic proliferation [43–45]. Thus, examination of CD11a, CD8α, and CD49d T cell phenotypes faithfully and durably identifies infection- or vaccination induced, pathogen-specific CD8 and CD4 T cells. (2) endogenous T cell responses can be studied without knowledge of specific *Plasmodium* antigens/epitopes or MHC class I or MHC class II restriction elements; and (3) any combination of inbred or

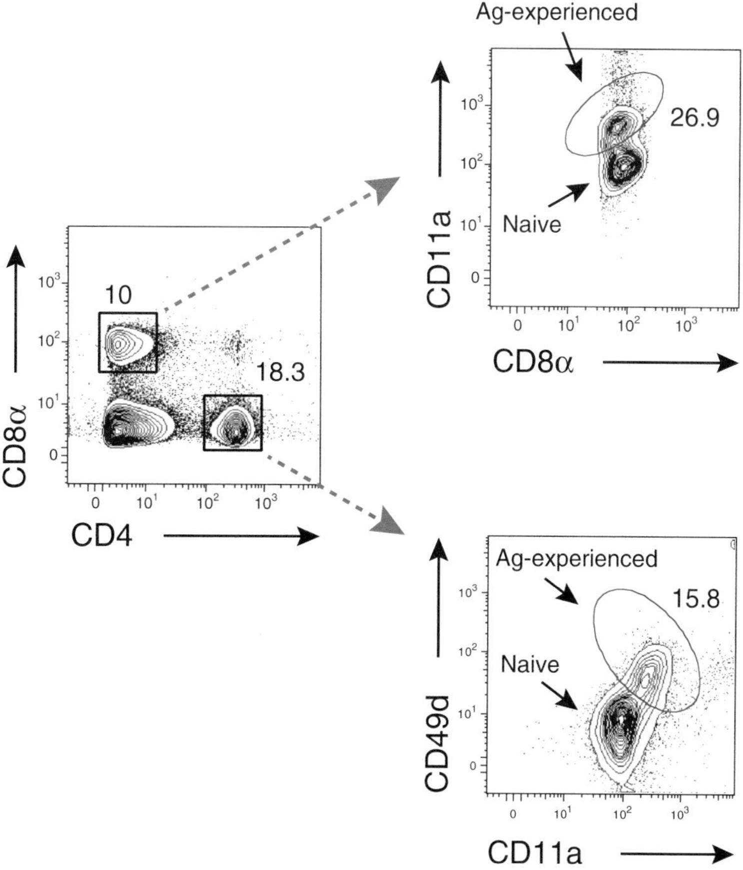

Fig. 2 The spleen from a C57BL/6 mouse was collected 7 days after vaccination with 20,000 *Plasmodium yoelii* radiation attenuated sporozoites (*Py*-RAS). Flow cytometric analyses were conducted to determine the fraction of CD8 and CD4 T cells that were activated by the whole attenuated parasite vaccine and recruited into the anti-*Plasmodium* immune response. Antigen-experienced CD8 T cells are $CD11a^{hi}CD8\alpha^{lo}$ and antigen-experienced CD4 T cells are $CD11a^{hi}CD49d^{hi}$ and are easily distinguished from naïve CD8 and CD4 T cells. *Numbers* refer to the fraction of cells within each defined population gate

outbred mouse strains and *Plasmodium* parasite species can be studied. Overall, these approaches allow for direct examination of the magnitude, kinetics, distribution, phenotype, and function of T cell responses to *Plasmodium* infection or preerythrocytic vaccination. These approaches also allow for longitudinal analyses of T cell responses through analyses of peripheral blood lymphocytes, and thus permit characterization of T cell responses in individual mice over time prior to parasite challenge studies.

The methods detailed below allow researchers to directly identify and interrogate CD4 and CD8 T cell populations induced by preerythrocytic vaccination and recovered from multiple tissues from the vaccinated host. Of note, methods for immunizing rodents with live attenuated *Plasmodium* parasite vaccine platforms have been previously covered [46, 47], so our chapter only describes methods for examining T cell responses induced by preerythrocytic vaccination. Such studies will continue to provide fundamentally important insight into the factors that determine the potent sterilizing immunity induced by preerythrocytic vaccines. This information can potentially guide improvement of current preerythrocytic vaccines as well as enhance the development of subunit vaccines that elicit similar populations of T cells. Defining the specific numerical and functional properties of T cells that determine protection will increase the likelihood of developing readily deployable vaccines in regions of the world where antimalarial vaccines are needed most.

2 Materials

2.1 Equipment

2.1.1 Isolation of Circulating Lymphocytes from Peripheral Blood

1. Heparinized Micro-Hematocrit capillary tubes.
2. 1.5 mL eppendorf tubes.
3. Hemocytometer for cell counting.
4. Trypan Blue (0.1 % solution in phosphate buffered saline (PBS)).
5. Light microscope with a 40× objective.
6. 20 μL, 200 μL, 1,000 μL pipettors and pipette tips.

2.1.2 Isolation of Lymphocytes from Spleen or Lymph Nodes

1. Scissors and forceps.
2. 15 × 60 mm (or 10 × 35 mm) tissue culture dishes.
3. Fine wire screen or 70 μm cell strainer.
4. Rubber-tipped plunger from 3 or 5 mL syringe.
5. 5 and 10 mL pipettes.
6. Drummond Pipette Aid.
7. Hemocytometer for cell counting.
8. Trypan Blue (0.1 % solution in PBS).
9. Light microscope with a 40× objective.
10. 20 μL, 200 μL pipettors and pipette tips.

2.1.3 Isolation of Lymphocytes from Liver

1. Scissors and forceps.
2. 15 × 60 mm tissue culture dishes.
3. Fine wire screen or 70 μm cell strainer.
4. Rubber-tipped plunger from 10 mL syringe.
5. 5 and 10 mL pipettes.

6. Drummond Pipette Aid.
7. Hemocytometer for cell counting.
8. Trypan Blue (0.1 % solution in PBS).
9. Light microscope with a 40× objective.
10. 20 μL, 200 μL pipettors and pipette tips.

2.1.4 Flow Cytometric Staining and Analyses of Lymphocytes

1. Refrigerated tabletop centrifuges with fixed-angle rotor for 1.5 mL eppendorf tubes and swinging bucket rotor and inserts to accommodate 15 mL tubes and 96-well plates.
2. Flow cytometer capable of exciting and detecting emissions from common fluorochromes such as fluorescein isothiocyanate (FITC), phycoerythrin (PE), peridinin chlorophyll protein (PerCP), allophycocyanin (APC), Pacific Blue (PacBlue), and allophycocyanin-cyanine 7 (APC-Cy7) (*see* **Note 1**).
3. Sterile 96-well flat bottom tissue culture plates or 5 mL round bottom flow cytometry tubes (BD Falcon, Fisher Scientific) (*see* **Note 2**).
4. Flow cytometric analysis software (e.g., FlowJo).

2.2 Reagents

2.2.1 Isolation and Staining of Lymphocytes from Peripheral Blood, Lymphoid Tissues and Liver

1. Complete RPMI-1640 medium: 500 mL of RMPI-1640, 50 mL heat-inactivated fetal bovine serum, 10 mM HEPES, 2 mM L-glutamine, 200 mg/mL gentamicin sulfate, 2 mM 2-mercaptoethanol, 100 U/mL penicillin, and 50 μg/mL streptomycin. Store sterile at 4 °C.
2. FACS staining buffer: 1 L of 1× PBS, 10 mL fetal bovine serum, 1 mL 20 % sodium azide. Store at 4 °C.
3. Red blood cell lysis buffer: 1 L of sterile water, 8.25 g NH_4Cl, 1 g $KHCO_3$, 0.037 g Na_2EDTA, adjusted to 7.2–7.4 pH with HCl. Filter-sterilized.
4. Cytofix (BD Biosciences) or other fixation agent. Store at 4 °C.
5. Anti-mouse-CD8α antibody (clone 53-6.7) (*see* **Note 3**).
6. Anti-mouse-CD4 antibody (clone GK1.5).
7. Anti-mouse-CD11a antibody (clone M17/4).
8. Anti-mouse-CD49d antibody (clone R1-2).
9. Anti-mouse-CD90 antibody (*see* **Note 4**).
10. Fixable cell viability dye (eBioscience) or fixable Ghost Dye (Tonbo) to discriminate between live and dead cells (*see* **Note 5**).
11. Anti-mouse-CD16/CD32 (clone 2.4G2) (*see* **Note 6**).
12. $CS_{252-260}$ or $CS_{280-288}$ MHC class I tetramer (*see* **Note 7**).

2.2.2 Isolation of Lymphocytes from Liver (Unique Reagents)

1. Ketamine or other drug to euthanize mouse.
2. Hanks' buffered salt solution (HBSS): 0.137 M NaCl, 5.4 mM KCl, 0.25 mM Na_2HPO_4, 0.44 mM KH_2PO_4, 1.3 mM $CaCl_2$, 1.0 mM $MgSO_4$, 4.2 mM $NaHCO_3$, 5 % fetal bovine serum, 12 mM HEPES buffer. Store sterile at 4 °C (*see* **Note 8**).
3. 35 % Percoll/HBSS solution (Percoll from GE Healthcare). Store sterile at 4 °C.

3 Methods

3.1 Isolation and Staining of Lymphocytes

This section describes the isolation and flow cytometric staining of lymphocytes recovered from the peripheral blood of mice immunized with preerythrocytic vaccines.

3.1.1 Measuring Responses in Peripheral Blood Tissue

1. Collect approximately 20–50 μL blood (*see* **Note 9**) from naïve or vaccinated mice (*see* **Note 10**) into 1.5 mL eppendorf tubes containing 0.5 mL of RPMI-1640 medium.
2. Centrifuge at 400 × *g* for 5 min at 4 °C in a refrigerated tabletop centrifuge.
3. Aspirate supernatant, suspend cells in 0.5 mL of red blood cell lysis buffer, vortex, and incubate at room temperature (RT) for ~3 min.
4. Add 0.9 mL of FACS buffer, spin at 400 × *g* for 5 min at 4 °C in a refrigerated centrifuge (*see* **Note 11** if doing functional analyses).
5. Aspirate supernatant, suspend pellet in 1.2 mL FACS buffer, and spin again at 400 × *g* for 5 min at 4 °C.
6. Aspirate supernatant, suspend pellet in appropriate volume of FACS buffer (*see* **Note 12**).
7. Add 100 μL of cell suspension into wells of flat-bottom 96-well plate (*see* **Notes 2** and **13**).
8. Centrifuge plate at 400 × *g* for 5 min at 4 °C in a tabletop centrifuge.
9. Decant or aspirate supernatants (*see* **Note 14**), lightly vortex plate to disrupt cell pellets.
10. Stain cells with appropriate staining cocktail(s):
    (a) If examining CS-specific CD8 responses using $CS_{252-260}$ (*P. berghei*) or $CS_{280-288}$ *P. yoelii* MHC class I tetramer, cell staining should be performed sequentially:
    - First, add 50 μL of the optimally titrated tetramer reagent, mix with pipetting and incubate at RT, 4 °C or on ice for 1 h (*see* **Note 15**).
    - Second, without washing cells directly add 100 μL of a cocktail of antibodies directed against cell surface

antigens. The surface antigen antibody cocktail should include anti-mouse-CD16/CD32 (clone 2.4G2), anti-mouse-CD8α, anti-mouse-CD11a, anti-mouse CD90; cell viability dye. If simultaneously examining CD4 T cells, the cocktail should also include anti-mouse-CD4 and anti-mouse-CD49d.

- Mix with pipetting and incubate the plate at 4 °C for 20–30 min.

(b) If examining total CD8 and CD4 T cells responses, all reagents are added simultaneously:

- Add 100 μL of a cocktail of antibodies directed against cell surface antigens. The surface antigen antibody cocktail should include anti-mouse-CD16/CD32 (clone 2.4G2), anti-mouse-CD8α, anti-mouse-CD11a, anti-mouse-CD4, anti-mouse-CD49d, anti-mouse CD90, and cell viability dye.
- Mix with pipetting and incubate the plate at 4 °C for 20–30 min.

11. Wash away unbound antibody and/or tetramer from wells by adding 150 μL of FACS buffer directly to wells containing staining cocktail, spin plate at 400 ×*g* for 5 min at 4 °C.
12. Decant or aspirate supernatants, lightly vortex plate, add 100 μL of Cytofix, and incubate at 4 °C for 7–10 min (*see* **Note 16**).
13. Wash away Cytofix from cells by adding 150 μL of FACS buffer directly to wells containing 100 μL of fixative, spin plate at 400 ×*g* for 5 min at 4 °C.
14. Decant or aspirate supernatants, lightly vortex, suspend cells in 180–200 μL of FACS buffer, then store cells at 4 °C protected from light until run on the flow cytometer.

3.1.2 Measuring Responses in Spleen or Lymph Node Tissue

This section describes the isolation and flow cytometric staining of lymphocytes recovered from secondary lymphoid tissues of mice immunized with preerythrocytic vaccines.

1. Harvest desired secondary lymphoid tissues using sterile scissors and forceps and place tissue into 15 mL conical containing 3 mL of RPMI-1640 medium.
2. Transfer the tissue and medium onto a fine mesh steel screen in a 15×60 mm (or 10×35 mm) tissue culture dish. Alternatively, transfer tissue and medium to a 70 μm cell strainer (*see* **Note 17**).
3. Push the tissue through the screen or filter using the head of plunger from a 3 or 5 mL syringe. Rinse the screen or filter with an additional 3 5 mL of RPMI 1640. Repeated pipetting of the suspension through the screen or filter is essential in

order to fully disrupt the tissue and create a single cell suspension. Rinsing screen or filter with fresh medium and combining fractions will enhance cell recovery.

4. Transfer the suspension from tissue culture dish to 15 mL conical and centrifuge samples at 400 × *g* for 5 min in 4 °C tabletop centrifuge.
5. Aspirate or decant supernatant. Suspend cells in 3 mL of red blood cell lysis buffer to the 15-mL conical, vortex, and incubate at RT for 30–60 s.
6. Add ~11 mL of FACS buffer (fill tube), centrifuge samples at 400 × *g* for 5 min in 4 °C tabletop centrifuge (*see* **Note 10** if performing functional analyses).
7. Aspirate or decant supernatant, suspend pellet, wash residual red blood cell lysis buffer from cells by adding 5 mL of FACS buffer and spin at 400 × *g* for 5 min at 4 °C.
8. Aspirate or decant supernatant, suspend pellet in 10 mL (for spleen cells) or 1–3 mL (for lymph node cells) of FACS buffer.
9. Determine total numbers of viable cells using hemocytometer, microscope with 40× objective, and Trypan Blue exclusion dye.
10. Adjust the cell concentration to 10–20 million viable cells/mL (*see* **Note 18**).
11. Add 100 μL of cell suspension into wells of 96-well flat-bottom plate (*see* **Notes 2** and **13**).
12. Centrifuge plate at 400 × *g* for 5 min at 4 °C in a tabletop centrifuge.
13. Decant or aspirate supernatants (*see* **Note 14**), lightly vortex plate to disrupt cell pellets.
14. Stain cells with appropriate staining cocktail(s):
    (a) If examining CS-specific CD8 responses using $CS_{252-260}$ or $CS_{280-288}$ MHC class I tetramer, cell staining should be performed sequentially:
    - First, add 50 μL of the optimally titrated tetramer reagent, mix with pipetting and incubate at RT, 4 °C or on ice for 1 h (*see* **Note 15**).
    - Second, without washing cells directly add 100 μL of a cocktail of antibodies directed against cell surface antigens. The surface antigen antibody cocktail should include anti-mouse-CD16/CD32 (clone 2.4G2), anti-mouse-CD8α, anti-mouse-CD11a, anti-mouse CD90; cell viability dye. If simultaneously examining CD4 T cells, the cocktail should also include anti-mouse-CD4 and anti-mouse-CD49d.
    - Mix with pipetting and incubate the plate at 4 °C for 20–30 min.

(b) If examining total CD8 and CD4 T cells responses, all reagents are added simultaneously:
   - Add 100 μL of a cocktail of antibodies directed against cell surface antigens. The surface antigen antibody cocktail should include anti-mouse-CD16/CD32 (clone 2.4G2), anti-mouse-CD8α, anti-mouse-CD11a, anti-mouse-CD4, anti-mouse-CD49d, anti-mouse CD90, and cell viability dye.
   - Mix with pipetting and incubate the plate at 4 °C for 20–30 min.

15. Wash away unbound antibody and/or tetramer from wells by adding 150 μL of FACS buffer directly to wells containing staining cocktail, spin plate at 400 × *g* for 5 min at 4 °C.
16. Decant or aspirate supernatants, lightly vortex plate, add 100 μL of Cytofix and incubate at 4 °C for 7–10 min (*see* **Note 16**).
17. Wash away Cytofix from cells by adding 150 μL of FACS buffer directly to wells containing 100 μL of fixative, spin plate at 400 × *g* for 5 min at 4 °C.
18. Decant or aspirate supernatants, lightly vortex, suspend cells in 180–200 μL of FACS buffer, then store cells at 4 °C protected from light until run on the flow cytometer.

3.1.3 Measurement of Responses in Liver Tissue

This section describes the isolation and flow cytometric staining of lymphocytes recovered from the livers of mice immunized with preerythrocytic vaccines.

1. Perfuse liver via portal vein with 10 mL of ice-cold HBSS. Remove the gall bladder.
2. Resect the liver and place in 50 mL conical containing 5 mL of ice-cold HBSS.
3. Transfer the tissue and medium onto a fine mesh steel screen in a 15 × 60 mm tissue culture dish. Alternatively, transfer tissue and medium to a 70 μm cell strainer (*see* **Note 17**).
4. Push the tissue through the screen or filter using the head of plunger from a 10 mL syringe. Rinse the screen or filter with an additional 10 mL of ice-cold HBSS. Repeated pipetting of the suspension through the screen or filter is essential in order to fully disrupt the tissue and create a single cell suspension. Rinsing screen or filter with fresh medium and combining fractions will enhance cell recovery.
5. Pass the liver cell suspension through a 70 μm cell strainer seated in a 50 mL conical. Rinse the filter with an additional 20 mL of ice-cold HBSS and combine fractions.
6. Centrifuge cells at 400 × *g* for 10 min at 4 °C in a tabletop centrifuge.

7. Aspirate or decant supernatant, and suspend cell pellet in 15 mL of RT 35 % Percoll/HBSS.
8. Centrifuge cells at 500 × *g* for 10 min at RT in a tabletop centrifuge. Important: Brakes should not be used on rotor.
9. Aspirate or decant supernatant and suspend cell pellet in 2 mL of red blood cell lysis buffer. Incubate for 3 min at RT. Add 12 mL of RPMI-1640 and transfer the entire cell suspension into a 15 mL conical.
10. Centrifuge cells at 400 × *g* for 5 min at 4 °C in a tabletop centrifuge.
11. Aspirate or decant supernatant, suspend pellet in 1 mL RPMI-1640 medium.
12. Determine total numbers of viable cells using hemocytometer, microscope with 40x objective, and Trypan Blue exclusion dye.
13. Adjust the cell concentration to 10–20 million viable cells/mL (*see* **Note 18**).
14. Add 100 μL of cell suspension into wells of 96-well flat-bottom plate (*see* **Notes 2** and **13**).
15. Centrifuge plate at 400 × *g* for 5 min at 4 °C in a tabletop centrifuge.
16. Decant or aspirate supernatants (*see* **Note 14**), lightly vortex plate to disrupt cell pellets.
17. Stain cells with appropriate staining cocktail(s):
    (a) If examining CS-specific CD8 responses using $CS_{252-260}$ or $CS_{280-288}$ MHC class I tetramer, cell staining should be performed sequentially:
        - First, add 50 μL of the optimally titrated tetramer reagent, mix with pipetting and incubate at RT, 4 °C or on ice for 1 h (*see* **Note 15**).
        - Second, without washing cells directly add 100 μL of a cocktail of antibodies directed against cell surface antigens. The surface antigen antibody cocktail should include anti-mouse-CD16/CD32 (clone 2.4G2), anti-mouse-CD8α, anti-mouse-CD11a, anti-mouse CD90; cell viability dye. If simultaneously examining CD4 T cells, the cocktail should also include anti-mouse-CD4 and anti-mouse-CD49d.
        - Mix with pipetting and incubate the plate at 4 °C for 20–30 min.

    (b) If examining total CD8 and CD4 T cells responses, all reagents are added simultaneously:
        - Add 100 μL of a cocktail of antibodies directed against cell surface antigens. The surface antigen antibody

cocktail should include anti-mouse-CD16/CD32 (clone 2.4G2), anti-mouse-CD8α, anti-mouse-CD11a, anti-mouse-CD4, anti-mouse-CD49d, anti-mouse CD90 and cell viability dye.

- Mix with pipetting and incubate the plate at 4 °C for 20–30 min.

18. Wash away unbound antibody and/or tetramer from wells by adding 150 μL of FACS buffer directly to wells containing staining cocktail, spin plate at 400 × *g* for 5 min at 4 °C.
19. Decant or aspirate supernatants, lightly vortex plate, add 100 μL of Cytofix and incubate at 4 °C for 7–10 min (*see* **Note 16**).
20. Wash away Cytofix from cells by adding 150 μL of FACS buffer directly to wells containing 100 μL of fixative, spin plate at 400 × *g* for 5 min at 4 °C.
21. Decant or aspirate supernatants, lightly vortex, suspend cells in 180–200 μL of FACS buffer, then store cells at 4 °C protected from light until run on the flow cytometer.

3.2 Analysis

This section describes the collection and analysis of flow cytometric data to determine the frequency of antigen-experienced effector and memory CD8 and CD4 T cells following preerythrocytic vaccination. This protocol does not describe how to properly compensate samples on a flow cytometer (*see* **Note 13**).

1. Using an analytical flow cytometer program, draw a population gate around viable lymphocytes using forward-area (FSC-A) and side-area (SSC-A) scatter parameters (*X*- and *Y*-axis, respectively). This population gate excludes cell debris (or small, likely dead cells) from further analysis.
2. Optional—If the flow cytometer is capable of analyzing forward width scatter (FSC-W), draw a population gate around single cell ("singlet") lymphocyte populations using forward width (FSC-W) and side-area scatter (SSC-A); this gate excludes cell doublets from further analysis.
3. Draw a population gate on lymphocytes that are negative for staining with viability dye reagents. This gate further excludes dead cells and enhances the quality and resolution of data for downstream analyses of T cell phenotype and function.
4. For CD8 T cell analyses, draw a population gate around CD8+ CD90+ cells by viewing CD8α staining on the *X*-axis, and CD90.2 staining on the *Y*-axis. Next gate on the antigen-experienced ($CD8\alpha^{lo}CD11a^{hi}$) CD8 T cells by examining CD8α expression and CD11a expression on the *X*- and *Y*-axis, respectively.
5. Optional—the fraction of $CD8\alpha^{lo}CD11a^{hi}$ CD8 T cells that are CS-specific can be determined by examining the fraction of

antigen-experienced CD8 T cells that bind the MHC class I tetramer by viewing CD8α on the *X*-axis and tetramer on the *Y*-axis (Figs. 1 and 2).

6. For CD4 T cell analyses, draw a population gate around CD4+CD90+ cells by viewing CD4 staining on the *X*-axis, and CD90.2 staining on the *Y*-axis. Next gate on the antigen-experienced ($CD11a^{hi}CD49d^{hi}$) CD4 T cells by examining CD11a expression and CD49d expression on the *X*- and *Y*-axis, respectively (Fig. 2).
7. Additional parameters of T cell phenotype and function and be analyzed by including additional reagents in the cell staining cocktails, assuming the analytical flow cytometer can accommodate the extra channels required (i.e., appropriate lasers and filter sets).

4 Notes

1. The suggested protocol requires access to a flow cytometer capable of simultaneous detection of six or more colors. Examination of additional phenotypic or functional parameters will require more sophisticated cytometers with additional lasers and filter sets. Although not recommended, omitting the anti-mouse-CD90 antibody and/or live/dead reagents will permit examination of additional phenotypic or functional parameters using a 6-color cytometer.
2. Protocols described here utilize 96-well flat bottom plates for cell staining, which increases work efficiency and decreases reagent use. However, identical results can be obtained by processing, staining, and analyzing cells in 5 mL Falcon tubes designed to fit most commercial analytical flow cytometers.
3. Each antibody reagent should be individually titrated to determine optimal final concentrations. Specific fluorochrome conjugates for each antibody will be dictated by the capabilities of the analytical flow cytometer.
4. Including the anti-mouse-CD90 antibody will allow resolution between the T cells of interest and non-T cells expressing CD8α or CD4 (e.g., dendritic cells or macrophages). Although these contaminating subsets are relatively low frequency events, including anti-mouse-CD90 can be particularly helpful when examining T cell responses in lymph nodes, spleen, or liver. Commonly available mouse lines such as C57BL/6, BALB/c and outbred mice express the CD90.2 allele. Congenic lines are also available that express the CD90.1 allele. Monoclonal antibodies that distinguish between these two polymorphisms are available and highly specific for each molecule, so care should be taken when selecting a CD90 clone. We recommend

clone 53-2.1 for anti-mouse-CD90.2 and clone OX-7 for anti-mouse-CD90.1.

5. Regents that resolve between live and dead lymphocytes are particularly useful, as dead cells tend to nonspecifically bind fluorochrome-conjugated antibodies. These unwanted interactions can significantly increase background staining and nonspecific signals during flow cytometry. If fixatives are included in the protocol, care should be taken that the selected dye withstands fixation (e.g., 4 % paraformaldehyde).

6. Nonspecific binding of antibodies can be minimized by including an unconjugated anti-mouse-FcR (CD16/CD32) antibody (clone 2.4G2).

7. Fluorochrome-conjugated MHC class I (H-2K^d) tetramer reagents for detection of CS-specific CD8 T cells in vaccinated BALB/c mice are available from the NIH tetramer core (http://tetramer.yerkes.emory.edu) or MBL, Inc. (http://www.mblintl.com).

8. HBSS is utilized at two different temperatures in the protocol for isolating lymphocytes from the liver. Be sure to adjust an appropriate volume to RT prior to harvesting liver tissues.

9. The capillary tubes utilized by our laboratory hold approximately 70 μL of blood. The total volume of blood collected in any specific interval should not exceed that recommended by IACUC guidelines. Particular care and consideration should be given to the execution of longitudinal experiments designed to include multiple serial bleeds from individual mice.

10. If tracking T cell responses longitudinally in peripheral blood, all animals should be assayed prior to vaccination to determine the individual background frequencies of circulating CD8α^{lo}CD11a^{hi} CD8 T cells and CD11a^{hi}CD49d^{hi} CD4 T cells. Of note, the described approaches are not likely useful for evaluating T cells responses induced by vectored vaccines designed to target liver stage *Plasmodium* parasites, as the surrogate marker of T cell activation approaches will not distinguish between T cell responses directed against the viral vector versus the *Plasmodium* antigen encoded by the vector.

11. If performing functional studies prior to T cell staining, substitute RPMI-1640 medium for FACS buffer. FACS buffer contains sodium azide, which poisons electron transport in eukaryotic and prokaryotic cells. Sodium azide is highly toxic so care should be taken when handling any solution containing this compound.

12. The volume of FACS buffer in which peripheral blood lymphocytes are suspended is ultimately dictated by the number of distinct flow cytometric analyses that will be performed. For example, if two independent staining cocktails will be applied

to the cells, suspend the cells in a minimum of 200 μL of FACS buffer; if six independent stains will be performed, suspend the cells in 600 μL of FACS buffer, etc. We routinely recover more than 100,000 lymphocytes from 20 μL of whole blood when the sample is processed using protocols described above.

13. Be sure to set aside a sufficient number of cells for the compensation staining control reactions. Only 2,000–5,000 events are generally required for compensation reactions. An explanation of compensation is not discussed here but has been thoroughly described elsewhere [48].
14. A flick-of-the-wrist can be used to invert the plate to decant (eject) supernatants into a suitable waste receptacle. Alternatively, supernatants can be aspirated individually. Do not tap the plate on a solid surface or flick the plate more than once or the cells of interest will also be ejected from the wells.
15. MHC class I tetramer reagents must be titrated for optimal staining. The incubation temperature (e.g., RT, 4 °C or on ice) should also be determined empirically. Anti-CD8α antibody can interfere with tetramer binding to TCR on CD8 T cells, so antibodies directed against CD8α (and other surface antigens) should only be added after the initial tetramer incubation.
16. After surface staining, we routinely fix cells with 4 % paraformaldehyde fixative solution such as Cytofix (BD Biosciences). This can be particularly important to stabilize the staining reactions when samples will not be immediately run on the analytical flow cytometer.
17. The methods used to disrupt tissues to generate single cell lymphocyte suspensions via mechanical means are not critical. Here we have outlined two methods that are routinely used in our laboratory to create single cell suspensions from secondary lymphoid tissues and liver (wire mesh and 70 μm cell strainer). Investigators should empirically determine the optimal method for their experiments, choosing methods that yield the largest number of viable cells.
18. From our experience, we have found it is best to only plate one to two million cells in a well. Using a known number of cells and optimizing antibody concentrations through titration experiments will ensure that tetramer and antibody reagents are not limiting.

Acknowledgements

The authors would like to thank current members of the Butler Laboratory for their critical reading of the manuscript and many helpful discussions. Work in the Butler Laboratory is supported by the National Institute of Allergy and Infectious Diseases of the National Institutes of Health through grant number 5K22AI099070, the National Institute of General Medical Sciences of the National Institutes of Health through Grant Number 8P20GM103447, and the American Heart Association through grant number 13BGIA17140002.

References

1. Griffin JT, Hollingsworth TD, Okell LC, Churcher TS, White M et al (2010) Reducing Plasmodium falciparum malaria transmission in Africa: a model-based evaluation of intervention strategies. PLoS Med 7, e1000324
2. World Health Organization (2014) Malaria vaccine rainbow table. http://www.who.int/vaccine_research/links/Rainbow/en/index.html
3. Clyde DF (1975) Immunization of man against falciparum and vivax malaria by use of attenuated sporozoites. Am J Trop Med Hyg 24:397–401
4. Hoffman SL, Goh LM, Luke TC, Schneider I, Le TP et al (2002) Protection of humans against malaria by immunization with radiation-attenuated Plasmodium falciparum sporozoites. J Infect Dis 185:1155–1164
5. Epstein JE, Tewari K, Lyke KE, Sim BK, Billingsley PF et al (2011) Live attenuated malaria vaccine designed to protect through hepatic CD8(+) T cell immunity. Science 334:475–480
6. Seder RA, Chang LJ, Enama ME, Zephir KL, Sarwar UN et al (2013) Protection against malaria by intravenous immunization with a nonreplicating sporozoite vaccine. Science 341:1359–1365
7. Spring M, Murphy J, Nielsen R, Dowler M, Bennett JW et al (2013) First-in-human evaluation of genetically attenuated Plasmodium falciparum sporozoites administered by bite of Anopheles mosquitoes to adult volunteers. Vaccine 31:4975–4983
8. Roestenberg M, Teirlinck AC, McCall MB, Teelen K, Makamdop KN et al (2011) Long-term protection against malaria after experimental sporozoite inoculation: an open-label follow-up study. Lancet 377:1770–1776
9. Roestenberg M, McCall M, Hopman J, Wiersma J, Luty AJ et al (2009) Protection against a malaria challenge by sporozoite inoculation. N Engl J Med 361:468–477
10. Bijker EM, Bastiaens GJ, Teirlinck AC, van Gemert GJ, Graumans W et al (2013) Protection against malaria after immunization by chloroquine prophylaxis and sporozoites is mediated by preerythrocytic immunity. Proc Natl Acad Sci U S A 110:7862–7867
11. Belnoue E, Costa FT, Frankenberg T, Vigario AM, Voza T et al (2004) Protective T cell immunity against malaria liver stage after vaccination with live sporozoites under chloroquine treatment. J Immunol 172:2487–2495
12. Nussenzweig RS, Vanderberg J, Most H, Orton C (1967) Protective immunity produced by the injection of x-irradiated sporozoites of *Plasmodium berghei*. Nature 216:160–162
13. Tarun AS, Dumpit RF, Camargo N, Labaied M, Liu P et al (2007) Protracted sterile protection with *Plasmodium yoelii* pre-erythrocytic genetically attenuated parasite malaria vaccines is independent of significant liver-stage persistence and is mediated by CD8+ T cells. J Infect Dis 196:608–616
14. Nganou-Makamdop K, van Gemert GJ, Arens T, Hermsen CC, Sauerwein RW (2012) Long term protection after immunization with *P. berghei* sporozoites correlates with sustained IFNgamma responses of hepatic CD8+ memory T cells. PLoS One 7, e36508
15. Schmidt NW, Butler NS, Badovinac VP, Harty JT (2010) Extreme CD8 T cell requirements for anti-malarial liver-stage immunity following immunization with radiation attenuated sporozoites. PLoS Pathog 6, e1000998
16. Bijker EM, Teirlinck AC, Schats R, van Gemert GJ, van de Vegte-Bolmer M et al (2014) Cytotoxic markers associate with protection against malaria in human volunteers immunized With Plasmodium falciparum sporozoites. J Infect Dis
17. Butler NS, Schmidt NW, Harty JT (2010) Differential effector pathways regulate memory CD8 T cell immunity against *Plasmodium berghei* versus *P. yoelii* sporozoites. J Immunol 184:2528–2538
18. Cockburn IA, Tse SW, Zavala F (2014) CD8+ T cells eliminate liver-stage *Plasmodium berghei* parasites without detectable bystander effect. Infect Immun 82:1460–1464
19. Chakravarty S, Baldeviano GC, Overstreet MG, Zavala F (2008) Effector CD8+ T

lymphocytes against liver stages of *Plasmodium yoelii* do not require gamma interferon for antiparasite activity. Infect Immun 76:3628–3631

20. Frevert U, Moreno A, Calvo-Calle JM, Klotz C, Nardin E (2009) Imaging effector functions of human cytotoxic CD4+ T cells specific for Plasmodium falciparum circumsporozoite protein. Int J Parasitol 39:119–132
21. Keesen TS, Gomes JA, Fares RC, de Araujo FF, Ferreira KS et al (2012) Characterization of CD4(+) cytotoxic lymphocytes and apoptosis markers induced by Trypanossoma cruzi infection. Scand J Immunol 76:311–319
22. Purner MB, Berens RL, Nash PB, van Linden A, Ross E et al (1996) CD4-mediated and CD8-mediated cytotoxic and proliferative immune responses to Toxoplasma gondii in seropositive humans. Infect Immun 64:4330–4338
23. Renia L, Grillot D, Marussig M, Corradin G, Miltgen F et al (1993) Effector functions of circumsporozoite peptide-primed CD4+ T cell clones against *Plasmodium yoelii* liver stages. J Immunol 150:1471–1478
24. Oliveira GA, Kumar KA, Calvo-Calle JM, Othoro C, Altszuler D et al (2008) Class II-restricted protective immunity induced by malaria sporozoites. Infect Immun 76:1200–1206
25. Overstreet MG, Chen YC, Cockburn IA, Tse SW, Zavala F (2011) CD4+ T cells modulate expansion and survival but not functional properties of effector and memory CD8+ T cells induced by malaria sporozoites. PLoS One 6, e15948
26. Weiss WR, Berzofsky JA, Houghten RA, Sedegah M, Hollindale M et al (1992) A T cell clone directed at the circumsporozoite protein which protects mice against both *Plasmodium yoelii* and *Plasmodium berghei*. J Immunol 149:2103–2109
27. Sano G, Hafalla JC, Morrot A, Abe R, Lafaille JJ et al (2001) Swift development of protective effector functions in naive CD8(+) T cells against malaria liver stages. J Exp Med 194: 173–180
28. Sponaas AM, Cadman ET, Voisine C, Harrison V, Boonstra A et al (2006) Malaria infection changes the ability of splenic dendritic cell populations to stimulate antigen-specific T cells. J Exp Med 203:1427–1433
29. Stephens R, Albano FR, Quin S, Pascal BJ, Harrison V et al (2005) Malaria-specific transgenic CD4(+) T cells protect immunodeficient mice from lethal infection and demonstrate requirement for a protective threshold of antibody production for parasite clearance. Blood 106:1676–1684
30. Stephens R, Langhorne J (2010) Effector memory Th1 CD4 T cells are maintained in a mouse model of chronic malaria. PLoS Pathog 6, e1001208
31. Lau LS, Fernandez-Ruiz D, Mollard V, Sturm A, Neller MA et al (2014) CD8+ T cells from a novel T cell receptor transgenic mouse induce liver-stage immunity that can be boosted by blood-stage infection in rodent malaria. PLoS Pathog 10, e1004135
32. Chen YC, Zavala F (2013) Development and use of TCR transgenic mice for malaria immunology research. Methods Mol Biol 923:481–491
33. Schmidt NW, Butler NS, Harty JT (2011) Plasmodium-host interactions directly influence the threshold of memory CD8 T cells required for protective immunity. J Immunol 186:5873–5884
34. Schmidt NW, Podyminogin RL, Butler NS, Badovinac VP, Tucker BJ et al (2008) Memory CD8 T cell responses exceeding a large but definable threshold provide long-term immunity to malaria. Proc Natl Acad Sci U S A 105:14017–14022
35. Kumar KA, Sano G, Boscardin S, Nussenzweig RS, Nussenzweig MC et al (2006) The circumsporozoite protein is an immunodominant protective antigen in irradiated sporozoites. Nature 444:937–940
36. Mauduit M, Gruner AC, Tewari R, Depinay N, Kayibanda M et al (2009) A role for immune responses against non-CS components in the cross-species protection induced by immunization with irradiated malaria sporozoites. PLoS One 4, e7717
37. Berenzon D, Schwenk RJ, Letellier L, Guebre-Xabier M, Williams J et al (2003) Protracted protection to *Plasmodium berghei* malaria is linked to functionally and phenotypically heterogeneous liver memory CD8+ T cells. J Immunol 171:2024–2034
38. Jobe O, Lumsden J, Mueller AK, Williams J, Silva-Rivera H et al (2007) Genetically attenuated *Plasmodium berghei* liver stages induce sterile protracted protection that is mediated by major histocompatibility complex Class I-dependent interferon-gamma-producing CD8+ T cells. J Infect Dis 196:599–607
39. Krzych U, Dalai S, Zarling S, Pichugin A (2012) Memory CD8 T cells specific for plasmodia liver-stage antigens maintain protracted protection against malaria. Front Immunol 3:370
40. Zarling S, Berenzon D, Dalai S, Liepinsh D, Steers N et al (2013) The survival of memory CD8 T cells that is mediated by IL-15 corre-

lates with sustained protection against malaria. J Immunol 190:5128–5141

41. Boyman O, Sprent J (2012) The role of interleukin-2 during homeostasis and activation of the immune system. Nat Rev Immunol 12:180–190
42. Akue AD, Lee JY, Jameson SC (2012) Derivation and maintenance of virtual memory CD8 T cells. J Immunol 188:2516–2523
43. Butler NS, Moebius J, Pewe LL, Traore B, Doumbo OK et al (2012) Therapeutic blockade of PD-L1 and LAG-3 rapidly clears established blood-stage Plasmodium infection. Nat Immunol 13:188–195
44. Rai D, Pham NL, Harty JT, Badovinac VP (2009) Tracking the total CD8 T cell response to infection reveals substantial discordance in magnitude and kinetics between inbred and outbred hosts. J Immunol 183: 7672–7681
45. McDermott DS, Varga SM (2011) Quantifying antigen-specific CD4 T cells during a viral infection: CD4 T cell responses are larger than we think. J Immunol 187:5568–5576
46. Renia L, Gruner AC, Mauduit M, Snounou G (2013) Vaccination using normal live sporozoites under drug treatment. Methods Mol Biol 923:567–576
47. Vaughan AM, Kappe SH (2013) Vaccination using radiation- or genetically attenuated live sporozoites. Methods Mol Biol 923:549–566
48. Kalina T, Flores-Montero J, van der Velden VH, Martin-Ayuso M, Bottcher S et al (2012) EuroFlow standardization of flow cytometer instrument settings and immunophenotyping protocols. Leukemia 26:1986–2010

Chapter 3

Characterization of Liver CD8 T Cell Subsets that are Associated with Protection Against Pre-erythrocytic Plasmodium Parasites

Stasya Zarling and Urszula Krzych

Abstract

Murine models of malaria, such as *Plasmodium berghei* (Pb) and *Plasmodium yoelii* (Py), have been used for decades to identify correlates of protection associated with immunization using radiation-attenuated sporozoites (RAS). To date, RAS is the only known immunization regimen to consistently deliver 100 % sterilizing immunity and is considered the "gold standard" of protection against malaria. The ability to isolate lymphocytes directly from the liver of immune mice has facilitated the identification of correlates of protection at the site of infection. Liver CD8 T cells have been identified as a key factor in mediating protection against challenge with infectious Plasmodium sporozoites. Liver CD3 + CD8 T cells can further be divided into subsets based on the expression of specific surface molecules and the increase of CD8 effector memory (T_{EM}) cells (identified by the phenotype $CD44^{+}CD62L^{-}$) has been shown to mediate protection by releasing of IFN-γ while CD8 central memory (T_{CM}) cells ($CD44^{+}CD62L^{+}$) are important for maintaining long-term protection.

Identification of multiple CD8 T cell subsets present in the liver relies on the ability to detect multiple surface markers simultaneously. Polychromatic flow cytometry affords the user with the ability to distinguish multiple lymphocyte populations as well as subsets defined within each population. In this chapter we present a basic 9-color surface staining panel that can be used to identify CD8 T_{EM}, CD8 T_{CM}, short-lived effector cells (SLECs), and memory precursor cells (MPECs) as well as identify those cells which have recently undergone degranulation (surface expression of CD107a). This panel has been designed to allow for the addition of intracellular staining for IFN-γ on other available channels (such as PE) as is discussed in another chapter for analysis of functional CD8 T cell responses.

Key words Malaria, Flow cytometry, CD8 T cells, CD8 T cell subsets, Liver

1 Introduction

CD8 T cells are considered key effectors against pre-erythrocytic (PE) stage malaria infection. Evidence supporting the effector function of CD8 T cells is based on studies in human [1–3] and animal models of immunization with radiation-attenuated sporozoites (RAS) [4, 5] and genetically attenuated parasites (GAP) [6–8], both of which induce long-lasting protection.

Ashley M. Vaughan (ed.), *Malaria Vaccines: Methods and Protocols*, Methods in Molecular Biology, vol. 1325,
DOI 10.1007/978-1-4939-2815-6_3,

Mouse models of malaria such as *Plasmodium berghei* (Pb) or *P. yoelii* (Py) have been useful in characterizing antigen (Ag)-specific T cell responses required to mediate this prolonged protection. Our laboratory has been studying mainly CD8 T cell responses induced by *P. berghei* RAS. We have demonstrated that naïve CD8 T cells expand and differentiate into various subsets, including IFN-γ-producing effectors and memory subsets in mice exposed to multiple immunizations with *P. berghei* RAS. The formation and persistence of memory T cells with a reservoir of central memory cells allow for the conscription of IFN-γ-producing effector/effector memory cells during reinfections. This information is most crucial towards building a better understanding of the cellular and molecular events that occur during the induction and maintenance of protective immune responses by pre-erythrocytic stage antigens and ultimately towards planning and development of an effective anti-malaria vaccine.

The information in this chapter builds on observations concerning the *P. berghei* model of protective immunity gathered by the members of our laboratory over the past two decades. The *P. berghei* model allows for the dissection of CD8 T cell responses not only in immune organs but also in nonimmune organs, such as the liver. The importance of liver CD8 T cells is particularly underscored in the RAS model because the attenuated sporozoites that home to the liver continue to undergo aborted development and form a repository of pre-erythrocytic stage antigens, including sporozoite- and liver-stage antigens. The availability of these antigens is inextricably linked to the maintenance of memory CD8 T cells that assure a fast, effective, and specific response against reoccurring infections [4]. On the basis of the expression of TCR Vβ gene segments by CD8 T cells, we observed that CD8 T cells in the liver are reflected in the peripheral blood, although the number of these cells is much smaller than in the liver [9]. The *P. berghei* RAS model also lends itself to the dissection of other immunologic components, such as cytokines, that together with the depot of antigens from the partly developed parasites regulate the network of cellular responses needed for the maintenance of sterile protection.

Apart from liver T cells, we have also investigated antigen-presenting cells (APCs), such as $CD8\alpha^{+}cDC11c^{+}$ [10], Kupffer cells (KCs) [11], and the various cytokines that play a role in the induction as well as the maintenance of CD8 T cells [12, 13]. In many instances, studies involving liver APCs and cytokines were needed for a better understanding of the function of liver CD8 T cells in protection against pre-erythrocytic stage malaria. In this chapter we focus predominantly on the methods for characterizing liver CD8 T cell subsets by flow cytometry, the initial steps involving preparation of the liver, such as perfusion and isolation of liver mononuclear cells, have been covered in another chapter.

Most of our approaches described here are based on experiments that have been performed with *P. berghei* RAS in C57BL/6 mice; however, these approaches can be extended to other murine RAS and GAP Plasmodium species as well as to RAS or GAP simian models where liver samples could be easily obtained from biopsies. In addition, the methodologies described here could provide an initial step towards further studies, such as the detection of tetramer-binding CD8 T cells, gene expression by particular CD8 T cell subsets, and in vitro CD8 T cell interactions with other T cells or with various APCs. Importantly, because our approaches are based on the processes associated with the differentiation of CD8 T cells, including the induction of effector function and memory formation, they rely on the differentiation-related expression of cell surface markers by the different CD8 T cell subsets. Hence, these methodologies are also applicable to the various kinetics studies of CD8 T cell subset induction and/or apoptosis.

Following RAS immunization, the overall population of intrahepatic CD8 T cells significantly increases as compared to naïve mice and protection is linked to both increased CD8 effector memory (T_{EM}) and central memory (T_{CM}) cells. These two main CD8 T cell subsets are defined on the basis of the surface expression of CD44 and CD62L and occasionally CD45 and CD122. In addition, the use of KLRG-1 and CD127 (IL-7Rα) provides further characterization of CD8 T_{EM} cells as short-lived effector cells (SLECs) (KLRG-1^{hi} CD127^{lo}) and memory precursor cells (MPECs) (KLRG-1^{lo}CD127^{hi}) (Fig. 1). The combination of these markers, along with the expression of CD107a (LAMP-1), which is an indication of recent degranulation, provides a detailed functional characterization and subset composition of liver CD8 T cells following exposure to pre-erythrocytic parasites.

While the flow cytometry technique was developed nearly four decades ago [14–16], the recent expansion of available fluorochromes has made polychromatic flow cytometry for complex phenotyping much more accessible. With all of these new fluorochromes the complexity and importance of panel design have increased. First, when choosing fluorochromes it is necessary to consider not only the "brightness" of the fluorochrome, but also the level of expression of the cell surface marker that is being identified. Thus, "bright" fluorochromes should be used on low-expressing markers or populations, while "dim" fluorochromes may be used on discrete-expressing markers (i.e., those which are either positive or negative such as CD3, CD4, or CD8). Secondly, it is necessary to consider the instrument and laser availability; for example, maximize the use of lasers by avoiding the use of multiple fluorochromes on the blue laser while neglecting to use the violet or UV lasers.

Since fluorochromes do not emit signal at a discrete wavelength, but rather over a spectrum, it is possible for the emission of one fluorochrome to "spill over" into a neighboring channel.

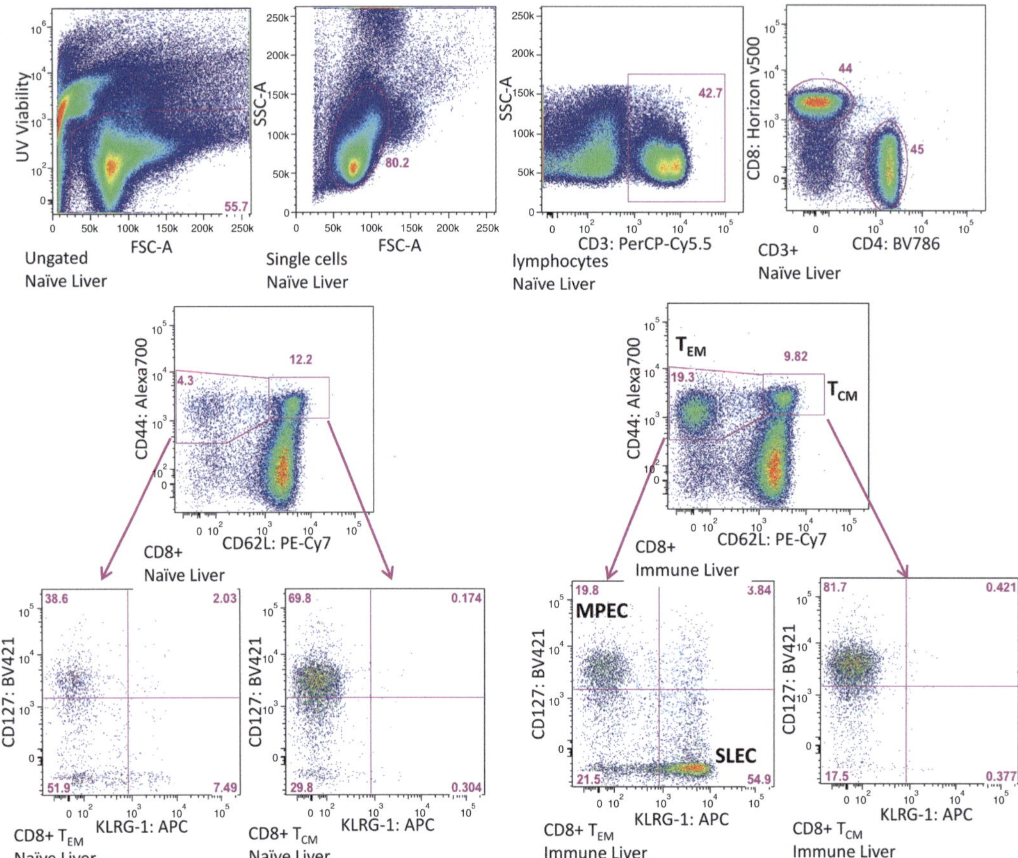

Fig. 1 Intrahepatic mononuclear cells were isolated from naïve C57BL/6 mice and C57BL/6 mice immunized with radiation-attenuated *Plasmodium berghei* sporozoites and stained according to the protocol as described

Compensation controls are important for calculating the amount of spillover into each channel that can be attributed to other fluorochromes used in the same panel. This is achieved by using single-stained controls for each fluorochrome. Data should be uncompensated when collected and can be compensated using analysis software based on single-stained control samples [17]. When the compensation is correctly set, the median fluorescence intensities (MFIs) of the positive and negative populations of the compensation control are similar to each other when viewed in other channels (e.g., the FITC-positive and -negative controls have a similar MFI when read in the PE channel) [18].

In addition to correctly calculating compensation, the inclusion of proper biological controls and fluorescence minus one (FMO) controls for markers of interest aids in correctly drawing gates to account for any "spillover" of other fluorochromes into the channel of interest which may not be evident in an unstained sample. Thus, gating on unstained samples may place the cutoff between positive and negative populations too low [17, 19].

Once the operator becomes familiar with the panel of fluorochromes used, FMO controls may not be necessary in every experiment, but they are always useful to include. Isotype controls may be used to determine any nonspecific binding of the antibody isotype and background fluorescence attributed to the fluorochrome. For markers with discrete populations, FMO controls are usually sufficient to determine gating: however if staining "sticky" cells such as dendritic cells, the marker of interest is expressed on a spectrum or if one is interested in a quantitative change in expression by MFI, isotype controls should be included as well. For the purposes of this protocol we include FMO controls for CD107a, KLRG-1, and CD127 to ensure proper gating during analysis.

2 Materials

Hanks' Basic Salt Solution (with calcium and magnesium) containing 2 % fetal bovine serum (FBS).

70 μM nylon cell strainer.

Percoll.

Red blood cell (RBC) lysis buffer.

Anti-mouse CD3:PerCP-Cy5.5 (clone 145-2C11).

Anti-mouse CD4:BV786 (clone GK1.5).

Anti-mouse CD8α:Horizon v500 (clone 53-6.7).

Anti-mouse CD44:Alexa700 (clone IM7).

Anti-mouse CD62L:PE-Cy7 (clone MEL-14).

Anti-mouse KLRG-1:APC (clone 2F1).

Anti-mouse CD127:BV421 (clone A7R34).

Anti-mouse CD107a:FITC (clone 1D4B).

Anti-mouse CD16/CD32 (FcR block, clone 2.4G2).

Live/dead blue fixable viability dye (Life Technologies).

Compensation control antibodies (anti-CD3, -CD4, or -CD8 labeled with each fluorochrome used).

Compensation beads (if using tandem dyes or insufficient number of cells).

FACS buffer: 1× phosphate-buffered saline (PBS), 2 % FBS.

96-Well V-bottom plate.

1.2 ml cluster tubes (Corning).

Formaldehyde.

BD LSR II, Fortessa or other multi laser flow cytometer equipped with UV laser.

FlowJo or other analysis software.

3 Methods

3.1 Isolation of Intrahepatic Mononuclear Cells

The details of liver perfusion and resection are described fully in another chapter. Isolation of liver intrahepatic mononuclear cells (IHMCs) has been described previously [20]. Briefly, following immunization with Pb RAS or challenge with Pb infectious sporozoites, mice are euthanized by CO_2 inhalation. After perfusion, liver lobes are placed in Hanks' Basic Salt Solution containing 2 % FBS and gently pressed through a 70 μM nylon cell strainer. The cell suspension is centrifuged at $60 \times g$ for 1 min. The supernatant is collected and centrifuged again at $450 \times g$ for 8 min. The cell pellet is then resuspended in PBS containing 37.5 % Percoll and centrifuged at $850 \times g$ for 30 min. The cell pellet is lysed of RBCs with RBC lysis buffer and subsequently washed twice in FACS buffer.

3.2 Antibody Staining Cocktail Preparation

1. For best results individual antibodies should be titrated for each marker-fluorochrome combination; the volumes listed here are generalized for the purpose of this protocol.
2. Calculate the total volume of each antibody needed for all samples.
   (a) 0.5–1 μl of each antibody per sample (*see* **Note 1**).
   (b) Add three extra samples to the total for CD3, CD4, CD8α, CD44, and CD62L for FMO controls (e.g., assume that you have ten samples; additionally add three FMO controls = 13 × 0.5 μl = 6.5 μl each of CD3, CD4, CD8α, CD44, and CD62L; 10 samples × 0.5 μl = 5 μl each of CD107a, KLRG-1, and CD127).
3. Calculate the total volume of FcR block (1 μl/sample) including FMO controls.
4. Calculate the total volume of viability dye (0.2 μl/sample) including FMO controls.
5. Calculate the volume of FACS buffer needed so that each sample and FMO control receives 100 μl total volume (100 μl × the number of samples – total volume of antibodies – total viability dye).
6. Combine FACS buffer, surface staining antibodies (except CD107a, KLRG-1, and CD127), viability dye, and FcR blocking antibody and mix well.
7. Remove 300 μl of the antibody mixture and set aside, add CD107a, KLRG-1, and CD127 antibodies to the remaining staining cocktail, and keep on ice.
   (a) Aliquot reserved 300 μl into 3 × 100 μl aliquots for FMO controls. Add CD107a, KLRG-1, or CD127 antibodies so that each FMO control lacks one antibody.

FMO 1: CD107a + KLRG-1.

FMO 2: CD107a + CD127.

FMO 3: KLRG-1 + CD127.

8. Keep staining cocktails on ice and protected from light until samples are ready for staining.

3.3 Sample Preparation

1. Aliquot 0.5–1.0 × 10^6 cells/sample in 96-well V-bottom plate; include three wells for FMO controls.
2. Aliquot 0.5–1.0 × 10^6 cells per well for compensation controls; include one well for each fluorochrome used as well as an unstained control (*see* **Note 2**).
3. Spin plate at 450 × *g* for 5 min at 4 °C, decant supernatant, and vortex to resuspend.
4. Wash cells with 200 μl/well FACS buffer. Spin at 450 × *g* for 5 min at 4 °C, decant supernatant, and vortex to resuspend.

3.4 General Surface Staining

1. Suspend all compensation control wells in 100 μl FACS buffer.
   (a) Heat kill 50 μl of viability compensation well @ 56 °C; approx. 3–5 min (place on ice before returning to well).
2. Add 1 μl/well of compensation antibody to the corresponding compensation wells.
   (a) For compensation controls CD4-conjugated antibodies work best, but CD3 and CD8 may be used as well to give defined positive and negative populations (*see* **Note 3**).
   (b) Add 0.2 μl of viability dye to viability compensation well.
3. Add 100 μl/well of surface stain antibody cocktail (prepared in Subheading 3.1) to sample wells. Cover plate with foil and incubate at 4 °C for 20 min.
4. Add 100–150 μl FACS buffer/well. Spin at 450 × *g* for 5 min at 4 °C, decant supernatant, and vortex to resuspend.
5. Wash with 200 μl/well FACS buffer, spin at 450 × *g* for 5 min at 4 °C, decant supernatant, and vortex to resuspend.

3.5 Analysis

1. *For analysis within 4 h:* Resuspend cells in 50 μl FACS buffer, transfer to 1.2 ml cluster tubes, and store at 4 °C in the dark until data collection on flow cytometer.
2. *For next-day analysis:* Resuspend cells in 100 μl/well 1–4 % formaldehyde in PBS, incubate for 20 min at 4 °C, and wash once with 100–150 μl FACS buffer. Resuspend in 50 μl FACS buffer, transfer to 1.2 ml cluster tubes, and store at 4 °C in the dark. Cells should be read within the next 3–4 days.

3. Follow established manufacturer or lab protocols for the particular instrument and software being used for data collection. If using a BD LSRII or Fortessa with FACSDiva software, start with voltages set according to daily CS&T settings and make adjustments as necessary prior to running samples (*see* **Note 4**).
4. A typical analysis is shown in Fig. 1.

4 Notes

1. CD127 staining typically requires a much larger volume of antibody than other markers to achieve good separation of populations; using >3 μl per sample will greatly improve final staining results.
2. May use splenocytes for compensation if available. Compensation beads are another option to use in place of cells if cell numbers are limited.
3. There should be one compensation control well per fluorochrome; these wells are single stained with each fluorochrome using CD3, CD4, or CD8 antibodies to give clear positive and negative populations for each fluorochrome. CD4 antibodies tend to work best for use as compensation controls. An unstained well should be included as well and may be used as a universal negative for compensation if any control does not give clear positive and negative populations. Alternatively, compensation beads can be included if cell numbers are limited or tandem dyes are being used. OneComp eBeads (eBiosciences) are specific for antibodies derived from mouse, rat, and hamster with both positive and negative populations included. When using tandem dyes, it is beneficial to use the same lot of antibody for your compensation control as well as sample staining as variations may occur between lots of conjugation; thus compensation beads can allow for bright and discrete staining of a marker which may not be expressed at high levels. Stain beads according to the manufacturer's specifications.
4. When setting voltages on the instrument start by viewing data for each single-stained compensation control on all detectors (in FACSDiva this is easily accomplished by viewing the Unstained Control tab). Adjust voltages so that the fluorochrome you are staining for is brightest in the detector for which it is stained and does not have spillover brighter in any other channel than the chrome specific for that channel (e.g., FITC is brightest in FITC and not brighter on PE than PE is on PE). Once the settings have been established, collect all compensation controls and then move on to samples (be sure that the voltage settings are the same for each PMT across all compensation controls or compensation cannot be correctly calculated).

Acknowledgement

The research described in this chapter was supported by the US Army Medical Research and Materiel Command. The views of the authors do not purport to reflect the position of the Department of the Army or the Department of Defense. Described procedures must be conducted under an IACUC-approved protocol in accordance with the Animal Welfare Act and the Guide for the Care and Use of Laboratory Animals (NRC, 2011).

The authors would like to thank the current Krzych lab members for their assistance with the performance of the assays.

References

1. Clyde DF, McCarthy VC, Miller RM, Hornick RB (1973) Specificity of protection of man immunized against sporozoite-induced falciparum malaria. Am J Med Sci 266:398–403
2. Clyde DF, Most H, McCarthy VC, Vanderberg JP (1973) Immunization of man against sporozoite-induced falciparum malaria. Am J Med Sci 266:169–177
3. Rieckmann KH, Beaudoin RL, Cassells JS, Sell KW (1979) Use of attenuated sporozoites in the immunization of human volunteers against falciparum malaria. Bull World Health Organ 57(Suppl 1):261–265
4. Berenzon D, Schwenk RJ, Letellier L, Guebre-Xabier M, Williams J, Krzych U (2003) Protracted protection to Plasmodium berghei malaria is linked to functionally and phenotypically heterogeneous liver memory CD8+ T cells. J Immunol 171:2024–2034
5. Guebre-Xabier M, Schwenk R, Krzych U (1999) Memory phenotype CD8(+) T cells persist in livers of mice protected against malaria by immunization with attenuated Plasmodium berghei sporozoites. Eur J Immunol 29:3978–3986
6. Khan SM, Janse CJ, Kappe SH, Mikolajczak SA (2012) Genetic engineering of attenuated malaria parasites for vaccination. Curr Opin Biotechnol 23:908–916
7. Butler NS, Schmidt NW, Vaughan AM, Aly AS, Kappe SH, Harty JT (2011) Superior antimalarial immunity after vaccination with late liver stage-arresting genetically attenuated parasites. Cell Host Microbe 9:451–462
8. Douradinha B, van Dijk M, van Gemert GJ, Khan SM, Janse CJ, Waters AP, Sauerwein RW, Luty AJ, Silva-Santos B, Mota MM, Epiphanio S (2011) Immunization with genetically attenuated P52-deficient Plasmodium berghei sporozoites induces a long-lasting effector memory CD8+ T cell response in the liver. J Immune Based Ther Vaccines 9:6
9. Lumsden JM, Cranmer MA, Krzych U (2010) An early commitment to expression of a particular TCRVbeta chain on CD8(+) T cells responding to attenuated Plasmodium berghei sporozoites is maintained following challenge with infectious sporozoites. Parasite Immunol 32:644–655
10. Jobe O, Donofrio G, Sun G, Liepinsh D, Schwenk R, Krzych U (2009) Immunization with radiation-attenuated Plasmodium berghei sporozoites induces liver cCD8alpha + DC that activate CD8 + T cells against liver-stage malaria. PLoS One 4, e5075
11. Steers N, Schwenk R, Bacon DJ, Berenzon D, Williams J, Krzych U (2005) The immune status of Kupffer cells profoundly influences their responses to infectious Plasmodium berghei sporozoites. Eur J Immunol 35:2335–2346
12. Zarling S, Berenzon D, Dalai S, Liepinsh D, Steers N, Krzych U (2013) The survival of memory CD8 T cells that is mediated by IL-15 correlates with sustained protection against malaria. J Immunol 190:5128–5141
13. Krzych U, Zarling S, Pichugin A (2014) Memory T cells maintain protracted protection against malaria. Immunol Lett 161(2):189–195
14. Bonner WA, Hulett HR, Sweet RG, Herzenberg LA (1972) Fluorescence activated cell sorting. Rev Sci Instrum 43:404–409
15. Herzenberg LA, Sweet RG, Herzenberg LA (1976) Fluorescence-activated cell sorting. Sci Am 234:108–117
16. Hulett HR, Bonner WA, Barrett J, Herzenberg LA (1969) Cell sorting: automated separation of mammalian cells as a function of intracellular fluorescence. Science 166:747–749

17. Herzenberg LA, Tung J, Moore WA, Herzenberg LA, Parks DR (2006) Interpreting flow cytometry data: a guide for the perplexed. Nat Immunol 7:681–685
18. Biosciences B (2009) Technical bulletin. An introduction to compensation for multicolor assays on digital flow cytometers. BD Biosciences, San Jose, CA
19. Perfetto SP, Chattopadhyay PK, Roederer M (2004) Seventeen-colour flow cytometry: unravelling the immune system. Nat Rev Immunol 4:648–655
20. Blom KG, Qazi MR, Matos JB, Nelson BD, DePierre JW, Abedi-Valugerdi M (2009) Isolation of murine intrahepatic immune cells employing a modified procedure for mechanical disruption and functional characterization of the B, T and natural killer T cells obtained. Clin Exp Immunol 155: 320–329

Chapter 4

Flow Cytometry-Based Assessment of Antibody Function Against Malaria Pre-erythrocytic Infection

Alyse N. Douglass, Peter G. Metzger, Stefan H.I. Kappe, and Alexis Kaushansky

Abstract

The development of new interventional strategies against pre-erythrocytic malaria is hampered by the lack of standardized approaches to assess inhibition of sporozoite infection of hepatocytes. The following methodology, based on flow cytometry, can be used to quantitatively assess *P. falciparum* sporozoite infection in vitro in medium throughput. In addition to assessing the efficacy of antibodies, this assay has a wide variety of applications for investigating basic science questions about the malaria liver stage. This approach is easily applied in a variety of laboratory settings, assesses the functionality of antibody responses against malaria sporozoites, and can be adapted for the limited quantities of sample which are typically available from clinical investigations.

Key words Malaria, Liver, Sporozoite, Flow cytometry

1 Introduction

A malaria vaccine that halts parasites at the clinically silent pre-erythrocytic stage of the life cycle would prevent both disease and transmission. To date, the most effective experimental vaccines to demonstrate long-standing sterile immunity in humans are the mosquito-bite administration of *r*adiation-*a*ttenuated *s*porozoites (RAS) [1] or administration of fully infectious parasites which are then killed by chloroquine (called *c*hloroquine chemo*p*rophylaxis with *Plasmodium falciparum* *s*porozoites, CPS) [2]. Protection is largely mediated by immunity directed at pre-erythrocytic stages as humans challenged with *P. falciparum* blood stages are not protected [2]. Historically, the hope for the widespread use of a live attenuated vaccine strategy has been limited by manufacturing and distribution constraints. However, these challenges have been partially overcome with the development of cryopreservation and aseptic mosquito production techniques [3]. Meanwhile, the only vaccine candidate to reach phase III trials, RTS,S, is a subunit

Ashley M. Vaughan (ed.), *Malaria Vaccines: Methods and Protocols*, Methods in Molecular Biology, vol. 1325, DOI 10.1007/978-1-4939-2815-6_4,

vaccine targeting the immunodominant protein on the surface of the sporozoite, *c*ircum*s*porozoite *p*rotein (CSP) [4]. RTS,S gives short-lived efficacy against clinical malaria in 30–50 % of patients [5], and protection is associated with anti-CSP antibody titer [6–8]. However, antibody titer cannot completely predict efficacy in any of the described vaccination strategies. Unlike subunit vaccines, live attenuated vaccine strategies likely elicit antibodies against a variety of targets in the pre-erythrocytic stages, further complicating the challenge of correlating antibody titer to protective efficacy. An accurate assessment of the functionality of vaccination-elicited antibodies could inform enhanced strategies to prevent malaria.

Recent experiments have demonstrated that prophylactic administration of anti-CSP monoclonal antibodies derived from a volunteer given RTS,S confers protection in a SCID-Alb-uPA mouse model which is repopulated with human hepatocytes [9]. Genetically attenuated vaccines in humans have also been shown to induce potent, blocking antibody responses in vitro [10]. However, the functional consequence of these antibodies in humans [10] remains unknown as volunteers from these trials have yet to be challenged [11]. Antibodies derived from volunteers immunized with CPS [12] and RAS [3, 13] regimens also produce functional antibodies which show partial protection against *P. falciparum* infection in vitro and in humanized mouse models [12].

While these data demonstrate the pivotal role antibodies play in mediating immunity to malaria, very little is understood about the relationship between antibody function and protection. Vaccine trials classically use enzyme-linked immunosorbent assay (ELISA) to quantify antibody titers and in turn correlate them with protection. While this assesses quantity of antibody responses, it does not identify functional quality or blocking potential. Furthermore, high antibody titers do not explain the variable and short-lived immunity [5] elicited by RTS,S, suggesting that antibody concentration alone is not predictive of immune function. Molecular parasitology has developed a variety of techniques and approaches to assess antibody functionality over the past several decades. Classically, functional assessment of anti-sporozoite antibody function is assessed via a "gliding assay" that monitors antibody inhibition of parasite motility on a glass slide [14]. This assay is both highly subjective and difficult to correlate with in vivo parasite activity. A more translatable approach, inhibition of sporozoite invasion (ISI), utilizes microscopy to count infected hepatocytes in vitro [15]. While ISI more closely assesses antibody inhibition of hepatocyte invasion, it is still subject to experimenter bias. Both the gliding assay and microscopy-based ISI are labor intensive, relying on visual microscopy of individual parasites. The capacity of sporozoites to wound cells can also be assessed [16] and may correlate to the parasite's capacity to leave the skin [17] or enter the liver parenchyma [17–19]. More recent assays involve bioluminescent imaging of liver-stage burden and determination of patency in live animals to establish antibody-mediated blocking of sporozoite invasion [20]. While this model is exquisitely sensitive and provides in vivo data, it remains low throughput due to the high cost of chimeric mice and transgenic parasites to assess antibody effects on *P. falciparum* invasion.

Here, we outline a flow cytometry-based assay to assess functionality of antibodies elicited after vaccination. In this case, functionality refers to both the ability of a sporozoite to wound a cell (also called "cell traversal" or "cell-wounding") and the sporozoite to invade a host cell (called "hepatocyte infection" or "cell-wounding"). Flow cytometry has been used to demonstrate concentration-dependent inhibition of sporozoite invasion by anti-CSP antibodies, and the protocol is highly reproducible and can be standardized across laboratories [21, 10]. Furthermore, it is designed to efficiently use small quantities of antibody or sera which make it well suited to assess functionality of antibodies collected during vaccine trials. The methods we describe may provide critical understanding about the characteristics of the antibody response required for protective immunization. We hope that these insights will facilitate the development of an effective pre-erythrocytic vaccine against malaria infection.

2 Materials

1. HC04 hepatoma cells (for *Plasmodium falciparum* infections [22]) or Hepa1-6 hepatoma cells (for *Plasmodium yoelii* infections, ATCC CRL-1830).
2. DMEM media supplemented with 10 % heat-inactivated fetal bovine serum (FBS), 200 IU/mL penicillin and 200 μg/mL streptomycin and 250 ng/mL amphotericin B (Fungizone).
3. 1× sterile phosphate-buffered saline (PBS).
4. 0.25 % Trypsin/EDTA.
5. *Plasmodium falciparum* 3D7 or *Plasmodium yoelii* 17XNL day 14–16 salivary gland sporozoites.
6. FITC-dextran 10,000 MW, anionic, lysine fixable (Invitrogen).
7. α-*Plasmodium falciparum* CSP monoclonal antibody (mAb) (clone 2A10) or α-*Plasmodium yoelii* CSP mAb (clone 2F6 [20]) conjugated to either Pacific Blue (Molecular Probes) or Alexa Fluor 647 (Molecular Probes), recommended stock concentration 1 mg/mL (*see* **Note 1**).
8. Cytofix/Cytoperm solution (BD Biosciences).
9. Perm/wash solution (BD Biosciences) + 2 % bovine serum albumin (BSA).

10. 5 mM EDTA in 1× PBS.
11. Filter-top fluorescence-activated cell sorting (FACS) tubes (Falcon).
12. Flow cytometer.
13. FACS analysis software.

3 Methods

3.1 Experimental Design and Assay Setup

Parameters in this assay can be modified depending on the overall goal of each experiment. Limiting amounts of parasites, sera, or test compound will influence the scale of the assay (i.e., 96-well vs. 24-well format) (*see* **Note 2**) and thus the number of parameters that can be assessed. The major components assessed in this assay are cell infection (percentage of cells that harbor intracellular parasites) and cell traversal (percentage of cells that have been wounded). When monitored in multiplex, parasites which have entered their host cells by productive invasion machinery as opposed to through cell wounding (traversal) can be distinguished. Specifically, a traversed cell is distinguished from an invaded cell by the presence of fluorescently labeled dextran that is added to the media during the invasion process as only cells which have compromised cell membranes from parasite traversal take up dextran during infection.

3.2 Required Controls

1. Unstained control—cells alone (no sporozoites or dextran).
2. Single-color controls—αCSP mAb staining only (contains parasites only), dextran only (contains parasites but no antibodies) (*see* **Note 4**).
3. Traversal control—dextran only (no parasites).
4. Appropriate sporozoite-treatment controls (we frequently use IgG, cytochalasin D, and *P. falciparum* αCSP 2A10 mAb; 2 μg/mL of *P. falciparum* 2A10 mAb gives ~80 % reduction of invasion [10, 20]).
5. Reference infection control—parasite and dextran without inhibition.

3.3 Protocol

1. One day prior to infection, seed plates with the appropriate number of cells per well (see Table 1).
2. On the day of infection, dissect the desired number of *Plasmodium* sporozoites from mosquito salivary glands using standard methodology (Table 1) (*see* **Note 5**). Keep on ice.
3. Make appropriate dilutions of the antibody/sera/compound to be tested in DMEM with 10 % FBS for the volume necessary for three wells, so each condition can be performed in triplicate (Table 1) (*see* **Note 6**).

Table 1
Quantities of cells and reagents to be used

Format of assay (*see* Note 2)	96-Well plate	24-Well plate	12-Well plate	6-Well plate
# Cells plated	0.1×10^6	0.3×10^6	0.6×10^6	1.2×10^6
Volume media/treatment	100 µL	250 µL	500 µL	1 mL
# Sporozoites	30,000	100,000	200,000	400,000
Volume PBS wash	200 µL	500 µL	1 mL	2 mL
Volume trypsin	100 µL	250 µL	500 µL	1 mL
Volume fix/perm	100 µL	100 µL	200 µL	200 µL
Volume 2 % BSA + perm/wash	80 µL	80 µL	160 µL	160 µL
Volume 5× antibody (in 2 % BSA + perm/wash)	20 µL	20 µL	40 µL	40 µL
Maximum parameters (i.e., infection, traversal, host cell viability)	1	2	3 (*see* **Note 3**)	4 (*see* **Note 3**)

4. Add 1 mg/mL FITC-dextran to each aliquot at this time to assess traversal (*see* **Note** 7).
5. Add *Plasmodium* sporozoites (enough for three wells) to each condition previously prepared in **step 3** (Table 1) (*see* **Note 8**). Incubate at room temperature for 15–25 min to activate the sporozoites.
6. Add the appropriate volume of media, parasite, dextran, and serum to each well (Table 1). Ensure that you have included the appropriate controls for compensation and untreated sporozoites.
7. Spin plate(s) at 500 × *g* for 3 min at room temperature to assist in sporozoite attachment to hepatocytes.
8. Transfer plate(s) to 37 °C, 5 % CO2 tissue culture incubator for 90 min.
9. Wash cells once with PBS, and then trypsinize with 0.25 % trypsin/EDTA (Table 1).
10. Inactivate trypsin with DMEM containing 10 % FBS, and then transfer cells to microcentrifuge tubes (Table 1).
11. Pellet cells at 1500 × *g* for 3 min and remove the supernatant.
12. Add Cytoperm/Cytofix solution to each tube and resuspend cells completely by pipetting up and down several times (Table 1). Incubate on ice for 15 min. Keep samples protected from light from this point forward.
13. Pellet cells at 1500 × *g* for 2 min and remove supernatant.
14. Resuspend cells in 200 µL PBS with 5 mM EDTA. At this point, the procedure can be paused for up to 1 week by storing cells at 4 °C in the dark.

15. Transfer samples to a 96-well V-bottom plate (*see* **Note 9**), apply a plate cover, and spin at 1500×*g* for 2 min. Remove supernatant.
16. Resuspend cells in 80 μL 2 % BSA in perm/wash buffer, apply a plate cover, and incubate at room temperature for 10 min while rotating.
17. Make a 5× stock (10 μg/mL) of the mAb to be used for staining. If assessing *P. falciparum* invasion use the *Pf*CSP 2A10 mAb; if assessing *P. yoelii* invasion, the *Py*CSP 2F6 mAb antibody is used. In both cases, we use a final concentration of 2 μg/mL mAb which has been conjugated to either Pacific Blue or Alexa Fluor 647.
18. Briefly spin the plate for 15 s at 500×*g* before adding 20 μL of the 5× antibody solution to designated wells (*see* **Note 8**). Apply a plate cover and incubate for 45 min on a rotator, protected from light.
19. Pellet cells at 1500×*g* for 2 min and remove the supernatant.
20. Resuspend the cells with 200 μL PBS+5 mM EDTA, pellet at 1500×*g* for 2 min, and remove the supernatant.
21. Resuspend cells in 200 μL PBS+5 mM EDTA and filter each sample through a 70 μm mesh into tubes that are compatible with your cytometer (*see* **Note 10**).
22. Samples can be run on any flow cytometer following filtration in the same FACS tubes, or a round-bottom 96-well plate if your cytometer has HTS capabilities.
23. When analyzing the FACS files, set gates for infection (αCSP signal) and traversal (FITC-dextran signal) (Fig. 1) (*see* **Note 11**).

4 Notes/Troubleshooting

1. Hybridomas for these mAbs were obtained from MR4 (*P. falciparum* CSP mAb 2A10) and Photini Sinnis and Fidel Zavala (*P. yoelii* CSP mAb 2F6).
2. When there are a large number of conditions to test, it is tempting to gravitate towards a 96-well plate format in order to increase throughput of the assay. With the low infection rate and sporozoite variability, the 96-well plate format will only provide consistent, statistically significant results for the total CSP-positive population or the Dextran-positive population, not both in combination. The minimum format for analyzing the effects on parasite traversal and invasion, however, is the 24-well plate format. Therefore, it is crucial to keep in mind that while we have successfully analyzed up to four parameters within the infected population with this assay, we were only able to do so in the largest format (six-well plates), which requires a substantial number of sporozoites.

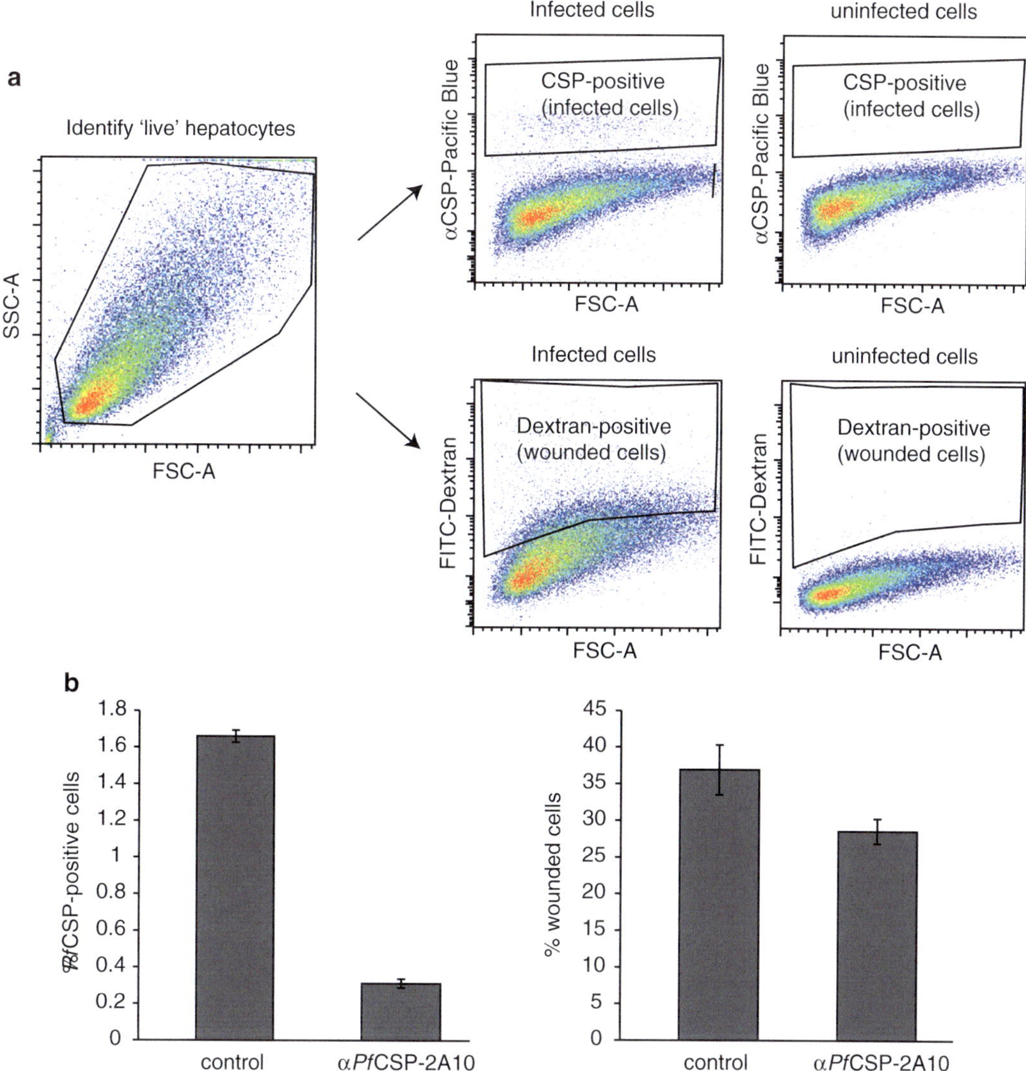

Fig. 1 Gating strategy for monitoring *P. falciparum* invasion and traversal in HC04 cells. HC04 hepatocytes are grown in culture and then infected with *P. falciparum* sporozoites in the presence of FITC-dextran. Cells are detached, fixed, permeabilized, and stained with a monoclonal antibody against circumsporozoite protein (CSP). (**a**) Infected cells are identified by flow cytometric analysis. HC04 cells are first identified by forward and side scatter and then assessed for staining with an antibody against *P. falciparum* CSP which has been conjugated to a Pacific Blue fluorophore. Wounded cells are identified in the FITC channel whereas CSP-positive cells are identified in the Pacific Blue channel. (**b**) Example dataset generated during inhibition of sporozoite invasion and traversal experiments. The αCSP monoclonal antibody 2A10 inhibits sporozoite invasion by approximately 80 % and traversal by approximately 25 %

3. This protocol does not describe in detail how to add parameters beyond infection and traversal rates. However, we have previously demonstrated that additional components such as host-cell apoptosis [23] and host DNA content [24] can be monitored using this approach. We expect that this approach

will allow for the multiplexing of many additional components, and thus have provided specifications for how to expand the platform to monitor additional numbers of infected cells.

4. Single-color controls are not required when only one parameter is being monitored.
5. An optimal infection will have one sporozoite for every three cells plated (MOI ~0.3).
6. It is best to test at least four different concentrations of the antibody/sera/compound (e.g., 1:10, 1:25, 1:100, and 1:250).
7. If you do not plan to include the assessment of traversal in your experiment, exclude the addition of dextran from all steps.
8. See Experimental Design section for a full list of control samples.
9. The volumes for each step remain the same if samples are stained in microcentrifuge tubes.
10. Press pipette tip to the surface of mesh firmly to make sure that cells are properly filtered.
11. The fitness of *Plasmodium* sporozoites can vary from week to week, even when maintained in the controlled laboratory setting, which will influence the infection rate observed in this assay. At 90 min post-infection, we generally observe ~1 % CSP-positive cells in the non-treated control infection.

References

1. Clyde DF, McCarthy VC, Miller RM, Hornick RB (1973) Specificity of protection of man immunized against sporozoite-induced falciparum malaria. Am J Med Sci 266(6):398–403
2. Bijker EM, Bastiaens GJ, Teirlinck AC, van Gemert GJ, Graumans W, van de Vegte-Bolmer M, Siebelink-Stoter R, Arens T, Teelen K, Nahrendorf W, Remarque EJ, Roeffen W, Jansens A, Zimmerman D, Vos M, van Schaijk BC, Wiersma J, van der Ven AJ, de Mast Q, van Lieshout L, Verweij JJ, Hermsen CC, Scholzen A, Sauerwein RW (2013) Protection against malaria after immunization by chloroquine prophylaxis and sporozoites is mediated by preerythrocytic immunity. Proc Natl Acad Sci U S A 110(19):7862–7867. doi:10.1073/pnas.1220360110
3. Seder RA, Chang LJ, Enama ME, Zephir KL, Sarwar UN, Gordon IJ, Holman LA, James ER, Billingsley PF, Gunasekera A, Richman A, Chakravarty S, Manoj A, Velmurugan S, Li M, Ruben AJ, Li T, Eappen AG, Stafford RE, Plummer SH, Hendel CS, Novik L, Costner PJ, Mendoza FH, Saunders JG, Nason MC, Richardson JH, Murphy J, Davidson SA, Richie TL, Sedegah M, Sutamihardja A, Fahle GA, Lyke KE, Laurens MB, Roederer M, Tewari K, Epstein JE, Sim BK, Ledgerwood JE, Graham BS, Hoffman SL (2013) Protection against malaria by intravenous immunization with a nonreplicating sporozoite vaccine. Science 341(6152):1359–1365. doi:10.1126/science.1241800
4. Gordon DM, McGovern TW, Krzych U, Cohen JC, Schneider I, LaChance R, Heppner DG, Yuan G, Hollingdale M, Slaoui M et al (1995) Safety, immunogenicity, and efficacy of a recombinantly produced Plasmodium falciparum circumsporozoite protein-hepatitis B surface antigen subunit vaccine. J Infect Dis 171(6):1576–1585
5. Agnandji ST, Lell B, Soulanoudjingar SS, Fernandes JF, Abossolo BP, Conzelmann C, Methogo BG, Doucka Y, Flamen A, Mordmuller B, Issifou S, Kremsner PG, Sacarlal J, Aide P, Lanaspa M, Aponte JJ, Nhamuave A, Quelhas D, Bassat Q, Mandjate S, Macete E, Alonso P, Abdulla S, Salim N, Juma O, Shomari

M, Shubis K, Machera F, Hamad AS, Minja R, Mtoro A, Sykes A, Ahmed S, Urassa AM, Ali AM, Mwangoka G, Tanner M, Tinto H, D'Alessandro U, Sorgho H, Valea I, Tahita MC, Kabore W, Ouedraogo S, Sandrine Y, Guiguemde RT, Ouedraogo JB, Hamel MJ, Kariuki S, Odero C, Oneko M, Otieno K, Awino N, Omoto J, Williamson J, Muturi-Kioi V, Laserson KF, Slutsker L, Otieno W, Otieno L, Nekoye O, Gondi S, Otieno A, Ogutu B, Wasuna R, Owira V, Jones D, Onyango AA, Njuguna P, Chilengi R, Akoo P, Kerubo C, Gitaka J, Maingi C, Lang T, Olotu A, Tsofa B, Bejon P, Peshu N, Marsh K, Owusu-Agyei S, Asante KP, Osei-Kwakye K, Boahen O, Ayamba S, Kayan K, Owusu-Ofori R, Dosoo D, Asante I, Adjei G, Chandramohan D, Greenwood B, Lusingu J, Gesase S, Malabeja A, Abdul O, Kilavo H, Mahende C, Liheluka E, Lemnge M, Theander T, Drakeley C, Ansong D, Agbenyega T, Adjei S, Boateng HO, Rettig T, Bawa J, Sylverken J, Sambian D, Agyekum A, Owusu L, Martinson F, Hoffman I, Mvalo T, Kamthunzi P, Nkomo R, Msika A, Jumbe A, Chome N, Nyakuipa D, Chintedza J, Ballou WR, Bruls M, Cohen J, Guerra Y, Jongert E, Lapierre D, Leach A, Lievens M, Ofori-Anyinam O, Vekemans J, Carter T, Leboulleux D, Loucq C, Radford A, Savarese B, Schellenberg D, Sillman M, Vansadia P (2011) First results of phase 3 trial of RTS,S/AS01 malaria vaccine in African children. N Engl J Med 365(20):1863–1875

6. Kester KE, Cummings JF, Ockenhouse CF, Nielsen R, Hall BT, Gordon DM, Schwenk RJ, Krzych U, Holland CA, Richmond G, Dowler MG, Williams J, Wirtz RA, Tornieporth N, Vigneron L, Delchambre M, Demoitie MA, Ballou WR, Cohen J, Heppner DG Jr (2008) Phase 2a trial of 0, 1, and 3 month and 0, 7, and 28 day immunization schedules of malaria vaccine RTS, S/AS02 in malaria-naive adults at the Walter Reed Army Institute of Research. Vaccine 26(18):2191–2202. doi:10.1016/j.vaccine.2008.02.048
7. Kester KE, Cummings JF, Ofori-Anyinam O, Ockenhouse CF, Krzych U, Moris P, Schwenk R, Nielsen RA, Debebe Z, Pinelis E, Juompan L, Williams J, Dowler M, Stewart VA, Wirtz RA, Dubois MC, Lievens M, Cohen J, Ballou WR, Heppner DG Jr (2009) Randomized, double-blind, phase 2a trial of falciparum malaria vaccines RTS, S/AS01B and RTS, S/AS02A in malaria-naive adults: safety, efficacy, and immunologic associates of protection. J Infect Dis 200(3):337–346. doi:10.1086/600120
8. White MT, Bejon P, Olotu A, Griffin JT, Riley EM, Kester KE, Ockenhouse CF, Ghani AC (2013) The relationship between RTS, S vaccine-induced antibodies, CD4(+) T cell responses and protection against Plasmodium falciparum infection. PLoS One 8(4), e61395. doi:10.1371/journal.pone.0061395
9. Foquet L, Hermsen CC, van Gemert GJ, Van Braeckel E, Weening KE, Sauerwein R, Meuleman P, Leroux-Roels G (2014) Vaccine-induced monoclonal antibodies targeting circumsporozoite protein prevent Plasmodium falciparum infection. J Clin Invest 124(1):140–144. doi:10.1172/JCI70349
10. Finney OC, Keitany GJ, Smithers H, Kaushansky A, Kappe SH, Wang R (2014) Immunization with genetically attenuated P. falciparum parasites induces long-lived antibodies that efficiently block hepatocyte invasion by sporozoites. Vaccine 32(19):2135–2138
11. Spring M, Murphy J, Nielsen R, Dowler M, Bennett JW, Zarling S, Williams J, de la Vega P, Ware L, Komisar J, Polhemus M, Richie TL, Epstein J, Tamminga C, Chuang I, Richie N, O'Neil M, Heppner DG, Healer J, O'Neill M, Smithers H, Finney OC, Mikolajczak SA, Wang R, Cowman A, Ockenhouse C, Krzych U, Kappe SH (2013) First-in-human evaluation of genetically attenuated Plasmodium falciparum sporozoites administered by bite of Anopheles mosquitoes to adult volunteers. Vaccine 31(43):4975–4983. doi:10.1016/j.vaccine.2013.08.007
12. Behet MC, Foquet L, van Gemert GJ, Bijker EM, Meuleman P, Leroux-Roels G, Hermsen CC, Scholzen A, Sauerwein RW (2014) Sporozoite immunization of human volunteers under chemoprophylaxis induces functional antibodies against pre-erythrocytic stages of Plasmodium falciparum. Malar J 13:136. doi:10.1186/1475-2875-13-136
13. Epstein JE, Tewari K, Lyke KE, Sim BK, Billingsley PF, Laurens MB, Gunasekera A, Chakravarty S, James ER, Sedegah M, Richman A, Velmurugan S, Reyes S, Li M, Tucker K, Ahumada A, Ruben AJ, Li T, Stafford R, Eappen AG, Tamminga C, Bennett JW, Ockenhouse CF, Murphy JR, Komisar J, Thomas N, Loyevsky M, Birkett A, Plowe CV, Loucq C, Edelman R, Richie TL, Seder RA, Hoffman SL (2011) Live attenuated malaria vaccine designed to protect through hepatic CD8(+) T cell immunity. Science 334(6055):475–480. doi:10.1126/science.1211548
14. Stewart MJ, Nawrot RJ, Schulman S, Vanderberg JP (1986) Plasmodium berghei sporozoite invasion is blocked in vitro by sporozoite-immobilizing antibodies. Infect Immun 51(3):859–864

15. Renia L, Vigario AM, Belnoue E (2002) Inhibition of sporozoite invasion. The double-staining assay. Methods Mol Med 72:507–516. doi:10.1385/1-59259-271-6:507
16. Mota MM, Pradel G, Vanderberg JP, Hafalla JC, Frevert U, Nussenzweig RS, Nussenzweig V, Rodriguez A (2001) Migration of Plasmodium sporozoites through cells before infection. Science 291(5501):141–144. doi:10.1126/science.291.5501.141
17. Tavares J, Formaglio P, Thiberge S, Mordelet E, Van Rooijen N, Medvinsky A, Menard R, Amino R (2013) Role of host cell traversal by the malaria sporozoite during liver infection. J Exp Med 210(5):905–915. doi:10.1084/jem.20121130
18. Amino R, Giovannini D, Thiberge S, Gueirard P, Boisson B, Dubremetz JF, Prevost MC, Ishino T, Yuda M, Menard R (2008) Host cell traversal is important for progression of the malaria parasite through the dermis to the liver. Cell Host Microbe 3(2):88–96. doi:10.1016/j.chom.2007.12.007
19. Baer K, Roosevelt M, Clarkson AB Jr, van Rooijen N, Schnieder T, Frevert U (2007) Kupffer cells are obligatory for Plasmodium yoelii sporozoite infection of the liver. Cell Microbiol 9(2):397–412. doi:10.1111/j.1462-5822.2006.00798.x
20. Sack BK, Miller JL, Vaughan AM, Douglass A, Kaushansky A, Mikolajczak S, Coppi A, Gonzalez-Aseguinolaza G, Tsuji M, Zavala F, Sinnis P, Kappe SH (2014) Model for in vivo assessment of humoral protection against malaria sporozoite challenge by passive transfer of monoclonal antibodies and immune serum. Infect Immun 82(2):808–817
21. Kaushansky A, Rezakhani N, Mann H, Kappe SH (2012) Development of a quantitative flow cytometry-based assay to assess infection by Plasmodium falciparum sporozoites. Mol Biochem Parasitol 183(1):100–103. doi:10.1016/j.molbiopara.2012.01.006
22. Sattabongkot J, Yimamnuaychoke N, Leelaudomlipi S, Rasameesoraj M, Jenwithisuk R, Coleman RE, Udomsangpetch R, Cui L, Brewer TG (2006) Establishment of a human hepatocyte line that supports in vitro development of the exo-erythrocytic stages of the malaria parasites Plasmodium falciparum and P. vivax. Am J Trop Med Hyg 74(5):708–715
23. Kaushansky A, Metzger PG, Douglass AN, Mikolajczak SA, Lakshmanan V, Kain HS, Kappe SH (2013) Malaria parasite liver stages render host hepatocytes susceptible to mitochondria-initiated apoptosis. Cell Death Dis 4:e762. doi:10.1038/cddis.2013.286
24. Austin LS, Kaushansky A, Kappe SH (2014) Susceptibility to Plasmodium liver stage infection is altered by hepatocyte polyploidy. Cell Microbiol 16(5):784–795. doi:10.1111/cmi.12282

Chapter 5

Assessment of Parasite Liver-Stage Burden in Human-Liver Chimeric Mice

Lander Foquet, Philip Meuleman, Cornelus C. Hermsen, Robert Sauerwein, and Geert Leroux-Roels

Abstract

Humanized mice with a chimeric liver are a promising tool to evaluate the "in vivo" efficacy of novel compounds or vaccine-induced antibodies directed against the pre-erythrocytic stages of *Plasmodium falciparum*. The absence of human red blood cells in these humanized mice precludes the transition from liver to blood stage. The qPCR-based method described below allows for a sensitive and reliable quantification of parasite DNA in the chimeric liver following a challenge via infected mosquito bite or intravenous injection of sporozoites. With this method approximately 25 % of the total chimeric liver is examined and a single infected hepatocyte can be detected in the analyzed tissue. The use of appropriate species-specific probes can also allow for the detection of other *Plasmodium* species in vivo.

Key words Humanized mouse model, Malaria, *Plasmodium falciparum*, Sporozoite, Liver stage, In vivo, qPCR

1 Introduction

1.1 Background

Plasmodium berghei and other rodent models for malaria have a long history of being used to test new candidate vaccines [1] before entering the clinical phase of experimentally challenging healthy volunteers with *P. falciparum* [2]. However, significant differences between rodent and human biology and their respective species-specific parasites [3] necessitate the availability of alternative models to study *P. falciparum*. Humanized mouse models have been developed to study the interactions of pathogens with human hepatocytes in vivo [4, 5]. These models are based on the ability of immune-deficient mice with a severe liver disease to accept a graft of human hepatocytes. The liver disease is either acquired through the transgenic overexpression of urokinase-type plasminogen activator in uPA$^{+/+}$-SCID mice or a knockout of the fumarylacetoacetate hydrolase (FAH) enzyme in FRG (Fah$^{-/-}$Rag2$^{-/-}$IL2-Rg$^{-/-}$) mice [6–10]. The hepatocyte-specific expression of uPA probably results

Ashley M. Vaughan (ed.), *Malaria Vaccines: Methods and Protocols*, Methods in Molecular Biology, vol. 1325, DOI 10.1007/978-1-4939-2815-6_5, © Springer Science+Business Media New York 2015

in cleavage of its substrate plasminogen into active plasmin within the rough endoplasmic reticulum (RER). The ensuing proteolytic damage within the RER is most likely the cause of hepatotoxicity, which ultimately results in hepatocyte apoptosis and sever liver disease [11]. Plasminogen cleavage also results in hepatocyte growth factor (HGF) activation in the liver and remodeling of the liver's extracellular matrix. These two latter functions promote hepatocyte engraftment and repopulation. The FAH knockout results in a defect in the tyrosine catabolic pathway, which results in the accumulation of maleylacetoacetate and fumarylacetoacetate, upstream of the FAH blockade. Maleylacetoacetate and fumarylacetoacetate are highly reactive and unstable and break down into succinylacetone and succinylacetoacetate which are toxic and cause hepatocellular injury [12]. This toxicity can be prevented by oral administration of 2-(2-nitro-4-trifluoro-methylbenzoyl)-1,3-cyclohexanedione (NTBC), which blocks the tyrosine catabolism pathway upstream of the toxic metabolites [7].

Human donor hepatocytes are tolerated due to the immunodeficiency caused by the SCID mutation or the knockout of the Rag2 and IL2-Rγ genes in the FRG mouse. Human hepatocytes repopulate the mouse liver within the existing liver architecture and can represent over 90 % of all hepatocytes within a few months [6, 13].

Importantly, the human hepatocytes that reside in the liver of the chimeric mice display normal function and morphology [14]. These humanized mice can subsequently also be infected with *P. falciparum* sporozoites by intravenous (IV) injection or infected mosquito bite [15–18] and full parasite maturation in human hepatocytes can be achieved. Because emerging merozoites cannot infect murine erythrocytes, the ongoing infection cannot be monitored via a blood analysis [14]. To overcome this limitation, a large volume of human erythrocytes can be injected into the peritoneal cavity in order to humanize the red blood cell compartment of the mouse prior to the transition from liver to blood stage. The following day the chimeric mouse blood can be transferred to an in vitro environment for further analysis [16]. Alternatively the infectious burden of the liver can be examined before the parasites are released from the liver [19, 20].

The use of a transgenic parasite (NF54) that expresses a GFP-firefly luciferase fusion enables the measurement of bioluminescence in vivo [20]. This technique allows for a fast measurement of luciferase expression throughout parasite liver-stage development without sacrificing the animal. However, it necessitates the production of transgenic parasites and requires costly imaging equipment. The recently established clone NF135 [21] or other new field clones cannot be detected in vivo without performing this challenging genetic modification. Moreover, since *P. vivax* sporozoites can only be obtained by allowing mosquitoes to feed on patients infected with wild-type parasites, it will not be possible to apply bioluminescence for in vivo *P. vivax* liver-stage detection.

An alternative technique, described below, consists of extracting human, mouse, and parasite DNA from an infected chimeric liver and the use of qPCR for the detection and quantification of the liver parasite burden. This technique can be used with unmodified, wild-type *P. falciparum* and may equally be applicable to study infections with *P. vivax* or other parasites, when using the appropriate specific primer sets.

1.2 Basic Experimental Design

This protocol describes a method to detect liver-stage *P. falciparum* infections in mice with a human chimeric liver (Fig. 1). Humanized mice can be generated in-house or purchased from a specialized vendor [5]. Since the liver parasite burden can differ from animal to animal we recommend using at least three mice for each experimental condition. We encourage investigators to use mice matched for age, weight, and human albumin level, since the latter is a marker of human chimerism [22]. Mice can be infected by IV injection (tail vein or retro-orbital plexus) of sporozoites or via infected mosquito bites. A reliable mosquito bite challenge consists of 20 infected mosquitoes that are allowed to feed for 20 min. After being deposited in the skin, approximately 100 *P. falciparum* sporozoites from each mosquito bite cross the endothelium of the capillaries and travel to the liver where they traverse Kupffer cells and hepatocytes to finally invade a small number of the latter [23–25]. After the mosquito bites, an unknown number of sporozoites enter the bite site and lead to an unknown number of infected human hepatocytes. By allowing the parasites to replicate inside hepatocytes for 5 days, we are able to detect an infection with a high sensitivity

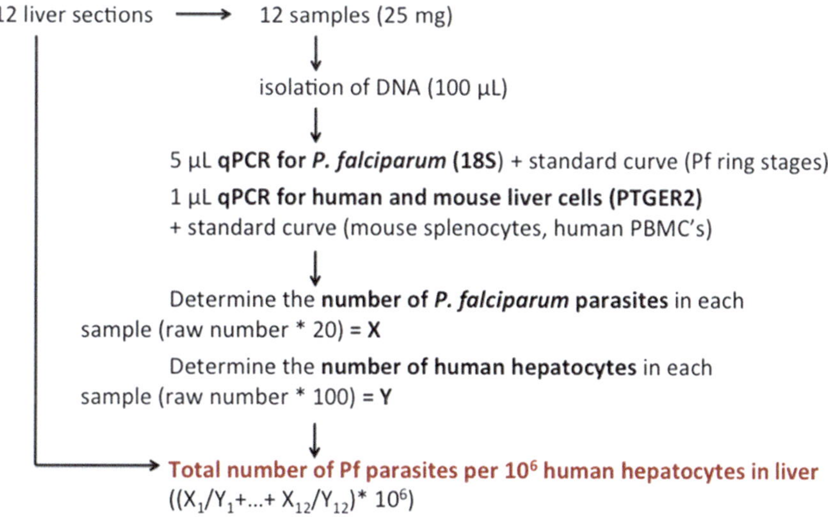

Fig. 1 Overview of assay procedures. Preparation of liver tissue sections, tissue fragmentation, DNA isolation, qPCR, and calculations to obtain a normalized determination of *P. falciparum* parasite numbers (*left panel*) in a humanized liver (*right panels*)

before merozoites leave the liver after 6–7 days. As it is not known how many parasite genomes are present in an infected hepatocyte after 5 days, we express the number of detected genomes as ring-stage equivalents [26]. To normalize for the varying numbers of human hepatocytes present in each mouse, we express the number of detected *P. falciparum* ring-stage equivalent copies per million human hepatocytes. Several approaches can be used to extract DNA from a humanized mouse liver. Homogenization of a whole liver, especially when it contains a few parasites (low DNA copy number), can lead to a strong dilution of the parasite DNA with the abundant mouse and human DNA and consequently to a loss of analytical sensitivity. Extraction of a single, randomly chosen liver tissue fragment (typically 25 mg for DNA extraction) may lead to a negative result by mere sampling error. Considering the low number of parasites that enter the liver and the unequal distribution of human hepatocytes throughout the organ it is easy to find a non-infected liver fragment. To avoid aforementioned errors based on sample dilution or sampling error, we proceeded with the collection of 12 samples (approximately 25 mg each) from the different liver lobes (Fig. 2). The resulting 300 mg of analyzed tissue represents about a quarter of the entire liver (1,200 mg), since chimeric uPA mice are frail and weigh on average only 12 g (*see* **Note 1**).

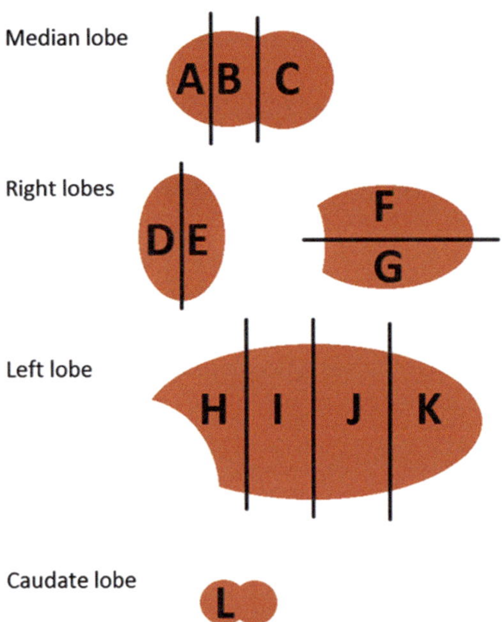

Fig. 2 Standardizing the sampling of humanized liver fragments. Five days post-infection, mice are euthanized by cervical dislocation. The livers are carefully removed and rinsed in PBS and 12 (24) standardized fragments (A–L) are prepared and placed in RNAlater until further analysis

2 Materials

2.1 Mosquito Bite Challenge in Humanized Mice and Enumeration of Sporozoites

1. Container with mosquito net top containing 20 *P. falciparum-infected* mosquitoes.
2. 70 % ethanol.
3. RPMI medium 1640 (1×) (Gibco, 52400-025).
4. 10 cm diameter Petri dishes.
5. Ice bucket/ice.
6. Glass tube and pestle.
7. Stereomicroscope for mosquito dissection.
8. Glass slides.
9. 23 gauge needle.
10. 27 gauge needle.
11. Hemocytometer.
12. Phase-contrast microscope.
13. Humid chamber.

2.2 Removal and Fixation of a Plasmodium-Infected Chimeric Mouse Liver

1. Dissection instruments.
2. 1 mL syringes.
3. 27 gauge needles.
4. Isoflurane mouth mask for mouse sedation.
5. Surgical platform.
6. 10 cm diameter Petri dishes containing PBS.
7. Microvette 500 μL EDTA tubes (Sarstedt, 20.1341).
8. RNAlater Stabilization Solution (Life Technologies, AM7021).
9. 1.5 mL tubes.

2.3 DNA Isolation from a Plasmodium-Infected Chimeric Mouse Liver

1. 1.5 mL tubes.
2. Precision scale to weigh 25 mg samples.
3. Scalpel and pincers.
4. High Pure PCR Template Preparation Kit (Roche, 11796828001) or similar.
5. Heating block.
6. Pipet tips (1 mL, 200 μL, 20 μL).
7. Centrifuge.

2.4 Parasite Detection and Quantification

1. 96-Well plates for qPCR.
2. qPCR machine (Lightcycler 480, Roche).
3. Pipet tips (1 mL, 200 μL, 20 μL).
4. DNA samples extracted from humanized mouse livers (100 μL).

5. Standard curve for parasite quantification: DNA samples from titrated *P. falciparum* ring stages (DNA from 1,000; 100; 10; 1; 0.5; 0.2 ring stages per reaction).
6. Standard curve for human or mouse quantification: DNA samples from human PBMCs and mouse cells (DNA from 10,000; 1,000; 100; 10 cells per reaction).
7. Forward/reverse 18S *P. falciparum* primers at a concentration of 10 μM from Hermsen et al. [26]. FAM-TAMRA probe for 18S *P. falciparum* at a concentration of 4 μM from Bijker et al. [27]. Forward/reverse common (human and mouse) primer at a concentration of 10 μM, FAM-BHQ1 human-specific probe at a concentration of 4 μM, and Cy5-BHQ2 mouse-specific probe at a concentration of 4 μM from Alcoser et al. [28].
8. Lightcycler 480 Probes Master (Roche, 04887301001).
9. Centrifuge.

3 Methods

An outline of the methodology is shown in Fig. 1.

3.1 Mosquito Bite Challenge in Humanized Mice and Enumeration of Sporozoites

1. Optional: Collect a pre-challenge blood sample from each mouse 1 h prior to mosquito bite challenge.
2. Prior to the bite challenge, dissect a sample of mosquitoes (at least 10) to enumerate the number of sporozoites present in each mosquito using standard techniques.
3. Sedate or immobilize the mouse on top of the container containing mosquitoes (*see* **Note 2**). Allow the mosquitoes to take a blood meal and lift the mouse every 2 min to interrupt mosquito feeding. This will result in more parasites being transferred to the mice (*see* **Note 3**).
4. After 20 min, the mouse is returned to its cage for recovery.
5. Kill mosquitoes by submerging in 70 % ethanol and wash in RPMI medium or PBS.
6. Using a stereomicroscope, count the number of mosquitoes that have taken a blood meal. Dissect the mosquitoes to ensure that a significant number were infected with sporozoites (*see* **Note 4**).

3.2 Removal and Fixation of a Plasmodium-Infected Chimeric Mouse Liver

1. Five days after the mosquito bite challenge, prepare to euthanize the mouse using standard methods.
2. Label 12 (or 24) 1.5 mL tubes and add 1 mL of RNAlater to store liver samples for DNA extraction.
3. Optional: For histology, label a 50 mL tube with 4 % formaldehyde for a sectioned piece of liver or prepare a tube for snap freezing a liver sample for cryosectioning.

4. Perform a cardiac puncture on the euthanized mouse (following standard protocol) or after inducing terminal anesthesia. This removes most of the blood from the liver (0.5–1 mL). This blood sample can be used to determine concentrations of relevant experimental variables (passively administered IgG, experimental drugs, liver function parameters, human albumin concentration, etc.).
5. Remove the whole liver and rinse in PBS.
6. Separate the different liver lobes and lay out in the following order: median lobe, anterior and posterior right lobe, left lobe, and caudate lobe (Fig. 2).
7. To obtain 12 (or 24) liver sections of approximately equal size, the median lobe is cut into three sections, both right lobes in two sections, the left lobe in four sections, and the small caudate lobe is kept as one fragment. Put every section in a 1.5 mL tube containing 1 mL RNAlater (Life Technologies) (*see* **Note 5**).
8. Optional: If a sample is necessary for histology, the center of the largest (left) lobe can be used. This leaves enough material to extract DNA from four (eight) 25 mg samples. Process this sample using standard protocols for fixation in formaldehyde or for snap freezing.
9. Store the liver sections in RNAlater overnight at 4 °C and transfer to the freezer for long-term storage or proceed to DNA extraction the next day.

3.3 DNA Isolation from a Plasmodium-Infected Chimeric Mouse Liver

1. Cut and weigh exactly 25 mg of each section and transfer to 12 (24) 1.5 mL tubes.
2. Add 40 μL proteinase K and 200 μL tissue lysis buffer from the kit to each sample and incubate for 2 h at 55 °C.
3. Add 200 μL binding buffer from the kit and incubate at 70 °C for 10 min.
4. Remove the insoluble tissue using a 1 mL tip and throw away; add 100 μL isopropanol to the remaining solution, vortex, and transfer to a DNA-binding column.
5. Follow the protocol from Roche, elute the DNA in 100 μL elution buffer at 70 °C, and continue immediately with the qPCR or store in the freezer at −20 °C.

3.4 Parasite Detection and Quantification

1. Prepare the master mix for parasite quantification: 20 μL containing 12.5 μL 2× buffer, 0.25 μL probe (10 μM), 1 μL of both the forward and reverse primer, and 5.25 μL PCR-grade water.
2. Prepare two reactions per sample: Add 20 μL of master mix and 5 μL DNA sample to a 96-well plate.
3. Add a standard curve of DNA extract from ring-stage parasites (e.g., 1,000; 100; 10; 1; 0.5; 0.2 copies per reaction) and elution buffer as a non-template control.

4. Centrifuge the 96-well plate during 3 min at 500×*g* RPM.
5. Run on a qPCR machine (e.g., Lightcycler 480) with the following settings:
   - Warm-up at 95 °C for 10 min.
   - 55 cycles of 15 s at 95 °C and 1 min at 60 °C.
6. Calculate the number of *P. falciparum* copies in 5 μL extract by the absolute quantification second derivative method.
7. To calculate the number of human hepatocytes present in the sample and the percentage of humanization, prepare a standard curve from DNA extracts from human cells (e.g., PBMCs) and mouse cells (e.g., spleen cells).
8. Perform a qPCR following the protocol described by Alcoser et al. [28]. Prepare the master mix: 10 μL 2× buffer, 1 μL of common forward and reverse primers, 1 μL of both human- and mouse-specific probes, and 5 μL PCR-grade water.
9. Prepare one reaction per sample: 19 μL master mix and 1 μL sample.
10. Add the standard curves of human and mouse DNA extract (10,000; 1,000; 100; 10; 1 copies per reaction) and elution buffer as non-template control.
11. Centrifuge the 96-well plate for 3 min at 500×*g*.
12. Run on a qPCR machine (Lightcycler 480) with the following settings:
    - Warm-up at 95 °C for 10 min.
    - 40 cycles of 15 s at 95 °C and 1 min at 60 °C.
13. Calculate the number of human and mouse cell copies in 1 μL extract by the absolute quantification second derivative method.
14. Multiply the total number (sum) of detected *P. falciparum* copies in the 12 (or 24) 5 μL extracts by 20; this is the total number of detected *P. falciparum* copies in the 12 (or 24) tissue fragments of 25 mg. Divide this number by the total number of human hepatocytes present in the 12 (or 24) 25 mg tissue fragments (number of human DNA copies per 1 μL multiplied by 100). By multiplying this number by 1,000,000 one is able to calculate the total number of ring-stage equivalents per million human hepatocytes (based on a 300 mg tissue sample).

    The final formula for this calculation is

$$\frac{\left(\text{Sum of parasites in the 12}\left(\text{or 24}\right) \textit{P. falciparum}\ \ 5.\text{.l}-\text{eluates}\right)\times 20}{\left\{\left(\text{Sum of human hepatocytes in the 12}\left(\text{or 24}\right)1.\text{.l}-\text{eluates}\right)\times 100\right\}}\times 10^{6}$$

15. To calculate the percentage of human hepatocytes, divide for each sample the number of detected human genomes (hepatocytes) by the total number of detected genomes (human and mouse). Because only approximately 60 % of the mouse liver cells are hepatocytes [29], the calculated average percentage (of 12 or 24 samples) has to be multiplied by 1.667 to determine the final percentage of humanization of the hepatocytes in the chimeric liver.

4 Notes

1. Unlike the SCID chimeric uPA mouse, the human liver-chimeric FRG mouse is robust in size and has a liver that is larger than its non-humanized counterpart. 24 samples should be taken from the FRG huHep mouse, two from each of the 12 liver sections.
2. Sedation is difficult for humanized uPA-SCID mice due to their frailty and small size whereas human-liver chimeric FRG mice can easily be sedated with isoflurane.
3. The abdomen of the mice can be shaven but in our hands this is not necessary to allow for mosquito feeding.
4. Because of the interrupted feeding, it is possible that the amount of blood taken is too small to see with the naked eye.
5. Human-liver chimeric FRG mouse livers are larger and larger tubes/greater volumes of RNAlater may be required.

References

1. Leitner WW, Bergmann-Leitner ES, Angov E (2010) Comparison of *Plasmodium berghei* challenge models for the evaluation of pre-erythrocytic malaria vaccines and their effect on perceived vaccine efficacy. Malar J 9:145
2. Sauerwein RW, Roestenberg M, Moorthy VS (2011) Experimental human challenge infections can accelerate clinical malaria vaccine development. Nat Rev Immunol 11(1):57–64
3. Macchiarini F et al (2005) Humanized mice: are we there yet? J Exp Med 202(10): 1307–1311
4. Meuleman P, Leroux-Roels G (2009) HCV animal models: a journey of more than 30 years. Viruses 1(2):222–240
5. Kaushansky A et al (2014) Of men in mice: the success and promise of humanized mouse models for human malaria parasite infections. Cell Microbiol 16(5):602–611
6. Meuleman P et al (2005) Morphological and biochemical characterization of a human liver in a uPA-SCID mouse chimera. Hepatology 41(4):847–856
7. Azuma H et al (2007) Robust expansion of human hepatocytes in Fah-/-/Rag2-/-/Il2rg-/-mice. Nat Biotechnol 25(8):903–910
8. Bissig KD et al (2007) Repopulation of adult and neonatal mice with human hepatocytes: a chimeric animal model. Proc Natl Acad Sci U S A 104(51):20507–20511
9. Vanwolleghem T et al (2010) Factors determining successful engraftment of hepatocytes and susceptibility to hepatitis B and C virus infection in uPA-SCID mice. J Hepatol 53(3): 468–476
10. Tateno C et al (2013) Morphological and micro-array analyses of human hepatocytes from xenogeneic host livers. Lab Investig 93(1):54–71
11. Braun KM, Sandgren EP (1998) Liver disease and compensatory growth: unexpected lessons from genetically altered mice. Int J Dev Biol 42(7):935–942

12. Grompe M et al (1993) Loss of fumarylacetoacetate hydrolase is responsible for the neonatal hepatic dysfunction phenotype of lethal albino mice. Genes Dev 7(12A):2298–2307
13. Wilson EM et al (2014) Extensive double humanization of both liver and hematopoiesis in FRGN mice. Stem Cell Res 13(3PA):404–412
14. Vaughan AM et al (2012) Development of humanized mouse models to study human malaria parasite infection. Future Microbiol 7(5):657–665
15. Sacci JB Jr et al (2006) *Plasmodium falciparum* infection and exoerythrocytic development in mice with chimeric human livers. Int J Parasitol 36(3):353–360
16. Vaughan AM et al (2012) Complete *Plasmodium falciparum* liver-stage development in liver-chimeric mice. J Clin Invest 122(10):3618–3628
17. Foquet L et al (2014) Vaccine-induced monoclonal antibodies targeting circumsporozoite protein prevent *Plasmodium falciparum* infection. J Clin Invest 124(1):140–144
18. Sack BK et al. (2013) A model for in vivo assessment of humoral protection against malaria sporozoite challenge by passive transfer of monoclonal antibodies and immune serum. Infect Immun. p. IAI. 01249-13
19. Foquet L et al (2013) Molecular detection and quantification of *Plasmodium falciparum-infected* human hepatocytes in chimeric immune-deficient mice. Malar J 12(1):430
20. Vaughan A et al (2012) A transgenic *Plasmodium falciparum* NF54 strain that expresses GFP-luciferase throughout the parasite life cycle. Mol Biochem Parasitol 186(2):143–147
21. Teirlinck AC et al (2013) NF135.C10: a new *Plasmodium falciparum* clone for controlled human malaria infections. J Infect Dis 207(4): 656–660
22. Tateno C et al (2004) Near completely humanized liver in mice shows human-type metabolic responses to drugs. Am J Pathol 165(1fb9c63d-0fa7-8bd3-eba4-7a81d8a986dc):901–913
23. Mota MM et al (2001) Migration of Plasmodium sporozoites through cells before infection. Science 291(5501):141–144
24. Rosenberg R et al (1990) An estimation of the number of malaria sporozoites ejected by a feeding mosquito. Trans R Soc Trop Med Hyg 84(2):209–212
25. Jin Y, Kebaier C, Vanderberg J (2007) Direct microscopic quantification of dynamics of *Plasmodium berghei* sporozoite transmission from mosquitoes to mice. Infect Immun 75(11):5532–5539
26. Hermsen CC et al (2001) Detection of *Plasmodium falciparum* malaria parasites in vivo by real-time quantitative PCR. Mol Biochem Parasitol 118(2):247–251
27. Bijker EM et al (2014) Sporozoite immunization of human volunteers under mefloquine prophylaxis is safe, immunogenic and protective: a double-blind randomized controlled clinical trial. PLoS One 9(11), e112910
28. Alcoser SY et al (2011) Real-time PCR-based assay to quantify the relative amount of human and mouse tissue present in tumor xenografts. BMC Biotechnol 11:124
29. Marcos R, Monteiro RA, Rocha E (2006) Design-based stereological estimation of hepatocyte number, by combining the smooth optical fractionator and immunocytochemistry with anti-carcinoembryonic antigen polyclonal antibodies. Liver Int 26(1):116–124

Chapter 6

Measurement of Antibody-Mediated Reduction of *Plasmodium yoelii* Liver Burden by Bioluminescent Imaging

Brandon K. Sack, Jessica L. Miller, Ashley M. Vaughan, and Stefan H.I. Kappe

Abstract

Antibodies against the infectious sporozoite stage of malaria have been shown to be effective in preventing infection of the liver and in mitigating the ensuing blood stage. However, only a handful of antibody targets have been vetted and shown to be successful in mediating in vivo protection. Even more limited are the means with which to measure how effectively antibodies can reduce the number of parasites establishing infection in the liver. Traditionally, only qPCR of infected mouse livers could accurately measure liver parasite burden. However, this procedure requires sacrifice of the animal and precludes monitoring of the ensuing blood stage infection. Herein we describe a method of accurately assessing antibody-mediated reduction of parasite liver burden by combining passive or active immunization of mice and mosquito bite challenge with luciferase-expressing transgenic *P. yoelii* parasites. This method is rapid, reliable and allows for observation of blood stage disease in the same animal. This model will prove integral in screening the efficacy of novel antibody targets as the search for a more effective malaria vaccine continues.

Key words Antibody, Humoral immunity, Malaria, Liver stage, Pre-erythrocytic, Bioluminescent imaging

1 Introduction

Historically, the majority of antibody (Ab)-based experimental vaccines for malaria control have been focused on the disease-causing blood stage parasite. As a result, the role of Abs in mediating protection at this stage has been well established and a number of stage-specific assays are available to measure the effects of Abs both in vitro and in vivo [1–4]. However, the pre-erythrocytic (skin to liver) stage of the parasite is an extremely attractive target for vaccine intervention given the low number of parasites at this stage and the lack of clinical symptoms during this stage. Data from clinical trials using live-attenuated sporozoites or a pre-erythrocytic subunit vaccine (RTS,S) have stoked this interest as

Ashley M. Vaughan (ed.), *Malaria Vaccines: Methods and Protocols*, Methods in Molecular Biology, vol. 1325, DOI 10.1007/978-1-4939-2815-6_6, © Springer Science+Business Media New York 2015

they both appear to rely heavily on anti-sporozoite Abs in mediating protection [5–9]. The RTS,S vaccine targets the major sporozoite surface protein, circumsporozoite protein (CSP), and this remains one of only a few sporozoite Ab targets identified to date. As the search for additional Ab targets intensifies, there will be a need to evaluate the ability of Abs to prevent the establishment of a parasite liver stage infection and subsequent blood stage infection in an efficient and physiologically relevant manner.

Currently, mouse models of malaria allow for noninvasive and accurate measurement of blood stage disease through either Giemsa-stained blood smears or flow cytometry [1, 2, 10–14]. Both of these methods, in addition to in vitro growth assays for *P. falciparum*, have allowed for extensive pre-clinical analysis of Ab-based interventions for blood stage malaria [15]. Prior to in vivo imaging, the only way to quantify parasite liver stage burden has been through labor-intensive counting of liver stage parasites via microscopy or by measuring liver parasite RNA using quantitative real-time PCR. While accurate, both of these methods require sacrifice of the animal, which precludes evaluation of the subsequent blood stage infection. Here, we describe an efficient and noninvasive method of assessing Ab-mediated inhibition of liver stage infection by challenging passively or actively immunized animals with a transgenic *P. yoelii* parasite that expresses a luciferase reporter [16]. This method is technically simple, accurate and does not require sacrifice of the animal—allowing for time course analysis of liver infection and for monitoring the ensuing blood stage infection.

1.1 Basic Experimental Design

Several bioluminescent malaria parasites exist for both *P. berghei* and the *P. yoelii* YM (lethal) strain [17–20]. However, the methods described here are optimized for a transgenic non-lethal *P. yoelii* XNL strain that expresses a GFP-luciferase fusion (Py-GFP-luciferase) [16]. Aside from non-lethality, this transgenic parasite has the advantage of being detectable at earlier time points of liver stage infection compared to similar transgenic parasites [17–20]. The parasite was generated by integrating a GFP-luciferase fusion-expressing construct into the dispensable *S1* locus [16]. The parasite develops normally and expresses luciferase throughout all stages of parasite development in both the mosquito and mouse [16]. Following intravenous injection of 10^5 sporozoites, parasite liver infection can be detected by in vivo bioluminescent imaging as early as 16 h with a peak between 42 and 48 h as the parasites begin the transition from the liver stage to the blood stage [16] (Fig. 1). Bioluminescent quantification of liver burden using this parasite has been shown to be as accurate as qPCR although not quite as sensitive at very low levels of infection. Thus, this system allows for a more efficient and immediate assessment of liver burden while enabling continued survival of the animal for monitoring of blood stage disease.

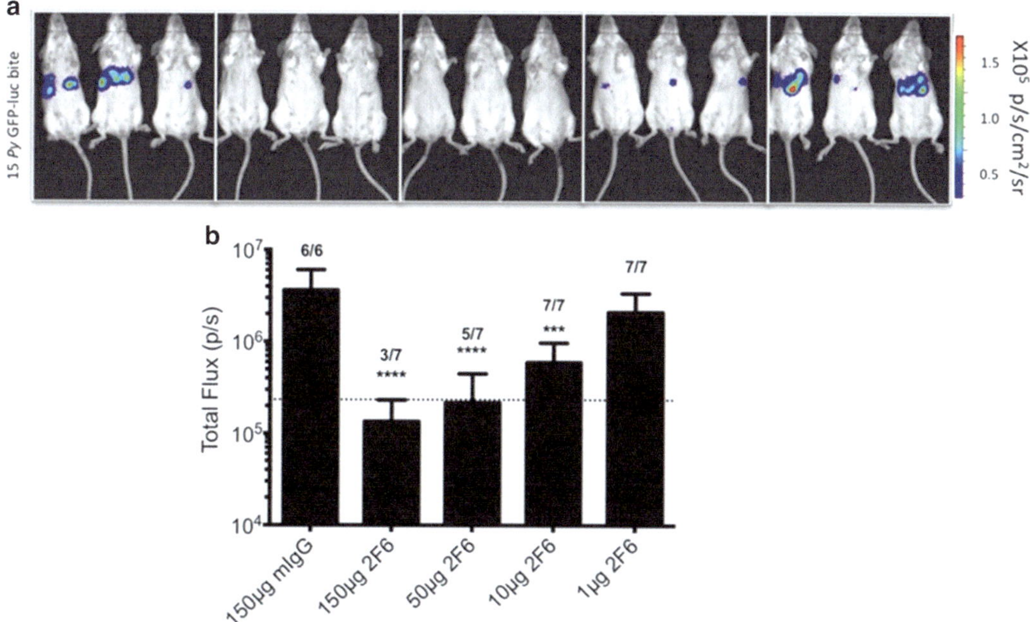

Fig. 1 Antibody-mediated inhibition following mosquito bite sporozoite challenge. Representative images (**a**) and quantification of liver burden (**b**) are shown from mice that were administered control antibody ("mIgG") or indicated doses of the anti-*P. yoelii* CSP monoclonal antibody (mAb) 2F6 prior to challenge by bite of 15 mosquitoes infected with *P. yoelii* expressing GFP-luciferase

Here, we describe how this method can be combined with active or passive immunization of animals to assess Ab-mediated inhibition of liver infection in mice. It is important to note that although inhibition of liver infection can be demonstrated with passive transfer of large doses of monoclonal Ab (mAb) followed immediately by intravenous sporozoite injection, detection of Ab-mediated reduction in liver infection is most sensitive when the challenge is performed via mosquito bite at least 16 h after passive transfer of Ab [21–24]. Using this methodology, it is possible to detect a wide range of inhibition of liver infection with subsequent follow up of blood stage infection (Fig. 1).

Passive transfer of mAb followed by mosquito bite infection and bioluminescent imaging has been rigorously verified as an effective means to detect Ab-mediated inhibition of liver infection [25]. Evaluation of Abs from other sources such as purified polyclonal Abs or serum containing polyclonal Abs against a particular target is also possible. Furthermore, the ability of serum containing Abs to multiple antigens (e.g., from mice immunized with live attenuated parasites) to inhibit liver infection has also been evaluated by this method [26]. However, passive transfer of serum substantially dilutes the Ab concentration and is limited by the amount that can be safely injected into a mouse. Thus, serum for passive transfer may not be available in sufficient quantities to mediate an observable effect especially in the case of serum from single antigen immunizations. In this case, it is preferable to actively immunize mice with a protein/peptide in adjuvant to elicit high-titer Abs in vivo. These immunized mice can then be depleted of $CD4^+$ and $CD8^+$ cells immediately prior to challenge to eliminate the possibility of T cells inhibiting liver infection. All of these methods are described in detail below.

2 Materials

2.1 Preparation of Immune Sera and Plasma

1. Attenuated live sporozoites or purified antigen in adjuvant (*see* Subheading 2.3).
2. 250 IU/mL heparin in phosphate buffered saline (PBS), pH 7.4.
3. 30 gauge needles.
4. 1 mL syringe.
5. Serum separator collection tubes (BD Microtainer, cat# 365956).
6. 1.5 mL microcentrifuge tubes.
7. Tabletop centrifuge.

2.2 Passive Transfer of Immune Sera/Ab

1. Immune sera or purified Ab (without sodium azide).
2. Purified antigen.
3. Adjuvant of choice.
4. Syringe appropriate for adjuvant method.
5. 27 gauge needles.
6. 1 mL 30 gauge insulin syringes.
7. 1.5 mL microcentrifuge tubes.
8. PBS.
9. Heat lamp.
10. Ethanol pads.
11. BALB/cJ mice.

2.3 Direct Challenge of Mice Actively Immunized with Peptide/Protein

1. Purified antigen in PBS.
2. Adjuvant of choice.
3. Syringe appropriate for adjuvant method.
4. 1 mL 30 gauge insulin syringes.
5. Anti-$CD4^+$ mAb (clone GK1.5).
6. Anti-$CD8^+$ mAb (clone 2.43).
7. PBS.

2.4 Py-GFP-luc Mosquito Bite Infection

1. Small cages suitable for mosquito containment.
2. Mouth aspirator (John W. Hock Company, model 612).
3. Day 14 Py-GFP-luc infected mosquitoes.
4. Xylazine.
5. Ketamine.

2.5 Bioluminescence Imaging

1. RediJect D-Luciferin (Perkin Elmer product # 760504, or equivalent).
2. 30 gauge needles.
3. 1 mL 30 gauge insulin syringes.
4. Black construction paper.
5. Isoflurane.
6. Isoflurane anesthesia system.
7. IVIS Lumina II animal imager (or equivalent).
8. Computer with Living Image software or equivalent.

3 Methods

3.1 Preparation of Immune Sera for Passive Transfer

1. Immunize 10 BALB/cJ mice with 2–3 doses of attenuated parasites or 3 doses of your antigen of choice in adjuvant at 2–4 week intervals (*see* **Note 1**). Mock immunize 10 mice as a control either with uninfected mosquito salivary gland extract or with an irrelevant protein in adjuvant.
2. Nine to fourteen days following the last immunization, euthanize the immunized mice by CO_2 asphyxiation and collect the mouse blood by cardiac puncture using a 27-gauge needle on a 1 mL syringe. Do not heparinize the syringe if serum (as opposed to plasma) is desired. Transfer the blood to a 1.5 mL microcentrifuge tube. Alternatively, serum separator tubes containing a gel matrix to separate cells from serum can be used (BD Microtainer tubes). In this case, transfer the blood immediately to these tubes and follow manufacturer's instructions for serum collection.
3. If plasma is preferred, coat the syringe with heparin by drawing 200 μL of heparin solution into the syringe and fully extending the plunger so the heparin comes into contact with the entire length of the syringe. Next, ensure that the heparin is in contact with the rubber of the plunger by holding the syringe vertical and tapping it until the all bubbles rise to the top. Fully depress the plunger, expelling excess air and heparin, leaving a small amount of heparin in the dead space between the plunger and needle.
4. Allow blood to clot for 30 min at room temperature. If collecting plasma, proceed directly to **step 6**.

5. Centrifuge clotted blood at 10,000 × *g* in a tabletop centrifuge for 10 min to separate serum.
6. The serum/plasma will separate as a supernatant above pelleted cells. Collect and pool (optional) serum from the 10 immunized mice. Store at −20 °C until use.

3.2 Passive Transfer of Immune Sera/Ab

1. If analyzing purified Ab, dilute Ab in PBS to desired concentration. If the Ab preparation contains sodium azide, this must be removed by standard dialysis/de-salting procedures. Do not dilute immune sera.
2. Load 1 mL insulin syringes with 30 gauge needles with 300 μL of undiluted immune sera or desired amount of diluted Ab (to a total volume of up to 300 μl). A good positive control should be included (*see* **Note 2**). Total Ab mass should be less than 500 μg.
3. A mock injection of species-matched (isotype-matched optional) Ab in a quantity matching the highest dose should also be administered. For serum passive transfer, an equal volume of serum from mock-immunized mice should be administered.
4. Inject the Ab/sera into the mice via the tail vein. To ease the injection process, the mouse should be pre-warmed with a heat lamp placed over a cage containing the mouse. The mouse is ready for injection when it begins to groom more often—a sign that the mouse is warm, making the tail vein dilated and easier to locate/inject. Wiping the mouse tail with an ethanol pad prior to injection will also bring the tail vein to the surface, enhance visualization of the vein, and ease injection.
5. Wait 16–24 h before proceeding to the challenge step (*see* **Note 3**).

3.3 Active Immunization and Challenge of Immunized Mice

1. Immunize at least 5 BALB/cJ mice per group with antigen in adjuvant or live attenuated parasites according to Subheading 3.1. Immunize an equal number of mice with an irrelevant antigen in adjuvant or mosquito salivary gland extract respectively.
2. At least 3 weeks following the final immunization, mice are ready to be challenged. Prior to challenge, it is wise to confirm the presence of serum Abs against the parasite or antigen by collecting a small amount of blood and analyzing via ELISA.
3. To deplete mice of T cells, prepare a solution of 0.5 mg/mouse of anti-$CD4^+$ (clone GK1.5) and 0.35 mg/mouse anti-$CD8^+$ (clone 2.43) Abs in a total of 200 μL of PBS per mouse.
4. Using a 1 mL syringe with a 30-gauge needle, inject 200 μL of the Ab cocktail intraperitoneally into each mouse.

5. Beginning at 6–12 h after administration of T cell depleting Abs, depletion can be confirmed by analyzing peripheral blood cells for the presence of $CD4^+$ and $CD8^+$ T cells using standard flow cytometry procedures.
6. Mice are ready for challenge 16–24 h after T cell depletion.

3.4 Py-GFP-luc Mosquito Bite Infection

1. Infect *Anopheles stephensi* mosquitoes with Py-GFP-luc gametocytes via an infectious blood meal using standard procedures [27].
2. On day 10 after mosquito infection, quantify mosquito infection rate by analyzing 10–12 mosquito midguts for the presence of oocysts (*see* **Note 4**).
3. On day 14 post mosquito infection, quantify mosquito salivary gland infection by dissecting 10–20 mosquitoes using standard procedures (*see* **Note 5**) [27].
4. Using a mouth pipette, transfer 15–20 mosquitoes into small containers modified with netting for housing mosquitoes, one per mouse to be infected (Fig. 2). Mosquitoes from different cages/infections can have varying levels of infection rates and salivary gland sporozoite numbers. If using mosquitoes from more than one starting cage, first transfer all mosquitoes into one cage and then aliquot into the bite cages to allow for equal distribution of mosquitoes, which may have varying infection rates between individual cages.
5. To improve the likelihood of mosquito feeding, starve mosquitoes 3–6 h prior to infection by removing the sugar pad or replacing the sugar pad with a pad soaked only in water.
6. Immediately prior to mosquito bite infection, mice must be anesthetized. To do this, the mice are injected intraperitoneally

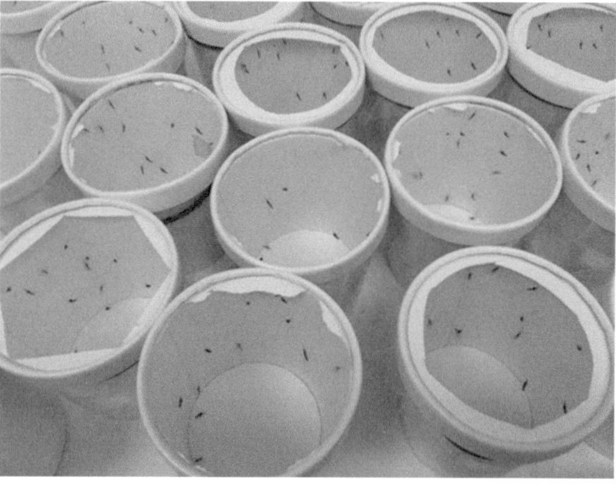

Fig. 2 Infected mosquitoes set up in small cages with a netting barrier to allow for a mosquito bite infection

with 8 μL/g body weight with a diluted Ketamine/Xylazine solution (1 mL Xylazine [20 mg/mL]+2 mL Ketamine [100 mg/mL]+13 mL sterile saline PBS) with a 1 mL insulin syringe.

7. Once mice are anesthetized (mice will be motionless, eyes open, slow but controlled breathing), place mice on small cages containing 15–20 mosquitoes, one mouse per cage. Begin timing infection and after 1 min, briefly lift each mouse from the top of the cage and replace to encourage mosquito bite probing (when sporozoites are injected) rather than feeding. After another minute (2 min after start of infection) rotate mice between different cages. This will minimize variation in mouse infection due to any cage-to-cage variation in mosquito bite infection. Repeat this lifting/rotating process for 10 min total. After 10 min, allow the mice to recover in a warm and humid environment to regain mobility before being returned to their cages.

3.5 Bioluminescent Imaging of Liver Stage Burden

1. Differences in liver stage burden are best assessed at the peak of liver infection, which is between 42–48 h for *P. yoelii* liver stage development. Thus, begin preparing for in vivo imaging during this time frame.
2. Thaw vials of RediJect D-luciferin (or equivalent luciferin) at room temperature in the dark in sufficient quantities to inject 100 μL/mouse.
3. If using mice with pigmented fur, it is necessary to shave the abdomen of the mouse with clippers in order to prevent absorption of light signal from the liver. It is necessary to shave the abdomen liberally, from the hip line to just above the rib cage vertically and mid-way to the back on each side.
4. Using a 1 mL syringe with a 30-gauge needle, intraperitoneally inject mice with 100 μL (or according to manufacturer's instructions) of luciferin 5–10 min prior to imaging. Bioluminescent output is constant between 5 and 20 min after injection, which allows for time to anesthetize and image mice. At this point, it is advised to inject mice in groups according to the number of mice to be imaged at once (typically 1–5, depending on imaging setup).
5. A piece of black construction paper can be used on the imaging surface for ease of cleaning following mouse imaging.
6. 2–3 min after luciferin injection, anesthetize mice using isoflurane in a box chamber at a flow rate according to the manufacturer's recommendations. Once mice are fully anesthetized, transfer to the imaging chamber of the bioluminescent imager.

7. Exact settings for each machine will vary, but using Living Image Software v3.0 with a Caliper Life Sciences in vivo imaging system (IVIS), consistent results can be obtained by acquiring images with a 10-cm-diameter field of view (FOV), a medium binning factor, and an exposure time of 2 min. Liver stage burden in control mice (infected following administration of mock Abs) should be visible at the anatomical site of the liver (*see* **Note 6**).
8. Immediately following imaging, return mice to their cage and monitor for quick recovery from isoflurane anesthesia.
9. Save the image of the mice according to software manufacturer's instruction.
10. Mice may now be monitored for effects on patency/parasitemia on days 3–21 via Giemsa-stained thin smear or flow cytometry using standard techniques.

3.6 Analysis of Liver Stage Burden

1. Quantitative analysis of bioluminescence can be performed by measuring the luminescence signal intensity utilizing the region of interest (ROI) settings of Living Image 3.0 software (XGI-8; Caliper Life Sciences). To measure the liver burden of each mouse, place ROIs of equal size (using copy and paste) around the area at the location of the liver for each mouse. Ensure each ROI within each image and between images/groups to be compared are of the same exact size. Liver burden is directly correlated with total flux values (in photons/second [p/s]) for each ROI and this value should be used for all comparisons of liver stage infection. Ensure the ROI's are measuring "radiance" which will display the total flux above each ROI.
2. Background flux can be determined by placing ROIs over the pelvis of each mouse where luminescence should be absent at 42–48 h post-infection. An example of ROI use for measuring liver burden and background can be seen in Fig. 3.

4 Notes

1. All animal experimentations must be approved by the relevant committees (for example, in the USA, such work is approved by the IACUC—the Institutional Animal Care and Use Committee) and personnel performing procedures on animals must receive appropriate training.
2. One example is a 150 μg/mouse dose of the anti-CSP repeat mAb (clone 2 F6) which is enough to reduce liver burden to background levels in BALB/cJ mice and prevent development of blood stage in ~50 % of mice.

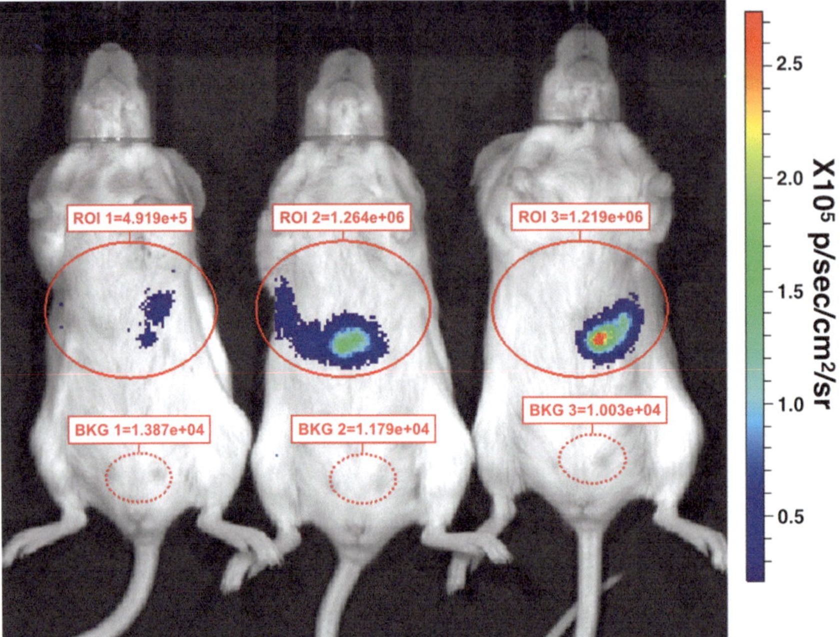

Fig. 3 Example of region of interest (ROI) placement for measuring liver stage burden and background luminescence

3. This allows for distribution of the antibody throughout the mouse tissue and greatly enhances the ability of antibodies to function in the skin. Failure to wait will result in decreased sensitivity of antibody activity [25].
4. In general, it is recommended to use mosquitoes from a cage that have an infection rate >50 % with the majority of mosquitoes harboring >10 oocysts per midgut.
5. Only use mosquitoes with an average of >10,000 sporozoites/mosquito for mosquito bite infection.
6. If there is no or low burden detectable, the exposure time can be increased to 5 min. Alternatively, the mice in question can be re-injected with luciferin to ensure there was not a problem with the luciferin injection.

Acknowledgements

We would like to thank the Center for Infectious Disease Research Center for Mosquito Production and Malaria Infection Research for their production of quality infected mosquitoes and parasites.

References

1. Boyle DB, Newbold CI, Smith CC, Brown KN (1982) Monoclonal antibodies that protect in vivo against Plasmodium chabaudi recognize a 250,000-dalton parasite polypeptide. Infect Immun 38(1):94–102
2. Majarian WR, Daly TM, Weidanz WP, Long CA (1984) Passive immunization against murine malaria with an IgG3 monoclonal antibody. J Immunol 132(6):3131–3137
3. Mlambo G, Kumar N (2007) A modified Plasmodium falciparum growth inhibition assay (GIA) to assess activity of plasma from malaria endemic areas. Exp Parasitol 115(2):211–214. doi:10.1016/j.exppara.2006.08.003
4. Grimberg BT (2011) Methodology and application of flow cytometry for investigation of human malaria parasites. J Immunol Methods 367(1–2):1–16. doi:10.1016/j.jim.2011.01.015
5. Kester KE, Cummings JF, Ofori-Anyinam O, Ockenhouse CF, Krzych U, Moris P, Schwenk R, Nielsen RA, Debebe Z, Pinelis E, Juompan L, Williams J, Dowler M, Stewart VA, Wirtz RA, Dubois MC, Lievens M, Cohen J, Ballou WR, Heppner DG Jr (2009) Randomized, double-blind, phase 2a trial of falciparum malaria vaccines RTS, S/AS01B and RTS, S/AS02A in malaria-naive adults: safety, efficacy, and immunologic associates of protection. J Infect Dis 200(3):337–346. doi:10.1086/600120
6. Chuang I, Sedegah M, Cicatelli S, Spring M, Polhemus M, Tamminga C, Patterson N, Guerrero M, Bennett JW, McGrath S, Ganeshan H, Belmonte M, Farooq F, Abot E, Banania JG, Huang J, Newcomer R, Rein L, Litilit D, Richie NO, Wood C, Murphy J, Sauerwein R, Hermsen CC, McCoy AJ, Kamau E, Cummings J, Komisar J, Sutamihardja A, Shi M, Epstein JE, Maiolatesi S, Tosh D, Limbach K, Angov E, Bergmann-Leitner E, Bruder JT, Doolan DL, King CR, Carucci D, Dutta S, Soisson L, Diggs C, Hollingdale MR, Ockenhouse CF, Richie TL (2013) DNA prime/Adenovirus boost malaria vaccine encoding *P. falciparum* CSP and AMA1 induces sterile protection associated with cell-mediated immunity. PLoS One 8(2):e55571. doi:10.1371/journal.pone.0055571
7. Epstein JE, Tewari K, Lyke KE, Sim BK, Billingsley PF, Laurens MB, Gunasekera A, Chakravarty S, James ER, Sedegah M, Richman A, Velmurugan S, Reyes S, Li M, Tucker K, Ahumada A, Ruben AJ, Li T, Stafford R, Eappen AG, Tamminga C, Bennett JW, Ockenhouse CF, Murphy JR, Komisar J, Thomas N, Loyevsky M, Birkett A, Plowe CV, Loucq C, Edelman R, Richie TL, Seder RA, Hoffman SL (2011) Live attenuated malaria vaccine designed to protect through hepatic CD8(+) T cell immunity. Science 334(6055):475–480. doi:10.1126/science.1211548
8. Seder RA, Chang LJ, Enama ME, Zephir KL, Sarwar UN, Gordon IJ, Holman LA, James ER, Billingsley PF, Gunasekera A, Richman A, Chakravarty S, Manoj A, Velmurugan S, Li M, Ruben AJ, Li T, Eappen AG, Stafford RE, Plummer SH, Hendel CS, Novik L, Costner PJ, Mendoza FH, Saunders JG, Nason MC, Richardson JH, Murphy J, Davidson SA, Richie TL, Sedegah M, Sutamihardja A, Fahle GA, Lyke KE, Laurens MB, Roederer M, Tewari K, Epstein JE, Sim BK, Ledgerwood JE, Graham BS, Hoffman SL (2013) Protection against malaria by intravenous immunization with a nonreplicating sporozoite vaccine. Science. doi:10.1126/science.1241800
9. Ewer KJ, O'Hara GA, Duncan CJ, Collins KA, Sheehy SH, Reyes-Sandoval A, Goodman AL, Edwards NJ, Elias SC, Halstead FD, Longley RJ, Rowland R, Poulton ID, Draper SJ, Blagborough AM, Berrie E, Moyle S, Williams N, Siani L, Folgori A, Colloca S, Sinden RE, Lawrie AM, Cortese R, Gilbert SC, Nicosia A, Hill AV (2013) Protective CD8+ T-cell immunity to human malaria induced by chimpanzee adenovirus-MVA immunisation. Nat Commun 4:2836. doi:10.1038/ncomms3836
10. Barkan D, Ginsburg H, Golenser J (2000) Optimisation of flow cytometric measurement of parasitaemia in plasmodium-infected mice. Int J Parasitol 30(5):649–653
11. Jimenez-Diaz MB, Rullas J, Mulet T, Fernandez L, Bravo C, Gargallo-Viola D, Angulo-Barturen I (2005) Improvement of detection specificity of Plasmodium-infected murine erythrocytes by flow cytometry using autofluorescence and YOYO-1. Cytometry A 67(1):27–36. doi:10.1002/cyto.a.20169
12. Hein-Kristensen L, Wiese L, Kurtzhals JA, Staalsoe T (2009) In-depth validation of acridine orange staining for flow cytometric parasite and reticulocyte enumeration in an experimental model using Plasmodium berghei. Exp Parasitol 123(2):152–157. doi:10.1016/j.exppara.2009.06.010
13. Gerena Y, Gonzalez-Pons M, Serrano AE (2011) Cytofluorometric detection of rodent malaria parasites using red-excited fluorescent dyes. Cytometry A 79(11):965–972. doi:10.1002/cyto.a.21119
14. Somsak V, Srichairatanakool S, Yuthavong Y, Kamchonwongpaisan S, Uthaipibull C (2012)

Flow cytometric enumeration of Plasmodium berghei-infected red blood cells stained with SYBR Green I. Acta Trop 122(1):113–118. doi:10.1016/j.actatropica.2011.12.010

15. Heppner DG (2013) The malaria vaccine–status quo 2013. Travel Med Infect Dis 11(1):2–7. doi:10.1016/j.tmaid.2013.01.006
16. Miller JL, Murray S, Vaughan AM, Harupa A, Sack B, Baldwin M, Crispe IN, Kappe SH (2013) Quantitative bioluminescent imaging of pre-erythrocytic malaria parasite infection using luciferase-expressing Plasmodium yoelii. PLoS One 8(4):e60820. doi:10.1371/journal.pone.0060820
17. Mwakingwe A, Ting LM, Hochman S, Chen J, Sinnis P, Kim K (2009) Noninvasive real-time monitoring of liver-stage development of bioluminescent Plasmodium parasites. J Infect Dis 200(9):1470–1478. doi:10.1086/606115
18. Ploemen I, Behet M, Nganou-Makamdop K, van Gemert GJ, Bijker E, Hermsen C, Sauerwein R (2011) Evaluation of immunity against malaria using luciferase-expressing Plasmodium berghei parasites. Malar J 10:350. doi:10.1186/1475-2875-10-350
19. Ploemen IH, Prudencio M, Douradinha BG, Ramesar J, Fonager J, van Gemert GJ, Luty AJ, Hermsen CC, Sauerwein RW, Baptista FG, Mota MM, Waters AP, Que I, Lowik CW, Khan SM, Janse CJ, Franke-Fayard BM (2009) Visualisation and quantitative analysis of the rodent malaria liver stage by real time imaging. PLoS One 4(11), e7881. doi:10.1371/journal.pone.0007881
20. Franke-Fayard B, Djokovic D, Dooren MW, Ramesar J, Waters AP, Falade MO, Kranendonk M, Martinelli A, Cravo P, Janse CJ (2008) Simple and sensitive antimalarial drug screening in vitro and in vivo using transgenic luciferase expressing Plasmodium berghei parasites. Int J Parasitol 38(14):1651–1662. doi:10.1016/j.ijpara.2008.05.012, S0020-7519(08)00221-X [pii]
21. Miller JL, Sack BK, Baldwin M, Vaughan AM, Kappe SH (2014) Interferon-mediated innate immune responses against malaria parasite liver stages. Cell Rep 7(2):436–447. doi:10.1016/j.celrep.2014.03.018
22. Vanderberg JP, Frevert U (2004) Intravital microscopy demonstrating antibody-mediated immobilisation of Plasmodium berghei sporozoites injected into skin by mosquitoes. Int J Parasitol 34(9):991–996
23. Vanderberg J, Mueller AK, Heiss K, Goetz K, Matuschewski K, Deckert M, Schluter D (2007) Assessment of antibody protection against malaria sporozoites must be done by mosquito injection of sporozoites. Am J Pathol 171(4):1405–1406. doi:10.2353/ajpath.2007.070661, Author reply 1406
24. Kebaier C, Voza T, Vanderberg J (2009) Kinetics of mosquito-injected Plasmodium sporozoites in mice: fewer sporozoites are injected into sporozoite-immunized mice. PLoS Pathog 5(4):e1000399. doi:10.1371/journal.ppat.1000399
25. Sack BK, Miller JL, Vaughan AM, Douglass A, Kaushansky A, Mikolajczak S, Coppi A, Gonzalez-Aseguinolaza G, Tsuji M, Zavala F, Sinnis P, Kappe SH, Adams JH (2014) Model for in vivo assessment of humoral protection against malaria sporozoite challenge by passive transfer of monoclonal antibodies and immune serum. Infect Immun 82(2):808–817. doi:10.1128/IAI.01249-13
26. Keitany GJ, Sack B, Smithers H, Chen L, Jang IK, Sebastian L, Gupta M, Sather DN, Vignali M, Vaughan AM, Kappe SH, Wang R (2014) Immunization of mice with live-attenuated late liver stage-arresting P. yoelii parasites generates protective antibody responses to pre-erythrocytic stages of malaria. Infect Immun. doi:10.1128/IAI.02320-14
27. Vaughan AM, Kappe SH (2013) Vaccination using radiation or genetically attenuated live sporozoites. Methods Mol Biol 923:549–566. doi:10.1007/978-1-62703-026-7_38

Chapter 7

Detection of *Plasmodium berghei* and *Plasmodium yoelii* Liver-Stage Parasite Burden by Quantitative Real-Time PCR

Alexander Pichugin and Urszula Krzych

Abstract

Direct detection and quantification of liver-stage Plasmodium parasites became possible with the development of quantitative real-time PCR (qPCR). Here we describe the measurement of parasite burden in the livers of mice infected with the rodent malaria species, *Plasmodium berghei* and *Plasmodium yoelii*. This method is based on detection of expression of parasite ribosomal 18S RNA and can serve as an endpoint to accurately evaluate the efficacy of vaccines targeting the preerythrocytic stages of malaria. This approach is fast and highly reproducible and allows quantification of liver-stage parasite burden in different mouse strains and different Plasmodium species after infection with a range of sporozoite challenge doses.

Key words Malaria, Liver-stage, Plasmodium, Real-time PCR, 18S ribosomal RNA, Parasite load

1 Introduction

The life cycle of malaria parasites is complex and includes different stages each with unique patterns of Plasmodium antigen expression. Probably the most attractive target for vaccine design is the preerythrocytic stages of infection because the number of parasites that are encountered at any one time is relatively small and it precedes asexual blood stage replication and the encompassing clinical symptoms of the disease. Quantification of parasitemia in the blood is being widely used not only to estimate efficiency of blood stage vaccines, but also as a surrogate endpoint for protection induced by preerythrocytic vaccine candidates [1]. However, vaccine failure at the blood stage does not assess a vaccine's ability to induce preerythrocytic immunity and antigens involved in preerythrocytic immunity are likely to be ideal candidates for multi-subunit vaccines that target preerythrocytic and blood stage parasites.

The quantification of preerythrocytic stages of *P. berghei* (Pb) and *P. yoelii* (Py) parasites in rats [2] and mice [3] was firstly developed on the basis of hybridization of synthetic oligonucleotide probes with parasite DNA or RNA. Further application of polymerase chain

Ashley M. Vaughan (ed.), *Malaria Vaccines: Methods and Protocols*, Methods in Molecular Biology, vol. 1325,
DOI 10.1007/978-1-4939-2815-6_7, © Springer Science+Business Media New York 2015

reaction (PCR) [4], quantitative-competitive reverse transcription PCR (RT-qPCR) [5] and, finally, quantitative real-time PCR (qPCR) [6, 7] made fast and direct measurement of malaria parasites possible in the blood and tissues, including the liver.

In addition to precise measurement of preerythrocytic vaccine efficacy per se, quantification of liver-stage parasite burden can be used for high-throughput screening of novel vaccine candidates. Haddad D. et al. described a model of partial protection after vaccination of mice with plasmid DNA encoding Plasmodium circumsporozoite protein (CSP) [8]. It is unlikely that plasmid DNA vaccination can induce sterile protection; however its production is cheap and less time-consuming when comparing its use to more robust vaccine platforms, such as adjuvanted proteins or viruses. This model of partial protection can be used for the discovery of protective malaria antigens by rapid testing of DNA vaccines.

In this chapter we outline the following steps for quantification of liver-stage parasite burden: harvesting of livers, isolation of total RNA, reverse transcription, and SYBR Green qPCR. The information is based on our own experience and previous published studies in which these techniques were first described [7, 9–12]. We followed the Minimum Information for Publication of Quantitative Real-Time PCR Experiments (MIQE) guidelines [13] to encourage better experimental practice and establish high reproducibility and accuracy of our qPCR assay.

2 Materials

All solutions used in these assays need to be prepared in nuclease-free water and only analytical grade reagents are to be used. All reagents need to be prepared and stored at room temperature (unless indicated otherwise). All waste disposal needs to be done diligently following waste disposal regulations.

2.1 Liver Harvesting and RNA Isolation Components

1. Phosphate buffered saline (PBS).
2. Scissors, tweezers, Styrofoam table, 10 mL syringes, 18 G needles.
3. Screw cap tubes, 2 mL.
4. Liquid nitrogen.
5. Omni Homogenizer with Hard Tissue Omni Tip™ Plastic Homogenizing Probes (Omni International, Kennesaw, GA).
6. TRIzol Reagent (Life Technologies, Frederick, MD). Store at 4 °C.
7. Falcon Round-Bottom Polypropylene Tubes 14 mL (Thermo Fisher Scientific, Rockville, MD).
8. Microcentrifuge tubes, 0.5 mL.
9. Microcentrifuge for 12,000 ×*g* spins.

10. Chloroform.
11. 2-propanol.
12. 75 % Ethanol.
13. RNase-Free DNase Set (QIAGEN). Store at 4 °C.

2.2 Reverse Transcription Components

1. High Capacity cDNA Reverse Transcription Kit (Applied Biosystems, Carlsbad, CA). Store at −20 °C.
2. MicroAmp® 8-Tube Strips, 0.2 mL (Applied Biosystems).
3. MicroAmp® Optical 8-Cap Strips (Applied Biosystems).

2.3 qPCR Components

1. MicroAmp® Fast Optical 96-Well Reaction Plates, 0.1 mL (Applied Biosystems).
2. MicroAmp® Optical Adhesive Film Covers (Applied Biosystems).
3. SYBR Green PCR Master Mix (Applied Biosystems). Store at 4 °C.
4. Primers: Pb 18S rRNA forward—AAGCATTAAATAAAGC GAATACATCCTTAC; Pb 18S rRNA reverse—GGAGATTGG TTTTGACGTTTATGTG [9]; Py 18S rRNA forward—GGGG ATTGGTTTTGACGTTTTTGCG; Py 18S rRNA reverse—AAGCATTAAATAAAGCGAATACATCCTTAT [10]; mouse β-actin forward—GGCTGTATTCCCCTCCATCG; mouse β-actin reverse—CCAGTTGGTAACAATGCCATGT; dissolve all primers in nuclease-free water at a concentration of 100 nmol/ mL. Store at −20 °C.

3 Methods

All procedures are to be performed on ice (unless indicated otherwise). The temperature in the microcentrifuge should be set at 4 °C. Extra reactions should be included in the calculations to provide excess volume for the loss that occurs during reagent transfers. All procedures with animals must be conducted under an IACUC-approved protocol in accordance with the Animal Welfare Act and The Guide for the Care and Use of Laboratory Animals (NRC, 2011).

3.1 Isolation of Total RNA from Mouse Liver

Use caution at all times to avoid introducing RNAse during liver processing—ensure all materials are RNAse free.

1. 40–42 h after the challenge (*see* **Note 1**) euthanize each experimental mouse with CO_2 and attach it to a Styrofoam board with the abdomen facing up. Spray mouse with 70 % alcohol. Peel off the skin to expose thorax and abdomen. Cut through abdominal muscle wall. Take intestines out of the abdominal cavity, and gently move up the large liver lobes. Locate and cut

inferior vena cava with scissors. Cut through the ribcage and diaphragm to expose the heart. Using syringe and needle perfuse liver with 10 mL PBS through the left ventricle of the heart (*see* **Note 2**).

2. Cut the liver out, making sure to fully remove the gall bladder, and place the whole liver into a 2 mL screw cap tube. Immediately freeze the liver in liquid nitrogen (*see* **Note 3**). Make sure to use cryogloves, goggles or a face shield when working with liquid nitrogen.
3. Add 5 mL of TRIzol to a 14 mL round-bottom tube on ice. Using clean scissors transfer the liver from the screw cap tube to the tube with TRIzol. Use the Omni Tip™ homogenizer with the probe for hard tissue to homogenize the liver (*see* **Note 4**). Transfer 1 mL of suspension to a 1.5 mL microcentrifuge tube. Incubate homogenized samples for 5 min at room temperature to permit the complete dissociation of nucleoprotein complexes.
4. Centrifuge samples at 12,000 × *g* for 10 min (*see* **Note 5**). Transfer 0.5 mL of the cleared supernatant to a 1.5 mL microcentrifuge with 0.5 mL fresh TRIzol. Add 0.2 mL chloroform. Shake the tube vigorously by hand for 15 s and then incubate at room temperature for 3 min. Cool on ice for 3 min. Centrifuge samples at 12,000 × *g* for 15 min.
5. Transfer the upper aqueous phase (~0.5 mL) to 1.5 mL microcentrifuge tube (*see* **Note 6**), and precipitate the RNA by mixing with 0.5 mL 2-propanol. Incubate the samples at room temperature for 10 min and centrifuge at 12,000 × *g* for 10 min. Remove the supernatant and wash the RNA pellet with 1 mL 75 % ethanol by vortexing, centrifuge at 12,000 × *g* for 5 min. Discard ethanol (*see* **Note 7**).
6. Leave the tubes containing the RNA open in a tissue culture hood for 15 min at room temperature to dry the RNA pellet. Add 175 μL nuclease-free water. Close the lid and leave the tubes on ice for 30–60 min. The RNA will be gel-like and is fully dissolved by pipetting.
7. Add 5 μL of RNAse-free DNase and 20 μL of RDD buffer from the RNAse-Free DNase Set to each tube, mix gently by pipetting. Incubate for 10 min at room temperature followed by 5 min at 75 °C in a heat block and then chill on ice (*see* **Note 8**). Determine the RNA concentration photometrically.

3.2 Reverse Transcription

For the preparation of samples for reverse transcription, use hygienic procedures to insure PCR amplification without contamination.

1. Thaw High Capacity cDNA Reverse Transcription Kit components on ice. Mix 2 μL 10× RT Buffer, 2 μL 10× RT Random Primers, 0.8 μL 25× dNTP Mix, 1 μL MultiScribe™ Reverse

Transcriptase and 4.2 μL Nuclease-Free Water per RNA sample. Pipette 10 μL of the mixture into the each tube of a microtube strip. Add RNA in 10 μL of water (*see* **Note 9**).

2. Seal the tubes with the caps, vortex and briefly spin down the contents by centrifugation to remove air bubbles. Program a thermal cycler: 10 min at 25 °C, 120 min at 37 °C, 5 s at 85 °C, 4 °C for ∞, total volume 20 μL. Place the samples into the thermal cycler, run reverse transcription (*see* **Note 10**). Measure the concentration of cDNA photometrically.

3.3 Quantitative Real-Time PCR (Absolute Quantification)

1. Prepare primer working solutions and DNA standards to build standard curves (*see* **Note 11**). Prepare serial dilutions of DNA standards in water to have 10^8, 10^7, 10^6, and 10^5 DNA molecules in 2 μL. Prepare primer working solutions for parasite 18S rRNA and mouse β-actin (reference gene). To do this, mix the forward primer, reverse primer, and water (1:1:18 ratio). Primers and DNA standards should be aliquoted and stored at −20 °C.
2. Thaw primers, cDNA samples, and DNA standards. Mix 12.5 μL 2×SYBR Green PCR Master Mix, 1.6 μL primer working solution and 8.9 μL Nuclease-Free Water per well. Mix thoroughly and pipette 23 μL of the mixture into the each well of MicroAmp® Fast Optical 96-Well Reaction Plate (*see* Table 1). Add template DNAs and sample cDNAs in 2 μL of water to individual wells in triplicate (*see* **Note 12**). Add 2 μL of water for "no template added" triplicate control wells. Use the cDNA resulting from reverse transcription of RNA from the liver of a naive mouse as a negative control.
3. Seal the plate with MicroAmp® Optical Adhesive Film Cover and spin down the contents by centrifugation at 300×*g* for

Table 1
Configuration of qPCR plate to determine Plasmodium liver-stage parasite burden[a]

Mouse β-actin		Py or Pb 18S rRNA	
Standard 10^8	Unknown sample 3	Standard 10^8	Unknown sample 3
Standard 10^7	Unknown sample 4	Standard 10^7	Unknown sample 4
Standard 10^6	Unknown sample 5	Standard 10^6	Unknown sample 5
Standard 10^5	Unknown sample 6	Standard 10^5	Unknown sample 6
No template added	Unknown sample 7	No template added	Unknown sample 7
Negative control	Unknown sample 8	Negative control	Unknown sample 8
Unknown sample 1	Unknown sample 9	Unknown sample 1	Unknown sample 9
Unknown sample 2	Unknown sample 10	Unknown sample 2	Unknown sample 10

[a]Each sample is carried out in triplicate

1 min to remove air bubbles. Place the plate in the appropriate instrument; program a thermal cycler (*see* **Note 13**). Use the following thermal cycling conditions: 15 min at 95 °C, 40 cycles with 95 °C for 20 s; 60 °C for 30 s, and 72 °C for 50 s. Set ROX as a passive reference dye (see specific instrument instructions for further details on passive dye usage).

3.4 Analysis of qPCR Data

1. For analysis, choose an automatic baseline and threshold determination (*see* **Note 14**). All quantitations are normalized to the host reference gene—mouse β-actin—to account for variability in the initial concentration of the cDNA, the quality of the total RNA and the conversion efficiency of the reverse transcription reaction.
2. Confirm the absence of nonspecific amplification by analyzing PCR products by agarose gel electrophoresis (optional). Generate a melting curve using real-time PCR system software.
3. Represent liver stage parasite burden as ratio of number of copies of Plasmodium 18S rRNA to number of copies of mouse β-actin (*see* **Note 15**).

4 Notes

1. Expression of parasite 18S ribosomal RNA in the livers of mice reaches its peak at 40–42 h after intravenous challenge with Pb or Py sporozoites. We recommend that you titrate the challenging dose for each particular model because correlation between number of sporozoites injected and expression of 18S rRNA might vary significantly depending on the mouse strain and Plasmodium species used (*see* Fig. 1). We find that titration curves usually represent sigmoid curves with Lag phase, Log phase, and Stationary phase. For the following mouse–parasite combinations we use sporozoite challenges between 10,000 and 40,000 per mouse: C57BL/6–Pb, CD1–Py, CB6F1–Pb, CB6F1–Py, and BALB/c–Py.
2. The liver can also be perfused with 10 mL PBS through the hepatic portal vein. The color of the liver should change from dark red to pale brown with a successful perfusion. If the liver does not completely perfuse, additional perfusion with PBS can be carried out.
3. Liver samples can be transferred from liquid nitrogen to −80 °C for up to 1 month before processing.
4. Make sequential 5 s pulses with 5 s intervals between them. Repeat the pulses until the liver tissue is completely homogenized (usually 3–5 pulses). Liver homogenates in TRIzol can

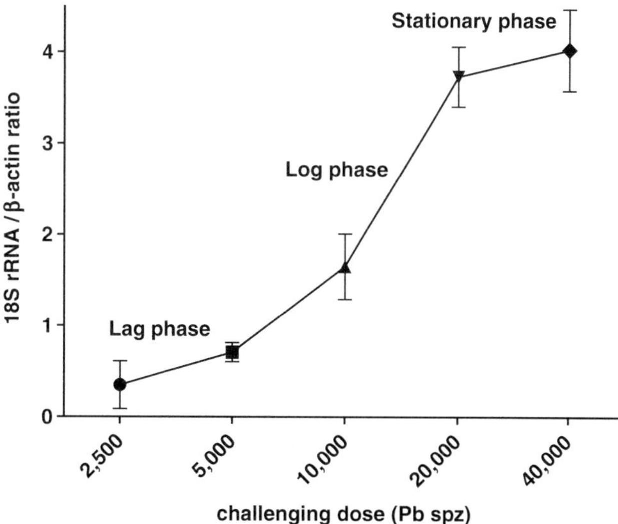

Fig. 1 Correlation between the challenging dose and expression of parasite 18S rRNA in the livers. C57BL/6 (B6) mice were challenged intravenously with different numbers of *P. berghei* sporozoites. Livers were harvested 40 h after the challenge. Liver stage parasite burden is presented as expression of Pb 18S rRNA normalized to mouse β–actin. Based on this curve, challenging dose of 20,000 Pb sporozoites has been chosen for B6/Pb model

be stored frozen at −80 °C up to 1 month before further processing.

5. This is an additional optional step for the samples with a high content of insoluble material which aids in its removal. After centrifugation aqueous supernatant contains the RNA. Do not perform this additional step if you are doing subsequent isolation of DNA from the same sample. In this case add 0.2 mL chloroform directly to a 1.5 mL microcentrifuge tube with 1 mL of liver homogenate in TRIzol after 3 min incubation at room temperature.
6. After centrifugation the sample contains a pellet of insoluble material, a red phenol–chloroform bottom phase, a thin white interphase, and a clear aqueous top phase. RNA is in the upper aqueous phase.
7. The RNA pellet can be stored in 75 % ethanol at −20 °C for up to 1 year or at 4 °C for up to 1 week. We find it convenient to pour away the 75 % ethanol and place the microcentrifuge tubes into a rack for 1 min, and then completely remove the rest of the ethanol with a 200 μL pipettor and tip. Make sure you don't lose the RNA pellet when pouring away the 75 % ethanol since the pellet does not stick to the bottom of the tube well.

8. RNA samples in water can be frozen and stored at −80 °C up to 1 year or used immediately for reverse transcription.
9. Do not overload the reverse transcription reaction with RNA. Use up to 2 μg of total RNA per 20 μL reaction. We find an optimal load of RNA is ~1 μg per reaction; dilute your RNA with Nuclease-Free Water if necessary.
10. cDNA samples can be stored at 4 °C for up to 24 h or up to 1 year at −20 °C.
11. Absolute quantitation compares the quantification cycle value (Cq) of unknown samples against a standard curve with known copy numbers. Plasmids containing cloned target sequences are commonly used as standards in quantitative real time PCR. It is also possible to use the products of amplification of genomic parasite DNA. Briefly, we run regular PCRs with Pb or Py 18S rRNA and mouse β-actin primers, elute the products from agarose gel, make serial dilutions and use these as a standards in qPCR.
12. 10–100 ng of cDNA template should be added to the qPCR reaction. Dilute the cDNA with Nuclease-Free Water if necessary. We usually make tenfold dilutions for all cDNA samples.
13. SYBR Green dye must be calibrated on your instrument. Refer to the appropriate instrument user guide to calibrate the instrument for SYBR Green.
14. The real-time PCR system software calculates baseline and threshold values for a detector based on the assumption that the data exhibit the "typical" amplification curve. A "typical" amplification curve has a plateau phase, linear phase, and exponential phase (geometric phase). We recommend reviewing all baseline and threshold values after analysis of the study data. If necessary, adjust the values manually as described in the appropriate instrument user guide.
15. We define protection as a reduction of parasite burden in the livers of experimental (vaccinated) mice compared to non-immunized (control) mice. Level of reduction of parasite load by particular antigen depends on many factors, such as vaccine platform, immunization schedule, and mouse–parasite combination.

Acknowledgement

This research was supported by the US Army Materiel Command. The views of the authors do not purport to reflect the position of the Department of the Army or the Department of Defense.

References

1. Limbach K et al (2011) Identification of two new protective pre-erythrocytic malaria vaccine antigen candidates. Malar J 10:65
2. Ferreira A et al (1986) Infectivity of Plasmodium berghei sporozoites measured with a DNA probe. Mol Biochem Parasitol 19(2):103–109
3. Arreaza G, Corredor V, Zavala F (1991) Plasmodium yoelii: quantification of the exoerythrocytic stages based on the use of ribosomal RNA probes. Exp Parasitol 72(1): 103–105
4. Hulier E et al (1996) A method for the quantitative assessment of malaria parasite development in organs of the mammalian host. Mol Biochem Parasitol 77(2):127–135
5. Lau AO, Sacci JB Jr, Azad AF (2001) Detection of Plasmodium yoelii stage mRNA in BALB/c mice. J Parasitol 87(1):19–23
6. Bell AS, Ranford-Cartwright LC (2004) A real-time PCR assay for quantifying Plasmodium falciparum infections in the mosquito vector. Int J Parasitol 34(7):795–802
7. Witney AA et al (2001) Determining liver stage parasite burden by real time quantitative PCR as a method for evaluating pre-erythrocytic malaria vaccine efficacy. Mol Biochem Parasitol 118(2):233–245
8. Haddad D et al (2004) Novel antigen identification method for discovery of protective malaria antigens by rapid testing of DNA vaccines encoding exons from the parasite genome. Infect Immun 72(3):1594–1602
9. Bhanot P et al (2003) Defective sorting of the thrombospondin-related anonymous protein (TRAP) inhibits Plasmodium infectivity. Mol Biochem Parasitol 126(2):263–273
10. Bruna-Romero O et al (2001) Detection of malaria liver-stages in mice infected through the bite of a single Anopheles mosquito using a highly sensitive real-time PCR. Int J Parasitol 31(13):1499–1502
11. Friesen J, Matuschewski K (2011) Comparative efficacy of pre-erythrocytic whole organism vaccine strategies against the malaria parasite. Vaccine 29(40):7002–7008
12. Schussek S et al (2013) Highly sensitive quantitative real-time PCR for the detection of Plasmodium liver-stage parasite burden following low-dose sporozoite challenge. PLoS One 8(10), e77811
13. Bustin SA et al (2009) The MIQE guidelines: minimum information for publication of quantitative real-time PCR experiments. Clin Chem 55(4):611–622

Part II

Mosquito Stages

Chapter 8

Membrane Feeding Assay to Determine the Infectiousness of *Plasmodium vivax* Gametocytes

Jetsumon Sattabongkot, Chalermpon Kumpitak, and Kirakorn Kiattibutr

Abstract

The evaluation of *Plasmodium vivax* gametocyte infectiousness by the membrane feeding assay is herein described. While *P. vivax* cannot be cultured and different parasite isolates may infect mosquitoes at different rates, the protocol described in this chapter identifies critical parameters to be considered when performing the assay such as methods for the preparation of the mosquitoes, the size of the blood cup, and the blood volume used. In previous studies the data have shown that the membrane feeding assay is useful for studies of parasite biology, and the effects of transmission blocking drugs and vaccines.

Key words Gametocyte infectiousness, *Plasmodium vivax*, Direct skin feed assay (DFA), Membrane feeding assay (MFA), Transmission blocking drugs, Transmission blocking vaccines

1 Introduction

Malaria gametocyte infectiousness in the natural population can be evaluated by feeding mosquitoes on gametocyte carriers. Feeding methods can be by direct contact of mosquitoes to the patient's arm (direct skin feeding assay, DFA), or collecting blood from patients and adding into glass feeders or blood cups covered with thin membranous material (membrane feeding assay, MFA) which mosquitoes can access the blood from. Depending on the parasite species and how the blood is prepared results for DFA and MFA can either be similar to or different from the same patient blood [1, 2]. Some isolates of *Plasmodium falciparum* parasites from patients can be routinely cultured in the laboratory and thus the membrane feeding protocol can be standardized, and is known as the standard membrane feeding assay (SMFA). As *P. vivax* can still not be cultured in the laboratory, parasites must be obtained directly from patients or gametocyte carriers in endemic areas. Advantages of MFA over DFA are that more mosquitoes can be used and the

Ashley M. Vaughan (ed.), *Malaria Vaccines: Methods and Protocols*, Methods in Molecular Biology, vol. 1325, DOI 10.1007/978-1-4939-2815-6_8,

comparison of gametocyte infectiousness to different vectors is also possible for each case of infected blood. The protocol described in this chapter has been used for *P. vivax* to evaluate gametocyte infectiousness, transmission blocking efficacy of vaccine candidates and efficacy of drugs in blocking sporogonic development [3–8]. There are factors that must be considered when working with the *P. vivax* MFA; (1) the duration that the gametocytes maintain their infectiousness after blood collection and before feeding to the mosquitoes, (2) the starvation period that each species of mosquito vector requires before blood feeding and (3) the correct age of the mosquitoes for the MFA. These parameters may vary in different settings. A small number of trials to identify the correct conditions is recommended. In our laboratory the mosquitoes (including *Anopheles dirus* and *An. minimus*) are either kept as a colony at the field site or transported to the field site before blood feeding.

2 Methods

2.1 Materials and Equipment

2.1.1 Materials

1. Human AB serum.
2. Sodium hypochlorite.
3. Phosphate buffer saline (PBS) pH 7.4.
4. RPMI.

2.1.2 Supplies

Brands or suppliers listed below are examples only, and any local brand supplier should suffice.

1. Glass feeders or blood cups (Somnunk Scientific, Bangkok, Thailand, www.coelenglastechniek.nl) (Fig. 1).
2. Transparent membrane Goldbeater membrane/Baudruche membrane. This membrane can be kept dry in the refrigerator for years.

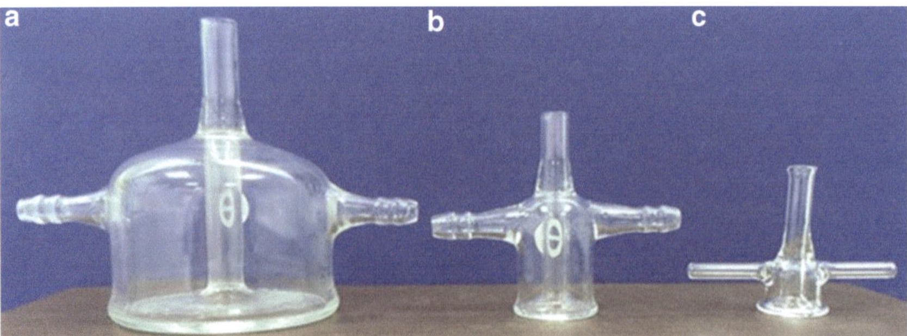

Fig. 1 Blood cups used for mosquito feeds. (***A***) A large cup with a diameter of 6 cm for ≤3 ml of blood. (***B*** and ***C***) are smaller cups with diameters of 2.5 cm and 1.7 cm for blood volume of ≤350 μl and ≤200 μl, respectively

3. Rubber Tubing, inner diameter 6.4 mm, outer diameter 9.6 mm.
4. Microcentrifuge tubes, 1.5 ml.
5. Pipette tips.
6. Filter paper #903 (Whatman).
7. Cryogenic vial, 1.8 ml (Corning).
8. Narrow stem transfer pipettes (Samco Scientific).
9. Paper towel or thin cloth.

2.2 Equipment

1. Benchtop centrifuge (Costar variable speed minicentrifuge).
2. Thermostatic circulator bath with pump or Immersion Bath Circulator (e.g., Model LCB-6D, Daihan Labtech Co., Ltd., Julabo ED Heating Immersion Circulator, etc.).
3. Mixer, Vortex-Genie, or equivalent.
4. Pipettors for 10, 20, 100, 200, and 1,000 μl pipette tips.

3 Procedure

3.1 Assembly of Membrane Feeding Apparatus

This should be done before blood samples are prepared.

1. Transparent membrane is cut into small square pieces, depending on the size of the blood cup (approx. 6×6 cm^2 for a large blood cup or 3×3 cm^2 for a small blood cup). Dipping the edge of the blood cup in PBS before attaching the membrane on the feeder will help the membrane to adhere to the edge of the blood cup. Fasten the membrane to the blood cup edge with a rubber band.
2. Before feeding, keep the membrane on the blood cup wet by soaking the membrane with PBS.
3. If many blood cups are going to be used per blood sample, connect each arm of the blood cup using rubber tubing (Fig. 2). One arm of the first blood cup and one arm of the last blood cup are connected to the tubing of the water bath circulator.
4. Turn on the water bath to check temperature, water circulation, and possible leakage of the water during circulation. The temperature should be set at 37–38 °C.

3.2 Sample Preparation and Membrane Feeding of Mosquitoes (See Note 1)

1. The blood volume used per cup will depend on the blood cup size. Please see Table 1 for recommended volumes. The blood volume should be enough to cover the surface of the membrane to ensure efficient blood feeding by the mosquitoes. Infected blood from patients can be collected either by venipuncture (for volumes of more than 300 μl) or finger prick (for

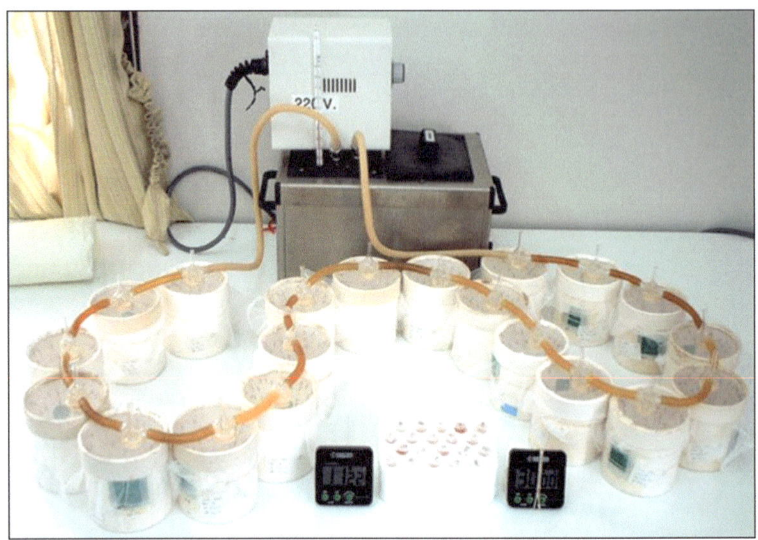

Fig. 2 Assembly of membrane feeding apparatus for the feeding of multiple mosquito cages

Table 1
The blood volume recommended for blood cup size

Blood cup shown in Fig. 1	Diameter (mm)	Minimum blood volume	Number of mosquitoes
A	60	≥3 ml	500–750
B	25	≥300 μl	50–100
C	17	≥200 μl	40–75

volumes ≤300 μl) into tubes with heparin, EDTA or other preferred anticoagulant. Infected blood should be kept at 37 °C by using a temperature controlled bag or by adding warm water to a Thermos flask. At the field laboratory the blood can be kept either in a water bath or an incubator before processing.

2. To remove the blood donor's plasma, the blood volume required for each experiment is transferred into microcentrifuge tube and centrifuged for 5 min at 1,396 × *g*. Plasma is collected for other studies or discarded. The packed blood cells are then washed once with an equal original blood volume of RPMI medium (without serum added). Repeat centrifugation step (*see* **Note 2**).

3. Add AB naïve serum as a control to avoid blood clotting, given the blood group of patients will vary. Additionally, serum for testing should be diluted 1:1 with AB naïve serum. Naïve or diluted test serum is added to aliquots of the washed packed

red blood cells to bring the volume back up to the initial blood volume transferred to the microcentrifuge tube. Keep microcentrifuge tubes containing the infected blood at 37 °C until the mosquitoes feed.

4. For the evaluation of transmission blocking vaccine candidate antibodies or drugs, after the appropriate addition of antibody or drug to naïve AB serum plus red blood cells, the blood samples are kept at 37 °C for 15 min before feeding to the mosquitoes. Gently vortex each tube before feeding to the mosquitoes. Transfer blood to the corresponding membrane feeder. Record the feeding time on a data sheet.
5. Once the blood feeding is completed, the membrane feeding apparatus is dismantled. The blood is removed and put in a double layered biohazard bag for disposing of infectious waste. The blood cup is treated with a 10 % Clorox solution and then cleaned with detergent and washed with 75 % ethanol before hygienic storage.

3.3 Mosquito Preparation Before and After Blood Feeding

1. There are two sizes of mosquito container, a large plastic container for 300–400 female mosquitoes (17 cm diameter 17 × 17 cm height) and a small paper cup for ≤100 females (9 cm diameter × 9 cm height). Each container is labeled with the date, total number of mosquito and species in each container and the membrane feeder number. Record the mosquito information on membrane feeding data sheet. For the mosquitoes (*An. dirus*, *An. minimus*, *An. campestris*) we find that the optimum starvation time is 6–12 h before feeding and 5–7 day old adult females are used in all experiments.
2. Position a container of mosquitoes under each of the membrane feeders (Figs. 2 and 3). Some laboratories cover the mosquito container with paper towels or a sheet of cloth

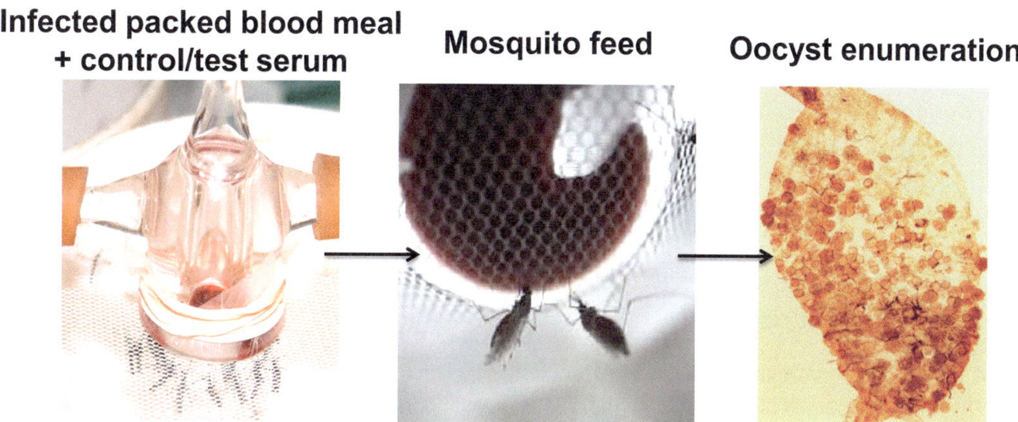

Fig. 3 The membrane feeding assay

during feeding to enhance the feeding rate of the mosquitoes. Allow mosquitoes to feed for 30 min.

3. After blood feeding, mosquitoes are allowed rest for a few hours before mosquitoes that did not blood feed are removed. Record the number of engorged mosquitoes on the mosquito container and data sheet (*see* **Note 3**).
4. After blood feeding, a cotton pad soaked with 10 % sucrose solution is put on each mosquito container for feeding purposes and replaced daily.
5. For transportation purposes, the mosquito container is packed within a closed container and should be kept at a temperature lower than 30 °C.

3.4 Parasite Examination in the Mosquito Midgut

1. Mosquitoes are examined for oocyst development on days 7–9 post blood feeding (Fig. 4). For gametocyte infectiousness studies, 50 % of the mosquitoes within each container are dissected for oocyst examination. If none of the mosquitoes carry oocysts, the remaining 50 % are dissected. The number of oocysts per mosquito and the range of oocyst size within each mosquito are recorded (*see* **Note 4**).
2. Sporozoite examination can be performed from day 14 onward (Fig. 4). If oocyst development is thought to be delayed, it is recommended that the midguts on day 14 onward mosquitoes are also checked to see if oocyst development has proceeded beyond that seen at days 7–9.

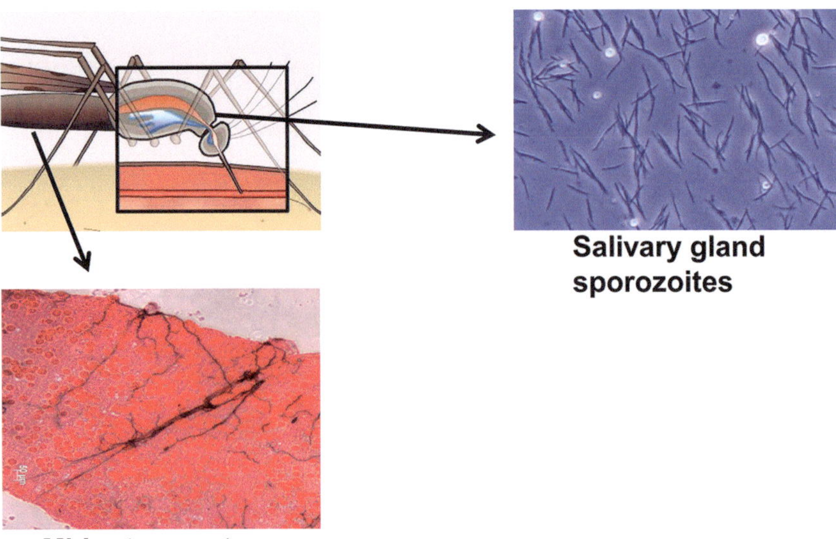

Fig. 4 Oocyst and sporozoite enumeration. Mosquito dissection after blood feeding for oocyst enumeration from the midgut is carried out on day 7–9 after blood meal and for sporozoite enumeration from the salivary glands on day 14–16

4 Notes

1. Handling of human sera and blood should be performed by trained staff with appropriate personal protective equipment and adequate safety precautions. Whole blood collected from patients can be added directly into blood cup or a plasma replacement can be substituted to reduce naturally blocking immunity from the donor or for evaluation of vaccines or drugs. The method described in this section is for plasma replacement.
2. Ensure that the surface of the packed cells is not removed as *P. vivax* parasites will be at the same level as the surface buffy coat after centrifugation. This will ensure that the parasites are not discarded with the buffer during the washing step.
3. All Infected mosquitoes must be accounted for during processing to ensure that there has been no mosquito escape as this will pose a risk of malaria infection in the laboratory.
4. It has been observed that some drugs did not reduce the average number of oocysts per mosquito but had an impact on the oocyst development and thus smaller oocysts were observed.

References

1. Sattabongkot J, Maneechai N, Phunkitchar V et al (2003) Comparison of artificial membrane feeding with direct skin feeding to estimate the infectiousness of Plasmodium vivax gametocyte carriers to mosquitoes. Am J Trop Med Hyg 69(5):529–535
2. Bousema T et al (2012) Mosquito feeding assays to determine the infectiousness of naturally infected Plasmodium falciparum gametocyte carriers. PLoS One 7(8), e42821
3. Ponsa N, Sattabongkot J, Kittayapong P, Eikarat N, Coleman RE (2003) Transmission-blocking activity of tafenoquine (WR-238605) and artelinic acid against naturally circulating strains of Plasmodium vivax in Thailand. Am J Trop Med Hyg 69:542–547
4. Sattabongkot J, Tsuboi T, Hisaeda H, Tachibana M, Suwanabun N, Rungruang T, Cao YM, Stowers AW, Sirichaisinthop J, Coleman RE, Torii M (2003) Blocking of transmission to mosquitoes by antibody to Plasmodium vivax malaria vaccine candidates Pvs25 and Pvs28 despite antigenic polymorphism in field isolates. Am J Trop Med Hyg 69:536–541
5. Malkin EM, Durbin AP, Diemert DJ, Sattabongkot J, Wu Y, Miura K, Long CA, Lambert L, Miles AP, Wang J, Stowers A, Miller LH, Saul A (2005) Phase 1 vaccine trial of Pvs25H: a transmission blocking vaccine for Plasmodium vivax malaria. Vaccine 23:3131–3138
6. Coleman RE, Polsa N, Eikarat N, Kollars TM Jr, Sattabongkot J (2001) Prevention of sporogony of Plasmodium vivax in Anopheles dirus mosquitoes by transmission-blocking antimalarials. Am J Trop Med Hyg 65:214–218
7. Hisaeda H, Stowers AW, Tsuboi T, Collins WE, Sattabongkot JS, Suwanabun N, Torii M, Kaslow DC (2000) Antibodies to malaria vaccine candidates Pvs25 and Pvs28 completely block the ability of Plasmodium vivax to infect mosquitoes. Infect Immun 68:6618–6623
8. Zhu G, Xia H, Zhou H, Li J, Lu F, Liu Y, Cao J, Gao Q, Sattabongkot J (2013) Susceptibility of Anopheles sinensis to Plasmodium vivax in malarial outbreak areas of central China. Parasit Vectors 6:176

Chapter 9

The Standard Membrane Feeding Assay: Advances Using Bioluminescence

Will J.R. Stone and Teun Bousema

Abstract

In preclinical development, the efficacy of agents with putative effects on *Plasmodium* transmission is determined using the standard membrane feeding assay (SMFA). Because the end-point of the SMFA is normally the enumeration of oocysts on the mosquito midgut, the assays reliance on mosquito dissections and microscopy makes it slow, labor-intensive, and subjective. Below, we describe a novel method of assessing the transmission of a *Plasmodium falciparum* strain expressing the firefly luciferase protein in the SMFA. The use of a transgenic parasite strain allows for the elimination of mosquito dissections in favor of a simple approach where whole mosquitoes are homogenized and examined directly for luciferase activity. Measuring the mean luminescence intensity of groups of individual or pooled mosquitoes provides comparable estimates of transmission reducing activity at 5–10-fold the throughput capacity of the standard microscopy based SMFA. This high efficiency protocol may be of interest to groups screening novel drug compounds, vaccine candidates, or sera from malaria exposed individuals for transmission reducing activity (TRA).

Key words SMFA, Mosquito feeding assay, Oocysts, Malaria, mosquitoes, Transmission reducing activity, Anopheles, *Plasmodium falciparum*, Infectivity, Luminescence

1 Introduction

Interventions that reduce the likelihood of humans with infectious malaria parasites seeding secondary mosquito infections are valuable components of malaria elimination campaigns [1, 2]. All drugs or vaccines that affect the asexual reproduction of *Plasmodium* life stages suppress transmission by limiting the number of parasites that develop into gametocytes; the life stages responsible for transmission from humans. In addition, drugs and vaccines can also specifically target mature transmission stages, gametocytes, or their transmissibility to mosquitoes. Only a limited number of antimalarial drugs have activity against gametocytes; these drugs include artemisinin derivatives [3], 8-aminoquinolines [4], and methylene blue [5]. With the renewed interest in malaria elimination, testing the activity of novel candidate drugs on gametocytes and their transmissibility is now widely advocated [6–9].

Ashley M. Vaughan (ed.), *Malaria Vaccines: Methods and Protocols*, Methods in Molecular Biology, vol. 1325, DOI 10.1007/978-1-4939-2815-6_9,

The development of transmission blocking vaccines (TBVs) is supported by the identification of immune markers of transmission reducing activity (TRA) among naturally exposed populations [10–15]. Antibodies to a handful of antigens expressed during the parasites sporogonic cycle in the mosquito have been shown to be able to interrupt this development to prevent mosquito infectivity [16], although it is evident that the full immune profile of naturally acquired transmission-reducing immunity remains to be explored.

The effect of any agent on *Plasmodium* transmission is determined by performing the standard membrane feeding assay (SMFA), in which mosquitoes are fed the putative transmission blocking agent along with a mixture of cultured *Plasmodium* gametocytes and blood. The outcome of the assay is the prevalence and intensity of parasites achieving successful sporogony in a sample of mosquitoes, which is determined by the quantification of *Plasmodium* oocysts on the dissected mosquito midgut. TRA is generally defined as the percentage reduction in mean oocyst intensity between test and control mosquitoes [17, 18]. Because the assay involves manually dissecting individual mosquitoes, and because of the requirement for large sample sizes to ensure precision in TRA estimates [17, 19], the SMFA in its current form is limited by labor-intensiveness and subjectivity [20, 21].

Transgenic *P. berghei* variants (PbGFPCON) have been used previously to increase the scalability of the SMFA. Though excellent correlations are described between *in silico* fluorescence based and manual oocyst counts [20, 22, 23], the technique requires all mosquito mid guts to be dissected and mounted prior to counting, so remains limited in scalability. Recently, a strain of *Plasmodium falciparum* expressing a fusion of the Green Fluorescent (GFP) and firefly Luciferase proteins, NF54HT-GFP-luc, was produced by Vaughan et al. [24]. This strain can be cultured in similar conditions and shows comparable growth patterns to the standard *P. falciparum* NF54 parasite strain. Importantly, NF54HT-GFP-luc was shown to express luciferase throughout the parasites life cycle, including all stages of the parasites sexual development in the mosquito [24]. Here, using cultured NF54HT-GFP-luc gametocytes, we present a luminescence based approach to SMFA evaluation that eliminates the need for mosquito dissections. Our previous assessments indicate that the luminescence assay performed on whole homogenized mosquitoes is equally or more sensitive than microscopy for infection detection, and that the mean luminescence intensity of groups of individual or pooled mosquitoes correlates closely with mean oocyst intensity in the same mosquito groups [25]. Variable productivity between concomitant oocysts [26, 27] limits the degree to which we can interpret actual oocyst number from luminescence intensity for individual mosquitoes. Therefore, for experiments requiring precise oocyst numbers, visualization and counting are still essential [20]. However, we suggest that because luciferase production reflects sporozoite proliferation more directly, luminescence intensity may provide a less abstract measure of TRA than oocyst intensity. Certainly, the assay is particularly suitable for studies where changes in oocyst size or maturation and not solely their presence are of interest [21].

The procedures involved in the SMFA have been described in detail elsewhere [28, 29]. It is not our intention to describe the already standardized methods of gametocyte culture, mosquito husbandry, and mosquito infection, but to provide a scalable alternative to microscopy for the determination of infection prevalence and TRA. Below, we provide a short summary of the methods involved in each step of the SMFA, with notes on details particularly relevant to our evaluation methodology.

1.1 Experimental Design

Our method involves assaying the luminescence intensity of homogenized individual or pooled mosquitoes, and utilizing this measure of luciferase activity as a proxy for mosquito infection intensity. Subheading 3.3 of the Methods describes how infection prevalence in groups of individual mosquitoes is determined using a cutoff based on the luminescence intensity of uninfected control mosquitoes. For the calculation of TRA, it is necessary to conduct separate mosquito feeds using the same gametocyte culture but with the addition of a neutral control (non-transmission blocking, and preferably isotypic). TRA may be calculated as the percentage reduction in mean luminescence intensity between each group of test mosquitoes and the control (Eqs. 1a and 1b). This method, transplanting mean oocyst intensity with luminescence intensity, is the most commonly used method of assessing the SMFA. Alternatively, when using individual mosquitoes, TRA may also be calculated from luminescence or oocyst outcomes using generalized linear mixed models (GLMMs). GLMMs incorporate the distribution of oocyst/luminescence counts from individual mosquitoes allowing for more robust analyses of TRA, and limiting the sample size necessary for achieving adequate statistical power [17]. Such analysis is not possible using the pooled mosquito assay, as only 2/3 observations will be recorded per cage.

$$\text{Microscopy based TRA \%} = \left(\frac{\text{Mean oocyst intensity of control mosquitoes} - \text{Mean oocyst intensity of test mosquitoes}}{\text{Mean oocyst intensity of control mosquitoes}} \right) * 100 \quad (1a)$$

$$\text{Luminesence based TRA \%} = \left(\frac{\text{Mean RLU of control mosquitoes} - \text{Mean RLU of test mosquitoes}}{\text{Mean RLU of control mosquitoes}}\right) * 100 \quad (1b)$$

With both the individual and pooled assay, the same numbers of mosquitoes should be sampled per cage as would be acceptable with oocyst detection (generally 25–50), however the increased scalability of the pooled method makes the evaluation of greater numbers of mosquitoes very feasible.

1.2 Gametocyte Culture

The NF54HT-GFP-luc parasite line is available upon request, and has been deposited at the Malaria Research and Reference Reagent Resource Center (MR4). Because parasite transfection was based on single strand crossover of the pEFGFP–luc plasmid, NF54HT-GFP-luc requires exposure to the selective agent WR99210 during culture to avoid reversion to wild type. Except for the addition of this selective agent, gametocyte culture for NF54HT-GFP-luc is no different than for the standard NF54 *P. falciparum* parasite line: Transgenic *P. falciparum* gametocytes (NF54HT-GFP-luc) (14-day culture, 0.3–0.5 % gametocytes, 2 % hematocrit) should ideally be obtained from an automated tipper system and prepared with packed red blood cells as previously described [24, 28, 29].

1.3 Mosquito Husbandry and the SMFA

Though the insertion of the GFP-Luciferase construct into the *Pf47* gene locus of NF54HT-GFP-luc was conducted under the assertion that the Pf47 protein was "dispensable," gene knockouts have since proven that the locus is essential for evasion of the mosquito immune system in *Anopheles gambiae,* but not in *A. stephensi* which lacks functional thioester containing protein 1 (TEP1) mediated immune mechanisms [30]. The NF54HT-GFP-luc *P. falciparum* strain is therefore restricted to experiments with *A. stephensi.* Though *A. gambiae* is the dominant vector for *P. falciparum* in Africa, the SMFA for *P. falciparum* transmission is generally conducted using the *A. stephensi* vector system, which is easier to breed and more permissive to infection.

For the SMFA, *Anopheles stephensi* should be reared as standard (30 °C and 70–80 % humidity, exposed to a 12/12 h day/night cycle). 3–5 day old mosquitoes should be fed on a glass membrane midi-feeder system containing 1.2 ml of the *P. falciparum* culture/reagent mix [28, 29]. Unfed and partially fed mosquitoes should be removed after feeding, and blood fed females should then be maintained at 26 °C and 70–80 % humidity. In each experiment, additional uninfected mosquitoes need to be assayed for the determination of infection positivity in test mosquitoes.

1.4 Infection Detection and Quantification Using Bioluminescence

Though oocyst detection by microscopy is possible from day 6 after initial infection [31] we advise waiting longer before conducting the luminescence assay to ensure optimal oocyst productivity. Luminescence intensity and the distinction between positive and negative mosquitoes increase from day 7 onwards [25]. Though oocyst productivity increases until their rupture at around day 10 post-infection (PI), thereafter becoming unpredictable due to sporozoite loss during hemolymph traversal, because of the increasing chance of mosquitoes becoming infectious to humans we suggest that day 9 PI is probably optimal for luminescence assessments. We suggest that the luminescence assay time point should generally be weighed on the aims of the study, but that day 7 PI is perhaps too early to sufficiently differentiate positive and negative mosquitoes.

Two variations on our standard method of luminescence based evaluation of mosquito infection are presented. These are as follows:

Individual mosquito assessments (*Subheadings 3.2 and 3.3*): Individual mosquitoes are homogenized and assayed, allowing for the determination of infection prevalence. The mean luminescence intensity of all mosquitoes in a sample is used as a proxy for mean oocyst intensity in the calculation of TRA. Though more objective, the speed of such assessments is not much in excess of microscopic oocyst detection.

Pooled mosquito assessments (*Subheadings 3.3 and 3.4*): For increased scalability, pools of mosquitoes may be homogenized and assayed together. The mean luminescence intensity of a predetermined number of repeat pools from each experimental group of mosquitoes is used for the calculation of TRA. Estimates of infection prevalence are not possible when pooling, but the scalability of the TRA assessments is increased 5–10 fold, depending on chosen sample numbers. Details of the timing of the pooled assay, with comparison to microscopy, are provided in the supplementary information of Stone et al. [25]. For each experimental feed, we find that the mean luminescence intensity of 3 pools of 5 or 10 is strongly correlated with mean luminescence intensity determined in the individual mosquito assay (Subheading 3.2) when these are carried out on separate mosquito samples from the same feeds. We also find that these measures provide TRA estimates that correlate strongly with TRA estimates made using standard oocyst counts.

2 Materials

2.1 Luminescence-Based SMFA Evaluation

1. CO_2 source for mosquito sedation.
2. Netted cages for mosquito collection.
3. Autoclavable pestles (Argos Technologies, Elgin, IL).
4. Handheld pestle rotator (Argos Technologies, Elgin, IL).

5. 1.5 ml conical bottom microcentrifuge tubes.
6. Grinding buffer: Phosphate buffered saline (PBS) pH 7.2, containing 1 % EDTA, 1 % Protease inhibitor cocktail solution (Protease Inhibitor Cocktail Kit [78410], Thermo Scientific, Waltham, MA).
7. 200 µl pipette tips.
8. Tube racks.
9. Ice trays.
10. Microcentrifuge.
11. 96-well clear bottomed plates (uClear black plates [655090], Greiner BioOne, Frickenhausen, Germany).
12. Plate rocker.
13. Luciferase assay buffer (Luciferase assay system [E152A], Promega, Madison, WI).
14. Luciferase assay substrate (Luciferase assay system [E151A], Promega, Madison, WI).
15. Multi-purpose plate reader (Synergy 2, BioTek, Winooski, VT).

3 Methods

3.1 Preparation of Reagents

1. Prepare fresh mosquito grinding buffer. Dispose of if unused after 24 h.
2. Remove luciferase assay buffer from storage at –20 °C, and allow to thaw to room temperature.

3.2 Determining Infection Prevalence and Intensity in Groups of Individual Mosquitoes

1. Prepare assay plate plans, including space for blank wells (assay substrates only) and negative controls on each plate. In each experimental run, at least the same number of uninfected negative control mosquitoes should be processed as for a single infectious feed (i.e., if 30 mosquitoes are processed from each infectious feed, at least 30 uninfected mosquitoes should be processed as negative controls, and assayed on the same plates. Because individual mosquito assays require numerous assay plates, uninfected controls should be spread out so that some are assayed on every plate).
2. Aliquot 48 µl of mosquito grinding buffer into microcentrifuge tubes (one tube per mosquito). Place tubes in racks (*see* **Note 1**), and store until ready for use at 4 °C.
3. Aliquot 12 µl of luciferase assay buffer into all assay plate wells according to plate plans. Store covered at room temperature (*see* **Note 2**).
4. Remove required number of mosquitoes from primary feeding cage into a smaller netted container.

5. Remove microcentrifuge tubes from the fridge into an ice-tray, and move the tray next to the mosquito cage on the bench-top.
6. Immobilize mosquitoes with CO_2.
7. Remove mosquitoes one by one into microcentrifuge tubes. As soon as a mosquito is placed in a tube, place a pestle on top, with enough pressure to ensure that the mosquito is submerged and killed (*see* **Note 3**).
8. Attach a handheld pestle rotator to the pestle, and homogenize the mosquito for approximately 5 s (*see* **Note 4**). Spin pestle at top of microcentrifuge tube to remove excess homogenate (*see* **Note 5**). After homogenization, remove pestle to a container for washing and autoclaving to allow reuse.
9. Repeat for all mosquitoes (*see* **Note 6**).
10. Pulse mosquito homogenates in a microcentrifuge for 15 s to remove residual homogenate from tube walls, and store in racks at 4 °C.
11. Remove homogenates from 4 °C, and using modified 200 μl pipette tips (*see* **Note 7**) mix and aliquot all mosquito homogenates separately from tubes into assay plate wells. 1–2 μl residual homogenate in the microcentrifuge tube is inevitable, but unavoidable (*see* **Note 5**). When entire assay plate is filled according to plate plan, cover and agitate gently on a rocker at room temperature for 30–45 min.
12. During the first plates incubation with luciferase assay buffer, reconstitute luciferase substrate according to the number of mosquitoes under analysis (60 μl per mosquito), and leave to equilibrate at room temperature in darkness (*see* **Note 8**). Additionally, ensure that the plate reader is on and warmed up, with settings appropriate for the luminescence assay (all wavelengths, 1 s measurement per well is sufficient).
13. With a multichannel pipette, add 60 μl luciferase substrate to every well (*see* **Note 9**). Place plate into plate reader immediately, shake for 5 s to mix (manually, if the machine is not capable of doing so during its program), and assay for luminescence intensity.

3.3 Data Processing

1. Name and store files with reference to assay date and plate plans.
2. Transfer all raw data (from an entire experiment) into a combined spread sheet, and calculate summary statistics, including mean blank well luminescence (from every plate). From each plate, the mean blank well value should be subtracted from all test well values (including uninfected mosquito controls) to correct for background luminescence.

3. A cutoff for infection positivity can be determined as the mean luminescence intensity of the corrected luminescence values for the uninfected controls (from every plate combined) plus five standard deviations (*see* **Note 10**).

3.4 Determining Infection Intensity in Groups of Pooled Mosquitoes

1. Prepare assay plate plans, including space for blank wells (assay substrates only) and negative control pools on each plate. Pool size and number should be decided in advance of all experiments. Here, we describe the preparation of 3 pools of 10 mosquitoes. In previous publications we have shown that 3 pools of 5 or 10 mosquitoes give similar results (*see* Subheading 1.4). In each experimental run, we suggest that at least the same number of uninfected negative control mosquitoes should be processed as for a single infectious feed (i.e., if 3 pools of 10 are processed from each feed, 3 pools of 10 uninfected mosquitoes should be processed as negative controls, and assayed on the same plates).
2. Aliquot 100 μl of mosquito grinding buffer into microcentrifuge tubes (one tube per pool). Place tubes in racks (*see* **Note 1**), and store until ready for use at 4 °C.
3. Aliquot 12 μl of luciferase assay buffer into all assay plate wells according to plate plans. Store covered at room temperature (*see* **Note 2**).
4. Remove required number of mosquitoes from primary feeding cage into a smaller netted container.
5. Remove microcentrifuge tubes from the fridge into an ice-tray, and move the tray next to the mosquito cage on the bench-top.
6. Immobilize mosquitoes with CO_2.
7. Remove mosquitoes one by one into a microcentrifuge tube. As soon as 10 mosquitoes are placed in a tube, place a pestle on top, with enough pressure to ensure that all mosquitoes are killed (*see* **Note 3**).
8. Attach a handheld pestle rotator to the pestle and homogenize the mosquitoes for approximately 10–15 s (*see* **Note 4**). Spin pestle at top of microcentrifuge tube to remove excess homogenate (*see* **Note 5**). After homogenization, remove pestle to a container for washing and autoclaving to allow reuse.
9. Total volume of mosquito grinding buffer per mosquito should be kept at 48 μl, as for the individual mosquito assay. After homogenisation, for pools of 10 mosquitoes, add additional mosquito grinding buffer to a total volume of 480 μl (380μl additional buffer). For pools of 5 mosquitoes, add additional mosquito grinding buffer to a total volume of 240 μl (140 μl additional buffer). Repeat for all mosquito pools (*see* **Note 6**).
10. Pulse mosquito homogenates in a microcentrifuge for 15 s to remove residual homogenate from tube walls, and store in racks at 4 °C.

11. Remove homogenates from 4 °C, and using modified 200 µl pipette tips (*see* **Note 7**) mix and aliquot at least three samples of 48 µl from each pooled homogenate into assay plate wells (*see* **Note 5**). When entire assay plate is filled according to plate plan, cover and agitate gently on a rocker at room temperature for 30–45 min.
12. During the first plates incubation with luciferase assay buffer, reconstitute luciferase substrate according to the number of mosquitoes under analysis (60 µl per mosquito), and leave to equilibrate with room temperature in darkness (*see* **Note 8**). Additionally, ensure that the plate reader is on and warmed up, with settings appropriate for the luminescence assay. Settings are as follows:
13. During the first plate's incubation with luciferase assay buffer, ensure that the plate reader is on and warmed up. Ensure that settings are appropriate for the luminescence assay (all wavelengths, 1 s measurement per well is sufficient).
14. With a multichannel pipette, add 60 µl luciferase substrate to every well (*see* **Note 9**). Place plate into plate reader immediately, shake for 5 s to mix (manually, the machine is not capable of doing so during its program), and assay for luminescence intensity.

4 Notes

1. When handling very large numbers of mosquitoes, it is easiest after addition of grinding buffer to microcentrifuge tubes to leave them open at 4 °C. It is therefore important that they be undisturbed, to minimize the risk of contamination.
2. Luciferase assay buffer is stored at −20 °C, and though it does not freeze at this temperature it is very viscous, remaining so until fully equilibrated at room temperature. Because of its viscosity, special care should be taken to ensure accuracy with pipetting. Multichannel pipettes are useful here, but wastage in reservoirs is significant.
3. If homogenizing all mosquitoes from a cage at once, we find it easiest to remove all mosquitoes to their tubes, placing a pestle into each tube in turn to immediately to kill the mosquito. Homogenization can then be initiated at the convenience of the technician. This also avoids time wastage due to CO_2 immobilization, which requires repetition every few minutes.
4. Manual homogenization is not truly standardizable; however, it quickly becomes apparent how long it takes for a mosquito to become homogenized. We find that 5 s is long enough to ensure an even mixture when homogenizing single mosquitoes, with no large body parts remaining intact. Mosquitoes differ in

size, so this may differ by 1 or 2 s either way. Some flexibility should be allowed here, but it is important that mosquitoes are not homogenized excessively. We have conducted studies using automated bead beating devices that show that high temperature/friction has a limiting effect on luciferase activity, which is why we advise caution.

For mosquito pools, longer homogenization is necessary to achieve the same consistency. For pools of 5 we advise approximately 10 s homogenization, while for pools of 10 mosquitoes, 15 s is adequate.

5. An additional consideration for the homogenization process is loss of material on the pestle. After homogenizing the mosquito, we spin the pestle in the empty upper half of the microcentrifuge tube to remove residual homogenate. We find that if any debris does remain on the pestle, this tends to be the harder and larger portions of the mosquito carcass (i.e., parts of leg). Though this and the process of pipetting homogenates from tubes to assay wells mean that a small amount of homogenate may not be assayed, our results on the sensitivity of this assay for the detection of low intensity infections (*see* Subheading 3.3) indicate that this has no detrimental effect.

   As only a portion (three aliquots) of each pool is assayed, homogenate loss is not an issue for pooled mosquitoes, so no additional measures need to be taken after homogenization. However, if the entire homogenate is required, the pestle may be rinsed into the same microcentrifuge tube while making the homogenate up to volume (48 μl grinding buffer per mosquito). For pools of 5 mosquitoes pestles can be rinsed with 140 μl of additional buffer, and for pools of 10 pestles can be rinsed with 380 μl. Our previous results indicate that there is remarkable consistency in luminescence read-outs between separate aliquots from the same mosquito pools [25].

6. As discussed in **Note 1**, and Subheading 1.4, the individual luminescence assay in the form described here does not represent a major increase in throughput over mosquito dissections. To increase scalability (for example if assessing enough mosquitoes to require two or more assay plates) it is generally useful if two technicians are available. After homogenization of enough mosquitoes to fill one assay plate, a second technician can then immediately prepare these homogenates for lysis, while the remaining cages of mosquitoes are homogenized.

   However, this is not essential, as the protease inhibitors in the grinding buffer are stable at room temperature for 24 h. By ensuring that mosquitoes are stored at 4 °C after homogenization, a single technician could perform homogenization and the assay sequentially, over a suitable timeframe.

7. Because homogenates contain mosquito debris, pipetting using standard tips is not efficient (blockage is common, and leads to

wastage of the homogenate, and time). Before beginning the assay, whenever convenient, we find it useful to cut the first half centimeter off a group of 200 pipette tips, to widen the opening and allow unimpeded transfer of mosquito homogenates.

Another option would be to spin down the mosquito homogenates to form a pellet, then remove only the supernatant using standard pipette tips to the assay plate. We find that this works equally well, but in the interest of time and standardization we have more often chosen to use the whole mixed homogenate.

8. Luciferase substrate should be kept in total darkness except during pipetting, and should ideally be used on the day of reconstitution (though freezing once for reuse is acceptable).
9. Because of the time sensitive reaction of the Luciferase enzyme once in contact with substrate, a multichannel pipette is essential here. Pipetting should be left until immediately prior to measurement. With a 1 s read per well, the time between substrate addition and assaying all wells in a 96 well plate should be just over 2 min. This is well within the stability range of the substrate we advise use of here. Other luciferase assay systems may have longer stability.
10. Previous results indicate that infection detection using individual mosquitoes is exceptionally robust at all levels of infection intensity. In experiments where almost half of all oocyst positive mosquitoes were in the 1–5 oocyst range ($n = 1350$), prevalence estimates made by microscopy and luminescence assay from separate mosquito samples were very similar (64.9 % and 67.7 % respectively), and adjustment of the luminescence based positivity threshold between the mean plus 3 and 10 SD had little impact on these prevalence estimates (66–68.8 %) [25].

References

1. Moonen B, Cohen JM, Snow RW et al (2010) Operational strategies to achieve and maintain malaria elimination. Lancet 376:1592–1603
2. Vannice K, Brown G, Akanmori B, Moorthy V (2012) MALVAC 2012 scientific forum: accelerating development of second-generation malaria vaccines. Malar J 11:372
3. Okell L, Drakeley C, Ghani A, Bousema T, Sutherland C (2008) Reduction of transmission from malaria patients by artemisinin combination therapies: a pooled analysis of six randomized trials. Malar J 7:125
4. Shekalaghe S, Drakeley C, Gosling R et al (2007) Primaquine clears submicroscopic *Plasmodium falciparum* gametocytes that persist after treatment with sulphadoxine-pyrimethamine and artesunate. PLoS One 2:e1023
5. Adjalley SH, Johnston GL, Li T et al (2011) Quantitative assessment of Plasmodium falciparum sexual development reveals potent transmission-blocking activity by methylene blue. Proc Natl Acad Sci 108:E1214–E1223
6. The malERA Consultative Group on Drugs (2011) A research agenda for malaria eradication: drugs. PLoS Med 8:e1000402
7. Delves M, Plouffe D, Scheurer C et al (2012) The activities of current antimalarial drugs on the life cycle stages of *Plasmodium*: a comparative study with human and rodent parasites. PLoS Med 9:e1001169
8. Delves MJ, Ruecker A, Straschil U et al (2013) Male and female Plasmodium falciparum mature gametocytes show different responses to antimalarial drugs. Antimicrob Agents Chemother 57:3268–3274

9. Bousema T, Churcher TS, Morlais I, Dinglasan RR (2013) Can field-based mosquito feeding assays be used for evaluating transmission-blocking interventions? Trends Parasitol 29:53–59
10. Outchkourov NS, Roeffen W, Kaan A et al (2008) Correctly folded Pfs48/45 protein of Plasmodium falciparum elicits malaria transmission-blocking immunity in mice. Proc Natl Acad Sci 105:4301–4305
11. Chowdhury DR, Angov E, Kariuki T, Kumar N (2009) A potent malaria transmission blocking vaccine based on codon harmonized full length *Pfs48/45* expressed in *Escherichia coli*. PLoS One 4:e6352
12. Wu Y, Ellis RD, Shaffer D et al (2008) Phase 1 trial of malaria transmission blocking vaccine candidates Pfs25 and Pvs25 formulated with montanide ISA 51. PLoS One 3:e2636
13. Ouédraogo AL, Roeffen W, Luty AJF et al (2011) Naturally acquired immune responses to Plasmodium falciparum sexual stage antigens Pfs48/45 and Pfs230 in an area of seasonal transmission. Infect Immun 79(12): 4957–4964
14. Bousema T, Sutherland CJ, Churcher TS et al (2011) Human immune responses that reduce the transmission of Plasmodium falciparum in African populations. Int J Parasitol 41:293–300
15. Roeffen W, Mulder B, Teelen K et al (1996) Association between anti-Pfs48/45 reactivity and *P. falciparum* transmission-blocking activity in sera from Cameroon. Parasite Immunol 18:103–109
16. Bousema T, Drakeley C (2011) Epidemiology and Infectivity of *Plasmodium falciparum* and *Plasmodium vivax* gametocytes in relation to malaria control and elimination. Clin Microbiol Rev 24:377–410
17. Churcher TS, Blagborough AM, Delves M et al (2012) Measuring the blockade of malaria transmission—an analysis of the standard membrane feeding assay. Int J Parasitol 42: 1037–1044
18. van der Kolk M, de Vlas SJ, Saul A, van de Vegte-bolmer M, Eling WM, Sauerwein W (2005) Evaluation of the standard membrane feeding assay (SMFA) for the determination of malaria transmission-reducing activity using empirical data. Parasitology 130:13–22
19. Miura K, Deng B, Tullo G et al (2013) Qualification of standard membrane-feeding assay with *Plasmodium falciparum* malaria and potential improvements for future assays. PLoS One 8:e57909
20. Delves M, Sinden R (2010) A semi-automated method for counting fluorescent malaria oocysts increases the throughput of transmission blocking studies. Malar J 9:35
21. Bell AS, Ranford-Cartwright LC (2004) A real-time PCR assay for quantifying *Plasmodium falciparum* infections in the mosquito vector. Int J Parasitol 34:795–802
22. Janse CJ, Franke-Fayard B, Mair GR et al (2006) High efficiency transfection of *Plasmodium berghei* facilitates novel selection procedures. Mol Biochem Parasitol 145: 60–70
23. Delves MJ, Ramakrishnan C, Blagborough AM, Leroy D, Wells TNC, Sinden RE (2012) A high-throughput assay for the identification of malarial transmission-blocking drugs and vaccines. Int J Parasitol 42:999–1006
24. Vaughan AM, Mikolajczak SA, Camargo N et al (2012) A transgenic *Plasmodium falciparum* NF54 strain that expresses GFP–luciferase throughout the parasite life cycle. Mol Biochem Parasitol 186:143–147
25. Stone WJR, Churcher TS, Graumans W et al (2014) A scalable assessment of Plasmodium falciparum transmission in the standard membrane feeding assay using transgenic parasites expressing GFP-luciferase. J Infect Dis. doi:10.1093/infdis/jiu271
26. Stone WJR, Eldering M, van Gemert G-J et al (2013) The relevance and applicability of oocyst prevalence as a read-out for mosquito feeding assays. Sci Rep 3
27. Zollner GE, Ponsa N, Garman GW et al (2006) Population dynamics of sporogony for *Plasmodium vivax* parasites from western Thailand developing within three species of colonized *Anopheles* mosquitoes. Malar J 5:68
28. Ponnudurai T, Lensen AHW, Van Gemert GJA, Bensink MPE, Bolmer M, Meuwissen JHET (1989) Infectivity of cultured *Plasmodium falciparum* gametocytes to mosquitoes. Parasitology 98:165–173
29. Ponnudurai T, Lensen AHW, Leeuwenberg ADEM, Meuwissen JHET (1982) Cultivation of fertile *Plasmodium falciparum* gametocytes in semi-automated systems. 1. Static cultures. Trans R Soc Trop Med Hyg 76:812–818
30. Molina-Cruz A, Garver LS, Alabaster A et al (2013) The human malaria parasite Pfs47 gene mediates evasion of the mosquito immune system. Science 340:984–987
31. Lensen AHW, van Druten J, Bolmer M, van Gemert GJA, Eling WM, Sauerwein R (1996) Measurment by membrane feeding of reduction in Plasmodium falciparum transmission induced by endemic sera. Trans R Soc Trop Med Hyg 90:20–22

Part III

Erythrocytic Stages

Chapter 10

Agglutination Assays of the *Plasmodium falciparum*-Infected Erythrocyte

Joshua Tan and Peter C. Bull

Abstract

The agglutination assay is used to determine the ability of antibodies to recognize parasite variant antigens on the surface of *Plasmodium falciparum*-infected erythrocytes. In this technique, infected erythrocytes are selectively labelled with a DNA-binding fluorescent dye and mixed with antibodies of interest to allow antibody–surface antigen binding. Recognition of surface antigens by the antibodies can result in the formation of agglutinates containing multiple parasite-infected erythrocytes. These can be viewed and quantified using a fluorescence microscope.

Key words Agglutination, Infected erythrocytes, *Plasmodium falciparum*, Variant surface antigens, PfEMP1, Malaria, Antibody, Naturally acquired immunity

1 Introduction

When *Plasmodium falciparum* parasites infect human erythrocytes, they insert parasite proteins into the infected erythrocyte surface. These proteins modify the immunological and cytoadhesive properties of the infected erythrocyte [1] and are targets of naturally acquired antibodies [2–5]. The major components of these proteins are variant surface antigens of the *P. falciparum* membrane protein 1 (PfEMP1) family, which undergo clonal antigenic variation and are extremely diverse [6, 7]. Thus, antibody recognition of antigens on the infected erythrocyte surface is usually variant specific, and antibodies that recognize one parasite isolate are often unable to recognize other isolates [8–11].

The agglutination assay was designed to test if antibodies in a plasma or serum sample of interest are able to recognize the surface antigens of erythrocytes infected by a particular parasite [8, 12, 13]. The assay is based on the fact that antibody recognition of similar or identical epitopes on multiple erythrocytes can lead to cross-linking of these cells to form agglutinates. The procedures for the agglutination assay are as follows: first, parasite-infected erythrocytes in a

Ashley M. Vaughan (ed.), *Malaria Vaccines: Methods and Protocols*, Methods in Molecular Biology, vol. 1325, DOI 10.1007/978-1-4939-2815-6_10, © Springer Science+Business Media New York 2015

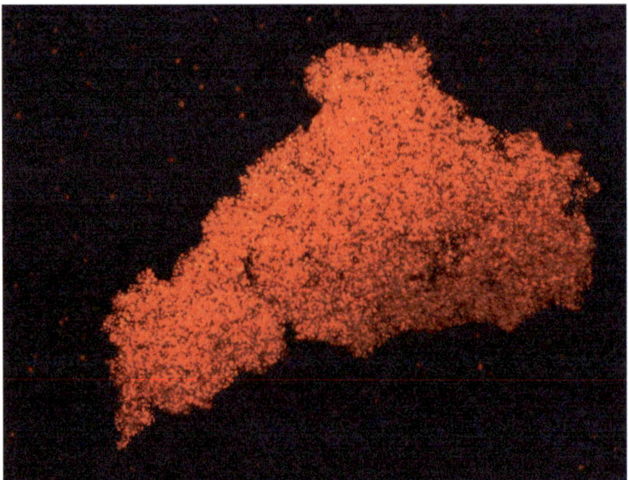

Fig. 1 An agglutinate stained with ethidium bromide in the individual agglutination assay. Agglutination was conducted on a culture-adapted parasite isolate using plasma from an adult from a malaria-endemic area

sample of interest are selectively stained with a DNA-binding fluorescent dye, which will not stain uninfected erythrocytes as they lack DNA. Next, the sample is rotated with serum or plasma (or any other antibody sample) of interest to allow antibody–surface antigen binding and agglutinate formation. Subsequently, the mixture is transferred onto a microscope slide, which is then examined under a fluorescence microscope. Agglutinates appear as fluorescent clusters of cells indicating recognition of surface antigens by antibodies in the serum (Fig. 1).

The agglutination assay was used to demonstrate an association between antibodies against the infected erythrocyte surface and protection [3] and to estimate of the in vitro rate of antigenic switching in *P. falciparum* [14]. Despite the advent of high-throughput flow cytometry as a parallel tool to measure antibody recognition of infected erythrocytes [15], the agglutination assay is still useful. First, it is unclear whether agglutination and flow cytometry measure recognition of the same epitopes, as flow cytometry detects simple antibody-antigen binding but agglutination involves cross-linking of multiple cells, which may require higher affinity interactions or those that are directed towards parts of the surface antigens that are flexible enough to allow cross-linking. Second, analysis of identical samples using these two approaches has not revealed a clear correlation [16, 17]. Third, the agglutination assay can be used to determine whether infected erythrocytes from different parasite samples are simultaneously recognized by the same or different antibody subsets (see the mixed agglutination assay—Subheading 3.3). Finally, when using polyclonal antibody samples for agglutination, the size of agglutinates provides an idea of the proportion of infected erythrocytes within a sample being recognized by the same subset of antibodies. These findings would be difficult to discern through flow-based approaches.

Nevertheless, the agglutination assay has limitations that may render it unsuitable for certain objectives. First, it is not as high-throughput as flow-based techniques, as the examination of slides using a microscope can be time-consuming. Second, agglutination is at best semiquantitative, as it is difficult to determine whether infected erythrocytes that are not part of agglutinates do not join such structures due to lack of antibody recognition or because of kinetic/mechanical reasons. Also, it is difficult to count the percentage of cells agglutinated, especially when large agglutinates are formed. Finally, the agglutination assay is much less effective for samples with low parasitemia (<0.5 %), which may be an issue when dealing with clinical parasite samples [12].

In this chapter, we describe two variations of the agglutination assay, the individual agglutination assay and the mixed agglutination assay. The individual agglutination assay is used to determine if a serum of interest has antibodies that can recognize surface antigens on infected erythrocytes from a single parasite sample. This assay can be done using a wet slide preparation, which requires immediate slide examination, or a fixed slide preparation, which allows slides to be stored and examined at a later date [18, 19]. The mixed agglutination assay (wet slide preparation only) is used to determine if a serum has antibodies that can simultaneously recognize surface antigens from different parasite samples [8].

2 Materials

Prepare all solutions at room temperature using deionized water. Make all media and culture the infected erythrocytes under sterile conditions. However, reagents used only on the day of the agglutination assay do not need to be sterile. Store all solutions at 4 °C unless stated otherwise.

2.1 Media

1. Roswell Park Memorial Institute (RPMI-1640) incomplete medium (RPMI-I): 0.2 % w/v glucose, 2 mM L-glutamine, 25 μg/mL gentamicin, 37.5 mM 4-(2-hydroxyethyl)-1-piperazineethanesulphonic acid 0.05 mg/mL hypoxanthine (dissolved in 1 M NaOH) in RPMI 1640. Remove 33 mL from a new 500 mL bottle of RPMI 1640. Add 5 mL 20 % w/v glucose, 5 mL 200 mM (100×) L-glutamine, 1.25 mL 10 mg/mL gentamycin, 18.75 mL 1 M HEPES, and 3 mL 8.4 mg/mL hypoxanthine in 1 M NaOH to the bottle (*see* **Note 1**). Mix thoroughly by inversion.
2. RPMI complete medium (RPMI-C): RPMI-I with 10 % blood group AB serum from malaria-naïve human donors. Heat-inactivate serum at 56 °C for 30 min. Add one volume of serum to nine volumes of RPMI-I. Mix thoroughly by inversion.

2.2 Infected Erythrocytes

1. Use either acute parasites from patients or culture-adapted parasites:
   (a) Acute parasites (*see* **Note 2**): Gently layer 5 mL of the patient's blood sample (or, if using erythrocytes after separation from plasma, up to 5mL of a 1:1 ratio of erythrocytes and RPMI-I) onto 3 mL of Lymphoprep in a 15 mL tube and centrifuge at 440 × *g* for 20 min (minimum acceleration and no brake) to remove peripheral blood mononuclear cells. Collect the erythrocyte pellet and rinse once with 10 mL of RPMI-I. Add a 1.5× pellet volume of RPMI-I (previously warmed to 37 °C) to resuspend the erythrocyte pellet. Next, mix an equal volume of Plasmion (Bellon, France) (previously warmed to 37 °C) and allow the tube to stand upright for 10 min at 37 °C. Discard the supernatant as it contains the granulocyte fraction. Rinse the erythrocyte pellet with 10 mL of RPMI-I and culture in RPMI-C to the mid- to late trophozoite stage in the same cycle (*see* **Notes 3** and **4**). Parasite cultures should be gassed with a sterile high-carbon dioxide gas mixture (92 % nitrogen, 5 % carbon dioxide, 3 % oxygen) and incubated at 37 °C.
   (b) Culture-adapted parasites: culture infected erythrocytes to the late trophozoite/early schizont stage in RPMI-C (*see* **Notes 3** and **4**), adding washed blood group O erythrocytes to adjust parasitemia whenever necessary (*see* **Note 5**). Parasite cultures should be gassed with a sterile high-carbon dioxide gas mixture (92 % nitrogen, 5 % carbon dioxide, 3 % oxygen) and incubated at 37 °C.
2. Culture-adapted parasites can be bulked up at the trophozoite stage, and cryopreserved in liquid nitrogen [20], but if this is done, each aliquot should be used on the same day it is thawed. Thawed parasites that were stored as mature trophozoites cannot be put back into culture.
3. The final parasitemia used in the assay should ideally be between 1 and 5 % for optimal results (*see* **Note 6**). When comparing the recognition of multiple parasite isolates, the parasitemia of each isolate should be adjusted to a constant level (e.g., 1 %) by the addition of a known number of uninfected washed blood group O erythrocytes at the start of the assay.

2.3 Components for Agglutination Assay: Wet Slide Preparation

1. RPMI-I (*see* **Note 7**).
2. Infected erythrocytes.
3. 96-well round-bottom microtiter plates.
4. 200 μg/mL ethidium bromide in RPMI-I (*see* **Note 7**): Use 200 μg/mL final concentration for the mixed agglutination assay [14], but dilute in RPMI-I to 10 μg/mL final concentration for the individual agglutination assay (*see* **Note 8**). [Ethidium bromide excitation: 510 nm; emission: 595 nm.]

5. 1 mg/mL stock DAPI (4,6-diamidino-2-methylphenylindole in dimethyl sulphoxide) (*see* **Note 8**). [DAPI excitation: 350 nm; emission: 470 nm.]
6. Petroleum jelly. Store at room temperature.
7. 18 mm square coverslips.
8. Glass microscope slides.
9. Fluorescence microscope that has a channel for DAPI (excitation wavelength ~350 nm) and ethidium bromide (excitation wavelength ~510 nm) and that detects fluorescence emissions at 470–600 nm.
10. Sera containing antibodies of interest (*see* **Note 9**).
11. Plate rotator: plates can be attached to rotating wheels or tube rotators.

2.4 Additional Components for Fixed Slide Preparation

1. Absolute methanol.
2. 5 μg/mL acridine orange in phosphate buffered saline (PBS) (*see* **Note 8**). [Acridine orange excitation: 500 nm; emission: 525 nm.]
3. Fluorescence microscope: the fluorescence channel that is used for ethidium bromide can also be used for acridine orange.

3 Methods

Perform all steps at room temperature unless stated otherwise. The agglutination assay does not have to be conducted under sterile conditions. All experiments should be carried out away from direct light to avoid excessive photobleaching of the fluorescent dyes. The procedure described herein is for a single experiment but can be adapted for multiple experiments as required.

3.1 Individual Agglutination Assay (Wet Slide Preparation)

1. Centrifuge the infected erythrocyte sample at 1,500 × *g* for 1 min.
2. Transfer the required volume of erythrocyte pellet into a tube with 10 μg/mL ethidium bromide in RPMI-I to give a 5 % hematocrit (pellet) (*see* **Notes 7** and **10**).
3. Resuspend the pellet thoroughly by pipetting up and down gently.
4. Add 10 μL of the infected erythrocyte suspension to a well of a 96-well round-bottom microtiter plate (*see* **Note 11**).
5. Add 2.5 μL of the serum of interest to the same well (*see* **Note 11**). A negative control must be included by adding 2.5 μL of serum from a malaria-naïve donor into a separate well containing 10 μL of the infected erythrocyte suspension (*see* **Note 12**). Similarly, a positive control should be carried

out by adding 2.5 μL of a malaria hyper-immune serum (known to cause agglutination) into a separate well containing 10 μL of the suspension.

6. Cover the plate with its lid and gently mix the contents of the well by swirling the plate (*see* **Note 13**).
7. Wrap the plate with aluminum foil and place it onto a plate rotator. Rotate the plate at a 45–60° angle at room temperature for 60 min (*see* **Note 14**).
8. Remove the plate from the rotator. Swirl the plate gently to resuspend the pellets and gently pipette the contents of each well onto a labelled microscope slide (*see* **Note 15**). If multiple slides are to be examined and blinding is necessary, the slides should be labelled in such a way as to enable blinding (*see* **Note 16**).
9. Gently place a coverslip with its edges previously lined with petroleum jelly onto the mixture (*see* **Note 17**).
10. Protect the microscope slide from light and transfer it to a dark fluorescence microscope room (*see* **Note 18**).
11. View the slide under bright field and then under fluorescence at 200× or 400×. Use a channel that allows fluorescence excitation at ~510 nm and fluorescence emission at ~595 nm.
12. Count the agglutinates, which will appear as fluorescent clusters of cells (Fig. 1) (*see* **Note 19** for counting tips).
13. The method of counting should include both the number and maximum size of agglutinates (Table 1). We suggest a counting scheme that assigns scores of 0–4 to each sample as follows (adapted from ref. 10):

    Size of agglutinates divided into four categories:

    Category A: 5–20 infected erythrocytes

    Category B: 21–50 infected erythrocytes

    Category C: 51–100 infected erythrocytes

    Category D: >100 infected erythrocytes

Table 1
Example of counting table for the individual agglutination assay

	Agglutinate size			
Sample	**5–20**	**21–50**	**51–100**	**>100**
1	𝍸 I	I		
2				

Final scores of 0–4 are awarded based on the number of agglutinates:

Score 0: <5 category A agglutinates

Score 1: 5–9 category A agglutinates

Score 2: ≥10 category A agglutinates or ≥1 category B agglutinate

Score 3: ≥5 category B agglutinates or ≥1 category C agglutinate

Score 4: ≥5 category C agglutinates or ≥1 category D agglutinate

3.2 Individual Agglutination Assay (Fixed Slide Preparation)

The wet slide preparation technique requires immediate slide examination to avoid rupture of infected erythrocytes. If agglutinates need to be counted on a different occasion (e.g., when a large number of slides is prepared), an alternative approach is to prepare fixed slides. This method involves post-agglutination staining and hence can only be used for the individual agglutination assay and not the mixed agglutination assay (*see* **Note 20**).

1. The individual agglutination assay is performed up to **step 8** as described in Subheading 3.1, except that the cells are resuspended in RPMI-I instead of 10 μg/mL ethidium bromide at **step 2** (*see* **Note** 7).
2. Gently spread the cells on the microscope slide in a circle with a 1–1.5 cm diameter using a 20–200 μL plastic pipette tip.
3. Allow the cells to dry at room temperature for 30 min (a hairdryer can be used to expedite drying).
4. Add absolute methanol to fix the cells for 1 min, allow the methanol to evaporate, and store the slides at room temperature (or at −80 °C if they are to be kept for >1 month) until microscopy is to be conducted.
5. For slide examination, stain with 13 μL of 5 μg/mL acridine orange in PBS.
6. Carry out **steps 9–13** of the previous section (Subheading 3.1) to complete the assay. The same fluorescence channel that is used for ethidium bromide can generally be used for acridine orange, but note that the optimal fluorescence emission for acridine orange (when bound to DNA) is at ~525 nm.

3.3 Mixed Agglutination Assay

1. This assay can be performed on two different infected erythrocyte samples.
2. Determine the parasitemia of each sample using flow cytometry or by counting from blood smears (*see* **Note 21**).
3. Centrifuge each infected erythrocyte sample at 1,500 × *g* for 1 min.
4. Transfer the required volume of pellet (*see* **Note 22**) into a new microcentrifuge tube containing a previously added 100× volume of dye (*see* **Note 23**). Separately stain the first sample

with 200 μg/mL ethidium bromide and the second with 5 μg/mL DAPI (*see* **Note 24**).

5. Wrap the tubes with aluminum foil and rotate at room temperature for 1 h to keep the pellets from settling (*see* **Note 25**).
6. Centrifuge the tubes at 1,500 × *g* for 1 min and remove as much of the dye as possible using micropipettes. Rinse the stained erythrocytes with RPMI-I five times (*see* **Note 7**). Each rinse consists of resuspending the erythrocyte pellet in a large volume of medium (at least 100× the volume of pellet), centrifuging at 1,500 × *g* for 1 min and removing as much medium as possible without disturbing the pellet (*see* **Note 26**).
7. Add a 50× pellet volume of RPMI-I and completely resuspend each pellet. Mix the two stained erythrocyte samples in a volume ratio to obtain equal parasitemia of both samples (*see* **Note 27**).
8. Centrifuge the parasite mixture at 1,500 × *g* for 1 min and remove most of the supernatant, leaving exactly 10 μL of supernatant per 0.5 μL of pellet.
9. Resuspend the pellet thoroughly and pipette 10 μL of the suspension into a well of a 96-well round-bottom microtiter plate (*see* **Note 11**).
10. Add 2.5 μL of the serum of interest to the well (*see* **Note 11**).
11. Carry out **steps 6–10** of the individual agglutination assay (Subheading 3.1) to complete this assay.
12. View the slide under bright field and then under fluorescence at 200× or 400× to count agglutinates (Table 2) (*see* **Note 28**). The presence of dual-color mixed agglutinates (Fig. 2) would signify simultaneous antibody recognition of the two different parasites, whereas the presence of two different types of single-color agglutinates (Fig. 3) would indicate distinct antibody subsets that recognize each parasite individually with no cross-reactivity (*see* **Note 29**).

Table 2
Example of counting table for the mixed agglutination assay

	Agglutinate size			
	5–20	21–50	51–100	>100
Orange (Ethidium bromide)	卌 I	I		
Blue (DAPI)				
Orange + Blue				

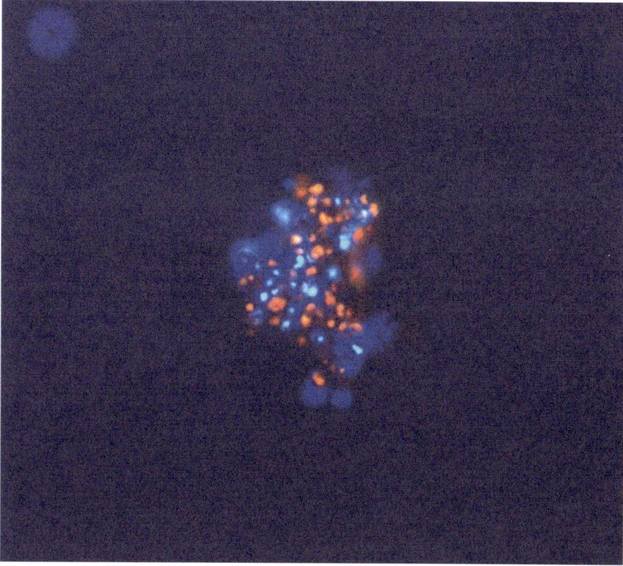

Fig. 2 An image of a mixed agglutinate captured using a single fluorescence channel. A culture-adapted parasite isolate was divided into two portions that were separately stained with DAPI (*blue*) or ethidium bromide (*orange*). Agglutination was conducted using plasma from an adult from a malaria-endemic area

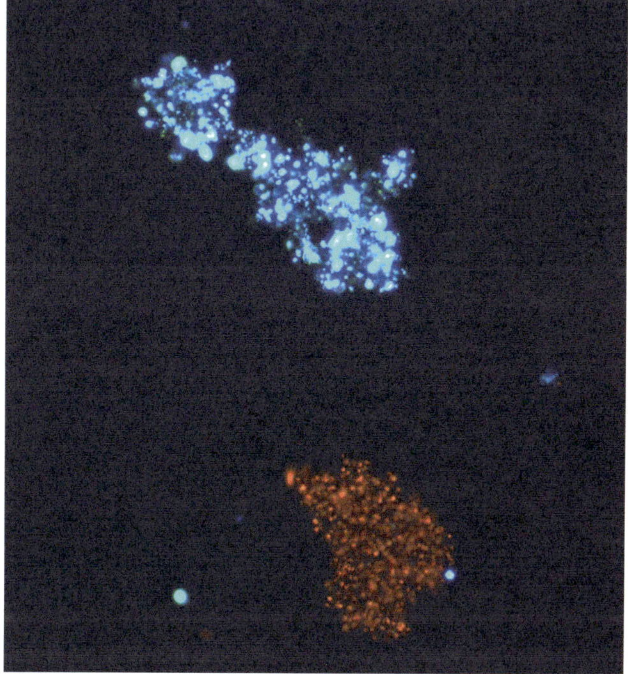

Fig. 3 An image of single-color agglutinates in a mixed agglutination assay captured using a single fluorescence channel. Two distinct parasite isolates were either stained with DAPI (*blue*) or ethidium bromide (*orange*). Agglutination was conducted using plasma from an adult from a malaria-endemic area

4 Notes

1. All ingredients for RPMI-I should be sterile-filtered if not commercially obtained as sterile reagents. All ingredients should be stored at 4 °C except for L-glutamine, which should be kept at −20 °C. The L-glutamine and hypoxanthine in NaOH should be made as single-use aliquots.
2. To avoid blood group-mediated agglutination, ensure that the patients' ABO blood group antigens will not be recognized by antibodies in the serum of interest. For instance, do not use serum from an individual with blood group A to agglutinate a parasite sample from an individual with blood group B.
3. Maximum agglutination generally occurs during the late trophozoite/early schizont stage [12].
4. Warm RPMI-C to 37 °C before using it for parasite culture.
5. Blood group O erythrocytes should generally be used for parasite culture (of culture-adapted parasites) to avoid blood group-mediated agglutination, unless the research question of interest requires the use of specific blood groups. If so, *see* **Note 2**.
6. Lower levels of parasitemia have been shown to result in the formation of smaller agglutinates [12]. The assay should be conducted with at least 1 % parasitemia (whenever possible) to give clear results.
7. PBS can be used as an alternative to RPMI-I to dilute ethidium bromide and to suspend and rinse infected erythrocyte pellets [12, 21].
8. Fluorescent dyes are light sensitive and should be stored at 4 °C in small tubes that are wrapped with aluminum foil to prevent photobleaching. Nevertheless, when in use during the assay, ethidium bromide, DAPI and acridine orange can be handled under dim lighting as they are relatively resistant to photobleaching. The working solutions should only be made in small amounts and used within a week. Stock solutions should be stored at −20 °C.
9. If plasma is to be used in agglutination assays this should be centrifuged at high speed (~16,000 × *g* for >10 min), followed by transfer of the supernatant to a new tube to remove residual platelets from the plasma. This should be done as platelets may mediate clumping of infected erythrocytes [22], which is a distinct phenomenon from antibody-mediated agglutination. Plasma or serum should also be heat-inactivated at 56 °C for 30 min to inactivate complement, which may also interfere with agglutination. Purified or monoclonal antibodies can also be used instead of sera if preferred.

10. It is preferable to make a suspension of infected erythrocytes and pipette equal volumes of the suspension into wells of a microtiter plate rather than transfer small volumes of pellet into each well, as the latter method will reduce the precision of the assay. A cell counter can be used to count and standardize the number of erythrocytes used in each assay.
11. To avoid bubble formation, do not push the pipette knob to the second stopping point during transfer of the fluorescent dye and serum into the microtiter plate well.
12. Match the negative control to the samples to be tested, i.e., use a plasma negative control for plasma samples and a serum negative control for serum samples. Examine an unblinded negative control first to determine the baseline level of non-specific agglutination, and include a blinded negative control with the samples to be examined.
13. One possible mixing method is to move the plate fairly rapidly using circular motions on a flat horizontal surface.
14. A longer rotation time generally results in the formation of larger agglutinates. An alternative to rotation is to secure the plate onto a shaker and shake gently [21].
15. Use pipette tips with larger apertures to prevent agglutinates from being disrupted upon ejection from the pipette tip. For instance, a 20–200 μL pipette tip is preferable to a 0.5–10 μL pipette tip. In our experience, agglutinates containing more than 10,000 cells can pass safely through the former with no observed disruption.
16. As the counting of agglutinates is only semiquantitative, if the experiment involves multiple slides with different expected results, it is essential to blind yourself from knowing the identity of each observed slide.
17. The petroleum jelly should be applied very thinly to the bottom four sides of the coverslip to prevent sample leakages and to provide space for the agglutinates (to avoid flattening them with the coverslip). This can be done by placing a very thin layer of petroleum jelly onto a flat surface, such as the bottom corner of a palm, and scraping that surface gently with each side of the coverslip.
18. Agglutinates should be scored immediately after slide preparation to minimize erythrocyte lysis. In our experience, leaving slides overnight at 4 °C for examination the following day sometimes results in some lysis. An alternative approach is to use a fixed slide preparation (Subheading 3.2).
19. General counting tips
    (a) Ensure that clusters of parasites identified as agglutinates under fluorescence have clear erythrocyte membranes when observed under bright field, as parasites (surrounded

by parasitophorous vacuole membranes) from lysed erythrocytes have a tendency to adhere and form clusters that look like agglutinates.

(b) Agglutinates tend to float and drift to the edges of the coverslip, and often cluster at one particular edge. Due to the bias in agglutinate distribution, it is essential to completely examine each slide rather than randomly select a specific number of fields to observe or count a predetermined number of cells.

(c) Due to their tendency to float, agglutinates are often slightly out of focus relative to unattached erythrocytes.

(d) An infected erythrocyte may contain more than one parasite but should only be counted as a single cell when determining agglutinate size. Hence, especially when determining the size of small agglutinates, constantly check bright field to ensure that agglutinate size is based on the number of infected erythrocytes and not the number of parasites.

20. An alternative to the fixed slide preparation method described here has been suggested in ref. [23].

21. To assess trophozoite parasitemia by flow cytometry, stain a small amount of pellet (~0.5 μL) with 100 μL of 10 μg/mL ethidium bromide in 0.5 % bovine serum albumin (BSA) in PBS for 10 min at room temperature. Rinse twice with 200 μL of 0.5 % BSA in PBS and resuspend the pellet in 200 μL of 0.5 % BSA in PBS. Set the flow cytometer to excite and detect fluorescence at the correct wavelengths for ethidium bromide (~510 nm and ~595 nm, respectively) and record the percentage of fluorescent cells. When assessing trophozoite parasitemia by a blood smear, count a total of 1,000 cells. It is essential to read multiple parts of the slide as trophozoites tend to have a heterologous distribution on glass slides.

22. When calculating the amount of pellet required for the mixed agglutination assay, keep in mind that the final amount required for each test is 0.5 μL of the pellet mixture. For example, if three mixed agglutination tests are being performed, a final pellet mixture of $0.5 \times 3 = 1.5$ μL is required. Assuming equal parasitemia, initially staining 1 μL of each pellet will lead to a final pellet mixture volume of 2 μL, which is sufficient for the assay.

23. We have tried staining with different dye volumes and have found that staining the parasite-infected erythrocytes with a dye volume 100× that of the erythrocyte pellet leads to increased breadth and intensity of staining compared to staining with a 20× volume or a 50× volume.

24. The high concentration of ethidium bromide (200 μg/mL) is helpful when using a ~350 nm excitation wavelength to observe both dyes in a single channel, but its concentration can be reduced to 10 μg/mL if it is observed separately from DAPI using ~510 nm excitation (*see* **Note 28**). Besides ethidium bromide and DAPI, acridine orange has been used by several groups to stain infected erythrocytes in agglutination assays [16, 18, 24]. However, in our hands, it stains infected erythrocytes multiple colors in a spectrum from green to orange. Hence, although acridine orange is suitable for the individual agglutination assay, it may be unsuitable for the mixed agglutination assay, which already involves two dyes of different colors.
25. Staining for a longer amount of time (e.g., 1 h) appears to increase breadth and intensity of staining compared to staining for a short time (e.g., 10 min). An alternative is to stain at 37 °C for 30 min.
26. Use a micropipette to remove the stain or rinse solution from each microcentrifuge tube. Initial liquid removal can be done using a larger micropipette, e.g., P1000, but removal of the final volumes of liquid should be done using a smaller micropipette, e.g., P10 or P200, to avoid accidental removal or disruption of the pellet.
27. Mixing liquid suspensions of each parasite rather than mixing pellets gives a more balanced mixture of the different parasites, which is critical for the mixed agglutination assay. The amounts mixed should be adjusted based on the initial parasitemia of each sample to give equal final parasitemias, e.g., if parasite A has double the parasitemia of parasite B, mix parasite A and B in a 1:2 ratio. To ensure accurate mixing, a cell counter can be used to determine the number of erythrocytes in each sample.
28. Ethidium bromide has a broad fluorescence excitation spectrum and can be excited at the same wavelength used to excite DAPI, i.e., ~350 nm (although this requires a higher concentration of ethidium bromide). Hence, both dyes can be viewed in a single channel if excitation is carried out at ~350 nm and a long-pass emission filter is used to allow capture of wavelengths from ~470 nm upwards. Alternatively, a microscope that can excite at different wavelengths consecutively (i.e., 350 nm and 510 nm) and obtain fluorescence images at different channels for image overlay can also be used.
29. If both mixed agglutinates and single-color agglutinates are seen, it is possible to estimate the degree of antigenic similarity between the two parasite samples based on the proportion of mixed agglutinates. Please refer to ref. [14] for details of the calculations required.

Acknowledgements

This work was supported by a Wellcome Trust Grant for a 4-Year Ph.D. in Infection, Immunology, and Translational Medicine (for J.T.).

This book chapter was published with permission from the director of KEMRI.

References

1. Rowe JA, Claessens A, Corrigan RA et al (2009) Adhesion of *Plasmodium falciparum*-infected erythrocytes to human cells: molecular mechanisms and therapeutic implications. Expert Rev Mol Med 11, e16
2. Aguiar JC, Albrecht GR, Cegielski P et al (1992) Agglutination of *Plasmodium falciparum*-infected erythrocytes from East and West African isolates by human sera from distant geographic regions. Am J Trop Med Hyg 47:621–632
3. Bull PC, Lowe BS, Kortok M et al (1998) Parasite antigens on the infected red cell surface are targets for naturally acquired immunity to malaria. Nat Med 4:358–360
4. Giha HA, Staalsoe T, Dodoo D et al (1999) Nine-year longitudinal study of antibodies to variant antigens on the surface of *Plasmodium falciparum*-infected erythrocytes. Infect Immun 67:4092–4098
5. Bull PC, Marsh K (2002) The role of antibodies to *Plasmodium falciparum*-infected-erythrocyte surface antigens in naturally acquired immunity to malaria. Trends Microbiol 10:55–58
6. Scherf A, Lopez-Rubio JJ, Riviere L (2008) Antigenic variation in *Plasmodium falciparum*. Annu Rev Microbiol 62:445–470
7. Chan J-A, Howell KB, Reiling L et al (2012) Targets of antibodies against *Plasmodium falciparum*-infected erythrocytes in malaria immunity. J Clin Invest 122:3227–3238
8. Newbold CI, Pinches R, Roberts DJ et al (1992) *Plasmodium falciparum*: the human agglutinating antibody response to the infected red cell surface is predominantly variant specific. Exp Parasitol 75:281–292
9. Forsyth KP, Philip G, Smith T et al (1989) Diversity of antigens expressed on the surface of erythrocytes infected with mature *Plasmodium falciparum* parasites in Papua New Guinea. Am J Trop Med Hyg 41:259–265
10. Bull PC, Lowe BS, Kortok M et al (1999) Antibody recognition of *Plasmodium falciparum* erythrocyte surface antigens in Kenya: evidence for rare and prevalent variants. Infect Immun 67:733–739
11. Iqbal J, Perlmann P, Berzins K (1993) Serological diversity of antigens expressed on the surface of erythrocytes infected with *Plasmodium falciparum*. Trans R Soc Trop Med Hyg 87:583–588
12. Marsh K, Sherwood JA, Howard RJ (1986) Parasite-infected-cell-agglutination and indirect immunofluorescence assays for detection of human serum antibodies bound to antigens on *Plasmodium falciparum*-infected erythrocytes. J Immunol Methods 91:107–115
13. Eaton MD (1938) The agglutination of *Plasmodium knowlesi* by immune serum. J Exp Med 67:857–870
14. Roberts DJ, Craig BAR et al (1992) Rapid switching to multiple antigenic and adhesive phenotypes in malaria. Nature 357: 689–692
15. Staalsoe T, Giha HA, Dodoo D et al (1999) Detection of antibodies to variant antigens on *Plasmodium falciparum*-infected erythrocytes by flow cytometry. Cytometry 35:329–336
16. Giha HA, Staalsoe T, Dodoo D et al (1999) Overlapping antigenic repertoires of variant antigens expressed on the surface of erythrocytes infected by *Plasmodium falciparum*. Parasitology 119:7–17
17. Warimwe G (2010) Studies on PfEMP1 expression in clinical isolates from Kenyan children with malaria. PhD thesis, Open University, UK
18. Bull PC, Kortok M, Kai O et al (2000) *Plasmodium falciparum*-infected erythrocytes: agglutination by diverse Kenyan plasma is associated with severe disease and young host age. J Infect Dis 182:252–259
19. Kinyanjui SM, Bull P, Newbold CI et al (2003) Kinetics of antibody responses to *Plasmodium falciparum*-infected erythrocyte variant surface antigens. J Infect Dis 187:667–674
20. Kinyanjui SM, Howard T, Williams TN et al (2004) The use of cryopreserved mature trophozoites in assessing antibody recognition of variant surface antigens of *Plasmodium falciparum*-infected erythrocytes. J Immunol Methods 288:9–18

21. Giha HA, Theander TG, Staalsø T et al (1998) Seasonal variation in agglutination of *Plasmodium falciparum*-infected erythrocytes. Am J Trop Med Hyg 58:399–405
22. Pain A, Ferguson DJP, Kai O et al (2001) Platelet-mediated clumping of *Plasmodium falciparum*-infected erythrocytes is a common adhesive phenotype and is associated with severe malaria. Proc Natl Acad Sci U S A 98:1805–1810
23. Mann EJ, Rogerson SJ, Beeson JG (2003) An alternative agglutination assay to measure antibodies to variant surface antigens of *Plasmodium falciparum*-infected erythrocytes. Trans R Soc Trop Med Hyg 97:717–719
24. Chattopadhyay R, Sharma A, Srivastava VK et al (2003) *Plasmodium falciparum* infection elicits both variant-specific and cross-reactive antibodies against variant surface antigens. Infect Immun 71:597–604

Chapter 11

Antibody-Dependent Cell-Mediated Inhibition (ADCI) of *Plasmodium falciparum*: One- and Two-Step ADCI Assays

Hasnaa Bouharoun-Tayoun and Pierre Druilhe

Abstract

The ADCI assay aims to measure the ability of parasite-specific antibodies, which by triggering blood monocytes, control *P. falciparum* parasite density. The assay relies on three easily accessible components: blood monocytes, immunoglobulins, and *P. falciparum* in vitro culture. Yet the reliability of results depends on the quality of the three above components, and therefore great care must be taken with each of them. We describe here different protocols for successfully carrying out the ADCI assay with emphasis on procedures and validation criteria necessary to ensure meaningful results.

Key words *P. falciparum*, ADCI, Cytophilic IgG, Monocytes, Fc gamma receptors

1 Introduction

Clinical experiments have shown that the Antibody-Dependent Cell-mediated Inhibition (ADCI) of *P. falciparum* is a major mechanism controlling malaria asexual blood-stages parasite density and thereby symptoms. Its relevance to clinical protection was previously established by ex vivo studies of material obtained during passive transfer of protection by immunoglobulin G (IgG) in humans, both by in vitro [1] and in vivo methods [2]. The corresponding ADCI *assay* was designed to reproduce the ADCI *mechanism* under in vitro conditions and thereby measure the ability of antibodies to inhibit the in vitro growth of *P. falciparum* blood stages in the presence of monocytes (MN).

Ashley M. Vaughan (ed.), *Malaria Vaccines: Methods and Protocols*, Methods in Molecular Biology, vol. 1325, DOI 10.1007/978-1-4939-2815-6_11, © Springer Science+Business Media New York 2015

Our studies have shown that antibodies that proved protective against *P. falciparum* are unable to inhibit parasite growth unless they cooperate with blood MN [3, 4]. It was also shown that antibodies that were not protective in vivo had no direct inhibitory effect on the parasite in the ADCI assay. Therefore, this assay is a means to discriminate protective from non-protective antibodies and to screen and identify target antigens. In the ADCI assay, IgG1 and IgG3 cytophilic antibodies, specific for merozoite surface antigens trigger MN to release a soluble mediator that blocks the division of surrounding intraerythrocytic parasites at the trophozoite stage [5].

The anti-parasite ADCI effect is (a) due to monokines or other soluble mediators released by MN which diffuse in the environment (blood or culture medium) and block the division of surrounding intraerythrocytic parasites at ring or trophozoite stage, which frequently appear as "crisis forms" or pycnotic trophozoites, preventing the cycle to resume and (b) triggered in MN when antibodies bridge merozoite surface antigen(s) via their heavy chain to Fc-gamma receptors on the MN surface [5, 6]. Consequently only the cytophilic antibodies of either IgG1 or IgG3 subclass can bind these receptors, while the non-cytophilic classes, IgG2, IgG4, and IgM are not efficient. In addition IgG2, IgG4, and IgM targeting the same antigens can compete out the binding of IgG1 and IgG3, and thereby inhibit ADCI. In vitro experiments and in vivo epidemiological studies have confirmed that as well as the titers of the IgG1 and IgG3 antibodies, it is also their balance, i.e., the ratio of cytophilic to non-cytophilic antibodies, in the blood as in the culture medium that is important to achieve a protective effect in humans and an ADCI anti-parasite effect in vitro [7].

We have found that the ADCI assay has several remarkable characteristics: (a) it requires the synergistic activation, or co-stimulation of both Fc gamma receptors FcγRIIa and FcγRIIIa (whereas FcγRI is not involved) [6]. This also implies that a very small number of effector MN in peripheral blood can exert this effect as only a small proportion express the FcγRIIIa receptor [8]; (b) a single merozoite per MN is sufficient to trigger optimal anti-parasitic activity; (c) only antigens, and no other parasite-derived factor, are required to trigger MN activation and a single antigen is as potent as the complex combination of antigens constituting the merozoite surface, provided they are bivalent, i.e., can bind at least two antibodies; (d) Very low antibody concentrations in the range of molecules having a hormonal effect, are effective [6] unlike antibodies with a direct neutralizing effect such as the growth inhibition assay (GIA), or mediating phagocytosis; (e) IgG3 subclass is more effective than IgG1 likely as it possesses a longer and more flexible hinge region; (f) only blood MN, but not differentiated MN, nor macrophages derived from MN, nor polymorphonuclear leukocytes (PMN), lymphocytes, or platelets, were found able to mediate an ADCI effect; (g) The MN function in ADCI is up regulated by TNF secreted by activated MN which thus has an autocrine effect [5].

The ADCI assay differs in several respects from the merozoite opsonization mechanism with which it is sometimes mistaken. The antibody promoted ingestion of either intraerythrocytic or free parasites (merozoites) by MN or macrophages is a common event which can be easily measured, but fundamentally differs from ADCI: (a) it involves predominantly the more abundant FcγRI receptors, whereas ADCI relies on FcγRIIa and FcγRIIIa, (b) it is mediated by all types of cells with phagocytic activity, MN, PMN, and above all differentiated MN and large tissue macrophages, whereas ADCI is not effective with the latter three, (c) from a pure arithmetic point of view the control of large parasite densities seen during IgG passive transfer cannot be explained by parasite opsonization, and in vitro the uptake of merozoites has little influence on the course of parasitemia, (d) the two-step ADCI assay demonstrate that MN do not act by a debris-removal type of activity, but in a more sophisticated manner where soluble mediators released by activated MN block many intraerythrocytic trophozoites in their development.

1.1 Implementing ADCI Assays in the Laboratory

The ADCI assay should not bear any particular difficulty to implement as it comprises of three components which are easily accessible and which preparation is of common practice in many laboratories, namely PBMC used to isolate blood MN, IgG and *P. falciparum* cultures. As for any cellular assay, care should be taken with the quality of each component, and rigorous conditions employed to yield meaningful results. We have established a series of criteria, listed in Table 1 to accept the results of a given ADCI assay as "meaningful" and therefore valid.

The major steps involved in the ADCI protocol are as follows:

1. Serum IgG preparation using ion exchange chromatography.
2. MN isolation from a healthy blood donor.
3. Preparation of *P. falciparum* parasites including synchronization and schizont enrichment.
4. Parasite culture in presence of antibodies and MN.
5. Specific Growth Inhibition assessed by microscopic observation or by flow cytometry analysis.

Table 1
ADCI assay performance requirements and key acceptance criteria

	Acceptance criteria for key assay components	Assay performance requirements
Parasite cultures quality *prior* to ADCI assay	*P. falciparum* cultures should show optimal speed of growth for the 8–10 days preceding the ADCI assay	Growth rate of parasite strain >6-fold in 48 h and >40× over 96 h
Quality of parasites prior to conducting ADCI assay	Satisfactory morphology, i.e., less than 5 % unhealthy—such as pycnotic forms	Schizont separation on gelatine every 4 days so as to seed fresh red blood cells with a minimal amount of infected culture and ensure that new culture contains a vast majority of fresh RBCs
Parasite stages at the start of the assay	Cultures should preferentially contain over 50–75 % of segmenters at the beginning of the ADCI assay	Asynchronous with a majority of mature forms (alternative is to use mature forms only obtained by separation on gelatine)
Parasite cultures during ADCI assay	The results of any ADCI assay must be excluded in case of suboptimal growth during the ADCI assay itself	Start ADCI assay at 0.5 % parasitemia, 2 % hematocrit Accept ADCI results only provided the cultures have shown >20× increase during the 72–96 h of the assay
Reactivity with Parasite antigen: This would only apply to antibodies directed against a limited number of antigens such as those elicited by some vaccine candidates	Recognition of parasite antigen by antibodies used in ADCI demonstrated using an alternative method (not ADCI) such as IFA and/or Western Blot	Demonstration of reactivity to parasite antigen required for conducting ADCI assays. Final antibody concentration in well should give positive signal in IFA when diluted 10× or preferably 100×

2 Materials

2.1 IgG Preparation Components

1. Tris buffer: 0.025 M Tris–HCl, 0.035 M NaCl, pH 8.8.
2. Phosphate buffered saline (PBS), pH 7.4.
3. Trisacryl GF-05-filtration column (Pall Life Sciences, USA).
4. DEAE-Ceramic Hyper DF column (Pall Life Sciences, USA) (*see* **Note 1**).
5. G25 Hitrap desalting column (GE Healthcare, Life Sciences, UK).
6. Amicon filters and tubes for protein concentration (Molecular weight cutoff: 50,000 kDa) (Merck Millipore, Germany).
7. Sterile Millex filters, 0.22 μm pore size (Merck Millipore, Germany).
8. UV Spectrophotometer.

2.2 Monocyte Preparation Components

1. Buffy coat or cytapheresis samples from a blood donor (large batches needed, *see* **Note 2**)
2. Ficoll Paque Plus (Sigma-Aldrich, Germany).
3. Hank's Balanced Salt Solution (HBSS) (Sigma-Aldrich, Germany).
4. RPMI 1640 culture medium prepared with glass distilled water (*see* **Note 3**), supplemented with 35 mM HEPES and 24 mM $NaHCO_3$.
5. Trypan blue exclusion dye to assess cell viability (Sigma-Aldrich, Germany).
6. Hemocytometer.
7. Dimethyl sulfoxide (DMSO) (Sigma-Aldrich, Germany).
8. Heat inactivated AB+ Human serum.
9. One milliliter cryogenic tubes (Nalgene, Thermo Scientific).
10. Naphtyl acetate esterase kit (Sigma-Aldrich) for MN number assessment.
11. Polystyrene 96-well flat bottom tissue culture plates (Costar, Corning, New York, USA).
12. Refrigerated centrifuge.
13. Incubator 37 °C humidified, 5 % CO_2.
14. Inverted light microscope.

2.3 Parasite Preparation Components

1. RPMI 1640 culture medium supplemented with 35 mM HEPES, 24 mM $NaHCO_3$, 7 μM hypoxanthine (CM).
2. Human Red Blood Cells (RBC) O+ group.
3. Ten percent AlbuMAX stock solution. Store at −20 °C.
4. Five percent sorbitol solution for parasite synchronization.
5. Type A porcine skin gelatin (Sigma-Aldrich) for schizont enrichment.
6. Fast modified Giemsa staining kit RAL 555 (RAL Diagnostics, France).
7. Reversible inhibitor of cysteine protease E64 (Sigma-Aldrich).
8. Percoll centrifugation medium (Sigma-Aldrich).

2.4 Flow Cytometry Analysis Components for Estimating the Number of Monocytes (Optional)

1. FITC conjugated anti-human CD14 monoclonal antibody (BD Biosciences).
2. PE conjugated anti-human CD32 monoclonal antibody (BD Biosciences).
3. PBS pH 7.4.
4. Fetal calf serum (FCS).
5. FACS tubes (BD Biosciences).

2.5 Flow Cytometry Analysis Components for the Detection of Infected RBC (Optional)

1. Dihydroethidium (Sigma-Aldrich) stock solution at 10 mg/ml in DMSO (store at −20 °C in the dark).
2. Thiazole orange dye (Sigma-Aldrich) stock solution at 1.5 mg/ml in methanol (store at −20 °C in the dark for a maximum of 2 months).
3. PBS pH 7.4.
4. Fetal calf serum.
5. FACS tubes (BD Biosciences).

3 Methods

3.1 IgG Preparation

IgGs are extracted from human sera (*see* **Note 4**) according to the following procedure:

1. Dilute the serum at a ratio 1:3 in Tris–HCl buffer.
2. Filter the diluted serum through a Trisacryl GF-05 gel filtration column previously equilibrated with Tris–HCl buffer. Ensure that the ratio of serum to filtration gel is 1 volume of undiluted serum to 4 volumes of GF-05 gel.
3. Pool the protein containing fractions.
4. Load over a DEAE-ceramic Hyper DF ion exchange chromatography column previously equilibrated with Tris–HCl buffer. Ensure that the ratio of serum to filtration gel is 1 volume of undiluted serum to 4 volumes of DEAE ceramic gel.
5. Collect fractions of 1 ml (or less depending on the column volume).
6. Measure the optical density (OD) of each fraction using a 280 nm filter (*see* **Note 5**).
7. Calculate the IgG concentration as follows:

$$\text{IgG concentration}\left(\text{mg}/\text{ml}\right)=\text{OD } 280\text{ nm}/1.4$$

8. Pool the fractions containing IgGs.
9. Concentrate the IgG solution using Amicon filters. Amicon filters are first soaked in distilled water for 1 h and then adapted to special tubes in which the IgG solution is added.
10. Centrifuge the tubes at $900\times g$ for 2 h at 4 °C. This usually leads to 25-fold concentration.
11. Perform a final step of gel filtration using a G25 column previously equilibrated with RPMI culture medium.
12. Collect the IgG fraction in RPMI culture medium.
13. Measure the optical density (OD) of each fraction using a 280 nm filter.

14. Calculate the IgG concentration.
15. Pool the fractions containing IgGs.
16. Sterilize the IgG preparation by filtration through 0.22 μm pore size sterile filters.
17. Store the sterile IgG solution at 4 °C for up to 1 month.
18. Validate the degree of purity of the IgG preparation by adding it at low concentration, e.g., 0.5–1.5 mg/ml to a parasite culture for 48 h and assess the absence of significant effect (<15 %) upon parasite growth as compared to control.
19. Store fractions of validated IgG at −20 °C in amounts corresponding to the volume needed for one assay. Thawed fractions should never be refrozen.

3.2 Monocyte Preparation

To reduce donor to donor variability batches made of large numbers of aliquots of Peripheral Blood Mononuclear cells (PBMC) are prepared from cytapheresis or buffy coat donors, cryopreserved and their efficacy assessed on one of the aliquots to validate the batch (*see* **Note 2**).

3.2.1 Preparation of Cryopreserved PBMC Aliquots

1. Dilute cytapheresis or buffy coat cells threefold in HBSS.
2. Carefully layer 2 volumes of diluted cytapheresis cells onto 1 volume of Ficoll Paque Plus solution in 50 ml conical tubes (maximum 20 ml of cell suspension per tube).
3. Centrifuge at 400 × *g* for 30 min at 20 °C.
4. Remove the PBMC layer at the Ficoll–plasma interface.
5. Add 45 ml of HBSS to the PBMC suspension.
6. Centrifuge at 400 × *g* for 10 min at 20 °C.
7. Carefully resuspend the pellet of PBMC in 45 ml of HBSS.
8. Centrifuge again. Repeat the washing step twice.
9. Finally centrifuge at 155 × *g* for 5 min at 4 °C to remove platelets that will remain in the supernatant.
10. Resuspend PBMC in 5 ml RPMI.
11. Calculate the cell concentration of the PBMC suspension: dilute a 20 μl sample of the cell suspension twofold in Trypan blue and count the number of viable cells using a hemocytometer.
12. Centrifuge the PBMC suspension at 250 × *g* for 10 min at 4 °C.
13. Prepare a solution of 20 % DMSO in heat inactivated AB+ human serum.
14. Resuspend PBMC at 30×10^6 cells/ml in heat inactivated AB+ human serum.
15. Add very slowly to the PBMC suspension an equal volume of the 20 % DMSO solution in human AB serum.

16. Aliquot the PBMC in cryogenic tubes (15×10^6 cells/ml/tube) and allow progressive slow cooling before final storage in liquid nitrogen.
17. Unfreeze an aliquot and process as described in Subheading 3.2.2 and then Subheading 3.4.1 or Subheading 3.4.2 with reference positive and negative sera so as to validate the remaining PBMC batch as satisfactory to perform ADCI assays (in our experience this procedure leads to the rejection of about 20–30 % of donors/preparations).

3.2.2 Monocyte Preparation from Cryopreserved PBMC

MN are isolated from PBMC using a negative selection method allowing the elimination of the non-MN subset of cells. We have observed that the more typical positive selection of MN using CD14-conjugated magnetic beads leads to activation of MN that can occasionally be deleterious to ADCI activity.

1. Before an ADCI test, thaw frozen PBMC by incubating the cryogenic tube in a 37 °C water bath for 10 min.
2. Resuspend the thawed cells in 45 ml of RPMI culture medium.
3. Repeat **step 11** of Subheading 3.2.1 to calculate the number of cells and assess cell viability.
4. Determine the number of MN in the PBMC suspension using the Naphtyl acetate esterase kit as recommended by the kit manufacturer.
5. Alternatively the number of MN can be determined using flow cytometry as follows:
   (a) Stain PBMCs with anti-CD14-FITC and anti-CD32-PE.
   (b) Wash cells once.
   (c) Run on a flow cytometer (excitation with a 488 nm laser).
   (d) Gate on all live cells on a SSC Lin/FSC Lin dot plot or density plot.
   (e) Display live cell population on a FL1 log/FL2 log dot or density plot (*FL1 channel corresponds to green emission and FL2 channel corresponds to yellow emission*).
   (f) Draw a gate around the double CD14+ CD32+ population.
   (g) Calculate percentage of CD14+ CD32+ cells in the live cell gate.
   (h) This percentage is equivalent to the percentage of MN in the PBMC vial.
6. Adjust the cell suspension to a concentration of 2×10^5 MN per 100 μl, with RPMI culture medium.
7. Distribute the PBMC suspension on polystyrene 96-well culture plates at 100 μl per well.
8. Incubate plates for 2 h at 37 °C, 5 % CO_2. During this incubation time, MN will adhere to the bottom of the plate wells.

9. Remove the non-adherent cells by carefully pipetting up and down with a pipette fitted with a 200 μl tip.
10. Wash the adherent MN 3 times by adding and thoroughly removing 200 μl of RPMI (*see* **Note 6**).
11. Add 30 μl of RPMI culture medium to each well.
12. Using an inverted microscope, control for the cell appearance and the relative homogeneity of cell distribution in the different wells (*see* **Note 7**).

3.3 Parasite Preparation

P. falciparum strains are cultivated in CM supplemented with 0.5 % AlbuMAX (*see* **Note 8**). Cultures should preferentially contain over 50–75 % of mature forms (segmenters) at the beginning of the ADCI assay. Alternatively, ADCI can be started with mature forms obtained from synchronized cultures (*see* **Note 9**).

Parasites are synchronized by sorbitol treatments as follows [9]:

1. Prepare a 5 % sorbitol solution in glass distilled water.
2. Centrifuge the asynchronous parasite culture suspension at 250 × *g* for 10 min at 20 °C.
3. Resuspend the pellet in the 5 % sorbitol solution. This will lead to selective lysis of schizont infected RBC without any effect on rings and young trophozoites.

When required, schizont infected RBC are enriched by flottation on porcine skin gelatin as follows:

1. Centrifuge the asynchronous parasite culture suspension at 250 × *g* for 10 min at 20 °C.
2. Resuspend the pellet in a 1 % solution of porcine skin gelatin type A in RPMI.
3. Incubate at 37 °C for 30 min. Schizont infected RBC will remain in the supernatant whereas trophozoite infected and uninfected RBC will sediment.
4. Carefully collect the supernatant and centrifuge at 250 × *g* for 10 min at 20 °C.
5. Prepare a thin smear from the pellet, stain and determine the parasitemia. Usually, synchronous schizont infected RBC are recovered at approximately 70 % parasitemia.

When a 2-step ADCI is performed, parasitophorous vacuole membrane-enclosed merozoites structures (PEMS) are prepared. PEMS containing each approximately 20 merozoites, are obtained using the reversible inhibitor of cysteine protease E64 as described [10]:

1. Allow synchronous parasite culture, 2 % hematocrit to grow in CM, 0.5 % AlbuMAX, until middle stage schizonts are obtained. Each schizont contains 5–7 nuclei.

2. Add freshly prepared E64 to the parasite culture at a final concentration of 10 μM.
3. Incubate for 8 h, and then enumerate PEMS on Giemsa-stained smears.
4. Separate PEMS by centrifugation at, 2,000 × *g* for 20 min on a 45 % (v/v) Percoll gradient.
5. Wash the harvested PEMS with CM to remove E64.

3.4 The ADCI Assay

The ADCI assay can be performed using two alternative protocols. The one-step assay consists of a 96 h culture of the parasites in presence of MN and specific antibodies. The two-step assay includes a short term activation of MN by incubation with antibodies and *P. falciparum* merozoites. The supernatant of activated MN is then transferred onto a parasite culture to assess its inhibitory effect. It is more complex at the MN stimulation stage, and more straightforward for measuring parasite growth inhibition.

3.4.1 One-Step ADCI Assay

1. Add 20 μl of antibody reagent (test IgG or serum, positive control, negative control IgG or AB+ serum) to the MN prepared as described in Subheading 3.2.2.
2. Control wells consist of the following:
   (a) MN and parasites with normal IgG (NIgG) prepared from the serum of a healthy donor with no history of malaria.
   (b) Parasite culture with IgG to be tested without MN.
   (c) Parasite culture alone without MN or any test reagent.
3. Incubate the plate at 5 % CO_2 (or candle jar) at 37 °C for 2 h. This step avoids alkaline pH stress for the parasites at low CO_2 tension.
4. Add to each well 50 μl of an asynchronous culture of *P. falciparum* at 0.5–1 % parasitemia and 4 % hematocrit in CM with 1 % AlbuMAX.
5. Transfer plate to 37 °C, 5 % CO_2 (or candle jar) for a total of 96 h.
6. After 48 h in culture, add 50 μl/well of CM containing 0.5 % AlbuMAX.
7. After 72 h in culture, add 50 μl/well of CM containing 0.5 % AlbuMAX.
8. After 96 h remove supernatant and prepare thin smears.
9. Alternatively, prepare thin smears on part of the culture and transfer the rest of the cultures to flow cytometry tubes (*see* **Note 10**) for staining with thiazole orange and dihydroethidium as follows (plan to have infected RBCs for unstained and single staining for use in compensations. *Tubes used for single staining can follow the procedure outlined below but replace dye by PBS+ 1 % FCS when relevant*).

(a) Prepare a working solution of dihydroethidium at 40 μg/ml in PBS by diluting the stock solution 1:250.

(b) Dispense infected RBCs or uninfected RBC (used as controls) into FACS tubes (this should be approximately 25–50 % of the RBC content of a single ADCI well).

(c) Add 100 μl of PBS to each tube containing RBCs from the culture plate.

(d) Add 100 μl of dihydroethidium at 40 μg/ml to each tube (the final concentration of dihydroethidium is 20 μg/ml).

(e) Incubate tubes at 37 °C in the dark for 20 min.

(f) Add 1.5 ml of PBS+ 1 % FCS to each tube.

(g) Prepare a thiazole orange working solution by diluting the thiazole orange stock solution 1:1,000 in PBS. Protect from light until use. Working solution should be discarded after use.

(h) Pellet RBCs and remove supernatant.

(i) Resuspend pellets in 200 μl of Thiazole Orange at 1.5 μg/ml.

(j) Incubate for 30 min at room temperature in the dark.

(k) Wash cells with 1.5 ml of PBS+ 1 % FCS and open a FSC log/SSC log dot plot or density plot.

(l) Gate on RBC events

(m) Open a FL1 log/FL2 log dot plot or density plot showing only the gated RBCs (*FL1 signal corresponds to thiazole orange emission and FL2 signal corresponds to dihydroethidium emission*).

(n) Perform compensations between FL1 and FL2 emissions using single stained infected RBCs.

(o) Compare non infected RBCs stained with both dyes with infected RBCs stained with both dyes.

(p) Draw gates including double positive cells; these are the parasite infected cells.

(q) Quantify the percentage of RBCs showing double staining in each culture. This should include all conditions on the plate including the RBCs without parasite.

(r) Record data from all well samples in the ADCI plate.

10. Score the percentage of infected RBC in each well.

3.4.2 Two-Step ADCI Assay

1. Add to each MN containing well 50 μl of PEMS suspension in CM + 0.5 % AlbuMAX at a MN to merozoite ratio of 1:2. Add the same amount of PEMS suspension to the MN-free control wells (*see* **Note 11**).
2. Incubate at 5 % CO_2 (or candle jar) at 37 °C for 3 h.

3. Collect supernatants, centrifuge at $600 \times g$ and distribute in a 96-well culture plate (*see* **Note 12**).
4. Add to each well 50 µl of an asynchronous culture of *P. falciparum* at 0.5–1 % parasitemia and 4 % hematocrit in CM with 0.5 % AlbuMAX.
5. Transfer plate to 37 °C, 5 % CO_2 (or candle jar).
6. After 72 h remove supernatant and prepare thin smears.
7. Alternatively, prepare thin smears on part of the culture and transfer the rest of the cultures to a flow cytometry tube for staining with thiazole orange and dihydroethidium and follow the procedure outlined in **step 9** of Subheading 3.4.1.
8. Score the percentage of infected RBC in each well.

3.4.3 Calculation of the ADCI Activity and Validity of the Test

The specific growth inhibitory index (SGI) takes into account the possible nonspecific inhibition by MN or inhibition by antibodies alone. It is calculated as follows:

$$\mathrm{SGI} = 100 \times \left[1 - \frac{(\text{parasitemia with MN and test reagent} / \text{parasitemia with test reagent})}{(\text{parasitemia with MN and NIgG} / \text{parasitemia with only NIgG})} \right]$$

Results from a given ADCI assay cannot be considered valid unless the assay fulfilled several validation criteria. These criteria are mainly related to the quality of the parasite culture before and during the ADCI experiment (*see* Table 1) (*see* **Note 13**).

4 Notes

1. Preparation of IgG by affinity chromatography with protein A is not effective as it does not isolate the cytophilic human IgG3 isotype. Affinity chromatography with protein G is not recommended as it requires a stringent low pH exposure to detach the Ig from protein G which can denature the IgG or at least affect their properties.
2. The quality of MN preparations varies substantially from one donor to another, in part due to genetic factors but mostly due to phenotypic variations, themselves related to external factors, a typical example being a viral, e.g., flu, infection. Therefore small preparations from individual donors would yield MN preparations with unpredictable behavior in the ADCI assay. The preparation of large batches of cryopreserved cells (either cryopreserved purified MN, or preferentially cryopreserved PBMC as the viability of MN is better following the thawing of PBMC) is one way to overcome this difficulty, as the quality of each batch can be analyzed on one of the cryopreserved aliquots to validate the remainder of the batch.

In theory, monocytic cell lines induced to express relevant Fc gamma receptors should overcome this difficulty but in practice they have proven difficult to handle and have not offered the desired reproducibility.

3. The quality of the water used to prepare the CM is important for the MN function in ADCI. We have observed that highly pure deionized water obtained by reverse osmosis, although adequate for parasite culture, lacks minerals required for MN function. Water that contains traces of minerals, such as glass-distilled water provides satisfactory MN function.
4. IgG prepared from sera must be tested as we have frequently observed a non antibody-dependent inhibition of parasite growth when unfractionated sera was used, generally due to the presence of oxidized lipids. When appropriately stored, whole sera can be used, provided it is not thawed and refrozen serially, and preferentially sealed under atmospheric CO_2.
5. If available, a NanoDrop Spectrophotometer can be used for direct measurement of IgG concentration.
6. Avoid touching and scraping the bottom of the wells with the pipette tip. Tilting the plate at an angle and sliding the pipette tip along the side of the well helps in the process.
7. Partial contamination of MN by lymphocytes is not a major concern as they usually promote parasite growth.
8. Use RPMI freshly made, or stored in fully filled containers, as pH is an issue and can lead to inhibition of ADCI activity.
9. *P. falciparum* cultures should show optimal speed of growth for the 8–10 days preceding the ADCI assay, with an over six-fold growth rate in 48 h.
10. The remarkable progress of FACS technology and the very large range of dyes that have been produced for other purposes offer a very wide range of possible combinations and protocols to measure parasite growth by cell sorting in bio-assays such as ADCI or GIA. However simple staining of DNA proved insufficient particularly when dealing with low parasitemia: a small number of non-infected, false positive RBCs are counted and not distinguished from early rings, e.g., either genetic material remaining from reticulocytes or altered RBCs carrying nucleic acids. In addition parasite cultures always contain a proportion of dead parasites that should be distinguished from live ones etc. Several methods have been proposed over time, those relying on the modification of the dye by live parasites being preferred. The thiazole orange and dihydroethidium combination proposed here has been validated in our experiments following double-blind assessment as compared to microscopy. Conversely tritiated hypoxanthine incorporation is not precise enough to reliably distinguish minor differences in SGI, nor

does two-site capture ELISA. Several other techniques have been proposed for estimating the number of infected RBC such as for example the use of fluorescent GFP-transfected parasites or computer assisted picture analysis.

11. Alternatively the 2-step ADCI assay can be performed using highly synchronous and very mature schizonts, which release merozoites within a short culture time and hence activate MN in the presence of test IgG.
12. Supernatants must be kept at 37 °C or at least at room temperature, since they will lose activity at 4 °C or lower temperatures.
13. If required, murine IgG can be tested in ADCI with human MN. The IgG2a isotype is able to bind to the human Fcγ receptors present on MN.

References

1. Bouharoun-Tayoun H, Attanath P, Sabchareon A, Chongsuphajaisiddhi T, Druilhe P (1990) Antibodies that protect humans against Plasmodium falciparum blood stages do not on their own inhibit parasite growth and invasion in vitro, but act in cooperation with monocytes. J Exp Med 172:1633–1641
2. Badell E, Oeuvray C, Moreno A, Soe S, van Rooijen N, Bouzidi A et al (2000) Human malaria in immunocompromised mice: an in vivo model to study defense mechanisms against Plasmodium falciparum. J Exp Med 192:1653–1660
3. Khusmith S, Druilhe P (1983) Cooperation between antibodies and monocytes that inhibit in vitro proliferation of Plasmodium falciparum. Infect Immun 41:219–223
4. Lunel F, Druilhe P (1989) Effector cells involved in nonspecific and antibody-dependent mechanisms directed against Plasmodium falciparum blood stages in vitro. Infect Immun 57:2043–2049
5. Bouharoun-Tayoun H, Oeuvray C, Lunel F, Druilhe P (1995) Mechanisms underlying the monocyte mediated antibody-dependent killing of P. falciparum asexual blood stages. J Exp Med 182:409–418
6. Jafarshad A, Dziegiel MH, Lundquist R, Nielsen LK, Singh S, Druilhe PL (2007) A novel antibody-dependent cellular cytotoxicity mechanism involved in defense against malaria requires costimulation of monocytes FcgammaRII and FcgammaRIII. J Immunol 178:3099–3106
7. Roussilhon C, Oeuvray C, Muller-Graf C, Tall A, Rogier C, Trape JF et al (2007) Long-term clinical protection from falciparum malaria is strongly associated with IgG3 antibodies to merozoite surface protein 3. PLoS Med 4, e320
8. Laurent L, Clavel C, Lemaire O, Anquetil F, Cornillet M, Zabraniecki L et al (2011) Fcgamma receptor profile of monocytes and macrophages from rheumatoid arthritis patients and their response to immune complexes formed with autoantibodies to citrullinated proteins. Ann Rheum Dis 70:1052–1059
9. Lambros C, Vanderberg JP (1979) Synchronization of Plasmodium falciparum erythrocytic stages in culture. J Parasitol 65: 418–420
10. Salmon BL, Oksman A, Goldberg DE (2001) Malaria parasite exit from the host erythrocyte: a two-step process requiring extraerythrocytic proteolysis. Proc Natl Acad Sci U S A 98:271–276

Chapter 12

A Robust Phagocytosis Assay to Evaluate the Opsonic Activity of Antibodies against *Plasmodium falciparum*-Infected Erythrocytes

Andrew Teo, Wina Hasang, Philippe Boeuf, and Stephen Rogerson

Abstract

Infection with *Plasmodium falciparum* parasites causes the majority of malaria-related morbidity and mortality. Constant exposure to the pathogen leads to the acquisition of antibodies and high levels of antibodies have been associated with clinical protection against malaria. A possible protective mechanism is the opsonization of parasites, or malaria-infected erythrocytes (IEs), for phagocytic clearance. Current assays use adherent or chemically differentiated THP-1 cells to evaluate opsonic antibodies in patients' samples, but these assays are often time consuming and damage the effector cells. We have developed a high throughput flow cytometry-based phagocytosis assay using undifferentiated THP-1 cells to quantify the opsonic activity against late stage *P. falciparum*-IEs. Opsonic antibodies bound to IEs promote their phagocytic uptake through Fcγ receptors found on THP-1 cells. Moreover, undifferentiated THP-1 cells do not express CD36, a surface scavenger receptor that promotes non-opsonic phagocytosis. This technical advance allows quantification of opsonic antibodies and is an important tool for the performance of large, population-based studies of malaria immunity, and to provide a significant increase in the statistical power for such studies.

Key words Malaria, Phagocytosis, Opsonizing, High throughput, Population-based studies

1 Introduction

Malaria, especially *Plasmodium falciparum* infection, remains a deadly infection that threatens young children, and women who are in their first and second pregnancies. In young children and pregnant women, this susceptibility is partly attributed to the ability of late-stage *P. falciparum* infected erythrocytes (IEs) to sequester within small blood vessels [1] or maternal blood spaces of the placenta to avoid splenic clearance [2], and in part is due to the lack of preexisting immunity against antigenically different IEs. Repeated exposure to malaria leads to the acquisition of antibodies that are protective against clinical malaria [3, 4]. Possible antibody-mediated protective mechanisms include inhibition of

Ashley M. Vaughan (ed.), *Malaria Vaccines: Methods and Protocols*, Methods in Molecular Biology, vol. 1325, DOI 10.1007/978-1-4939-2815-6_12, © Springer Science+Business Media New York 2015

adhesion of IEs [5] and the opsonizing of IEs for phagocytosis [6]. Adapting our previously established phagocytosis assay [6], here we present a novel high throughput method for measuring the relative opsonic activity of antibodies in serum or plasma using undifferentiated, pro-monocytic THP-1 cells [7].

2 Materials

2.1 Equipment

1. Hemocytometer.
2. Glass microscope slides.
3. Polypropylene 15 ml and 50 ml tubes.
4. Transfer pipettes.
5. Multichannel pipettor.
6. Micron filter 0.22 μm.
7. Centrifuge with a microtiter plate holder.
8. 75 cm^2 vented culture flask.
9. MACS separation CS column (Miltenyi Biotec) (Optional).

2.2 Cell Culture

1. Late-stage *P. falciparum* asexual in vitro blood stage parasite cultures.
2. Undifferentiated THP-1 cells.
3. THP-1 culture medium: Roswell Park Memorial Institute (RPMI) 1640 supplemented with 10 % heat-inactivated, 0.22 μm filtered fetal bovine serum (FBS), 1 % penicillin-streptomycin-glutamine (from a 100× stock solution) and 25 mM 4-(2-hydroxy-ethyl-1-piperazineethanesulfonic acid (HEPES)).

2.3 Reagents and Flow Cytometer

1. Sterile phosphate-buffered saline (PBS) at pH 7.4.
2. FACS buffer: PBS with 10 % FBS and 0.02 % sodium azide at pH 7.4. Can be stored at 4 °C.
3. FACS Lysing solution (BD Biosciences): diluted 1:10 in sterile distilled water. Make up on the day of experimentation.
4. 100 % methanol.
5. Ethidium bromide (EtBr) 1 mg/ml.
6. Giemsa's Azure Eosin Methylene Blue Solution diluted 1:10 in tap water (known as Giemsa stain).
7. Trypan blue in PBS at 0.4 %, 0.22 μm filtered.
8. Paraformaldehyde (PFA) at 2 % in PBS, filtered and stored at 4 °C.
9. A 40–60–80 % Percoll gradient. This is prepared using Percoll, 10× PBS, RPMI-HEPES and sorbitol, and stored at 4 °C. To make the gradients, dissolve 12 g sorbitol powder in 33 ml

of RPMI-HEPES using a magnetic stirrer. Once dissolved, filter through a 0.22 μM filter. Mix 180 ml Percoll with 20 ml of 10× PBS and aliquot this Percoll/PBS solution into three tubes as follows:

(a) For the 40 % solution: 44 ml Percoll/PBS and 45 ml RPMI-HEPES.

(b) For the 60 % solution: 67 ml Percoll/PBS and 22 ml RPMI-HEPES.

(c) For the 80 % solution: 89 ml Percoll/PBS.

Add 11 ml of sorbitol/RPMI-HEPES filtered solution into each tube for a 100 ml total and store at 4 °C (*see* **Note 1**).

10. Heat-inactivated newborn calf serum (NCS).
11. U-bottom 96-well plates (BD Biosciences) (*see* **Note 2**).
12. HyperCyt® Autosampler (IntelliCyt) attached to a CyAnADP analyzer (Beckman Coulter) (*see* **Note 3**).

3 Methods

3.1 Cell Culture

1. *Plasmodium falciparum* is cultured as previously described [8].
2. THP-1 cells are cultured in vented culture flasks in THP-1 culture medium and kept at a density below 5×10^5 cells/ml in a humidified incubator at 37 °C supplemented with 5 % CO_2 (*see* **Note 4**).

3.2 Phagocytosis Assay

3.2.1 Preparation

1. To NCS-coated U-bottom 96-well plates add 3.3 μl of test patient sample serum, positive control serum (pooled sera from 40 individuals previously demonstrated to have high surface reactivity against IEs) and two negative controls consisting of a no serum control and serum sample from six malaria naïve individuals (*see* **Note 5**). An alternative to using pooled positive human serum is to use rabbit anti-human IgG antibody at 900 μg/ml. Samples should be analyzed at minimum in duplicate.
2. IEs are purified from a synchronous in vitro culture at 5–8 % parasitemia of mid-late stage trophozoites. Harvest the culture by centrifuging at 350 × *g* for 4 min at room temperature (RT) and remove the supernatant. Resuspend the erythrocyte pellet in RPMI-HEPES at RT. Set up the Percoll gradient by layering 2 ml of each of the three Percoll solution in a 15 ml tube: 80 % first, followed by 60 % and then 40 %. Overlay the resuspended erythrocytes on the top 40 % gradient (*see* **Note 6**). Alternatively, IEs can be purified using a MACS separation column [9].
3. Centrifuge the gradient at 1,620 × *g* for 15 min at RT (brake low). Remove the supernatant and the 40 % layer and collect the IEs

resting between the 40 % and 60 % layer with a transfer pipette to a 50 ml tube (*see* **Note 7**). Wash thrice with RPMI-HEPES at 350 × *g* for 3 min at RT. Perform a purity check of the IEs pellet with Giemsa stain. To do this, make a thin blood smear of a fraction of the IEs on a microscope slide, fix with methanol, Giemsa stain and determine the % parasitemia by light microscopy. A good preparation usually has >90 % parasitemia (*see* **Note 8**).

4. Stain IEs with 10 μg/ml EtBr for 30 min in the dark at RT. Wash cells thrice with RPMI-HEPES at 350 × *g* for 3 min at RT. Determine the cell density using a hemocytometer. Briefly, resuspend the pellet of IEs in 2 ml RPMI-HEPES, add 5 μl of resuspended IEs to 995 μl RPMI-HEPES (1:200 dilution), then load 10 μl onto a hemocytometer. Adjust the IEs to a final cell density of 1.65×10^7 cells/ml (*see* **Note 9**).

3.2.2 Opsonization

1. Add 30 μl of the IEs suspension (5×10^5 IEs) into each well of the 96-well plate containing test or control plasma and agitate cells by gently tapping the side of the plate and incubate at RT in the dark for 1 h. Thirty minutes into the incubation, re-agitate the cells.
2. Using a multichannel pipettor, wash cells thrice with RPMI-HEPES. Pellet cells between washes at 350 × *g* for 3 min at RT.
3. Resuspend the cells in 50 μl of THP-1 medium and aliquot, in duplicate (25 μl/well of cell suspension) into new NCS-coated U-bottom 96-well plates.

3.2.3 Phagocytosis

While IEs are opsonizing, prepare the THP-1 cells.

1. Harvest THP-1 cells from a culture flask and centrifuge cells at 350 × *g* for 4 min at RT and discard the supernatant. Determine the cell density using a hemocytometer. Briefly, resuspend cells in 2 ml THP-1 medium, add 5 μl of the cell suspension into 95 μl 0.4 % Trypan blue (1:20 dilution), then load 10 μl onto hemocytometer (*see* **Note 10**). Adjust THP-1 cell density to 5×10^5 cells/ml using THP-1 medium.
2. Dispense 50 μl of the THP-1 cell suspension (2.5×10^4 cells) into each well of the plate containing the opsonized IEs. Gently tap the side of the plates to mix the cells, and incubate for 40 min at 37 °C in a CO_2-supplemented humidified incubator (*see* **Note 11**).
3. To stop the phagocytosis, centrifuge the plate at 350 × *g* for 5 min at 4 °C.
4. Discard the supernatant and add 75 μl FACS Lysing solution to each well for 10 min at RT to allow unphagocytosed IEs to lyse. Centrifuge at 350 × *g* for 3 min at 4 °C, discard super-

natant and wash thrice with FACS buffer. Pellet cells at $350 \times g$ for 3 min at 4 °C between washes.

5. Fix the THP-1 cells in 100 μl chilled 2 % PFA and store at 4 °C in the dark for at least 2 h before FACS acquisition. Final density is typically 3.5×10^5 cells/ml.

3.2.4 FACS Acquisition

1. Calibrate the flow cytometer using manufacturer-supplied calibration beads to ensure reproducibility of the experiment.
2. Resuspend cells with a multichannel pipettor prior to FACS acquisition. Load the plate onto a Hypercyt® Autosampler attachment for a CyAnADP flow cytometer, and acquire samples for 30 s at approximately 500 events/s (*see* **Note 12**). For users without an autosampler, ensure that the flow rate and acquisition time are sufficient to acquire a minimum of 2,500 THP-1 cells for each test sample.
3. Gate the THP-1 cells based on their forward and side scatter properties (*see* **Note 13**). Place a marker so that 5 % of THP-1 cells in the negative control (either no serum or naïve serum) are positive for EtBr fluorescence (Fig. 1) (*see* **Note 14**).
4. The percentage of THP-1 cells that have phagocytosed IEs is determined by subtracting the average percentage of $EtBr^+$ THP1-cells in the negative control from the average percentage

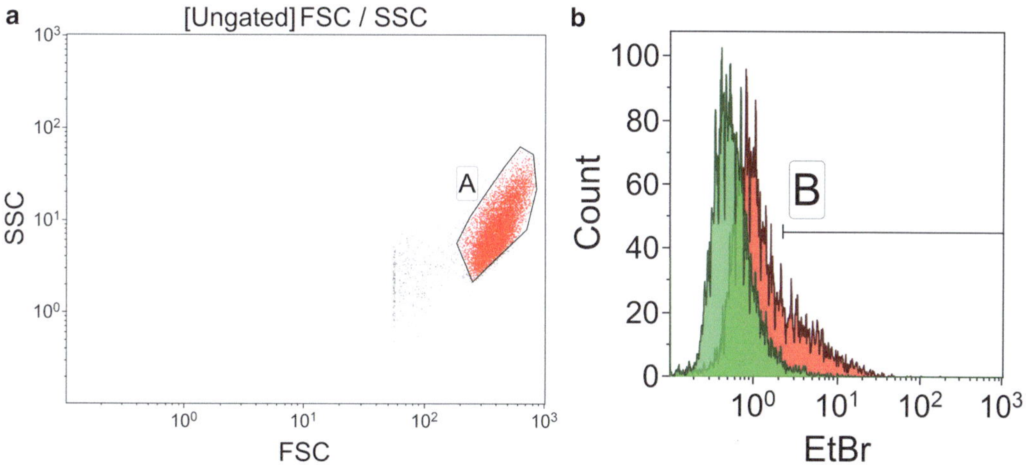

Fig. 1 FACS gating and analysis strategy. (**a**) Typical cytogram of THP-1 cells incubated with opsonized IEs. Acquired events are plotted according to their side scatter (SS) and forward scatter (FS) characteristics. Gate A separates THP-1 cells from cellular debris. (**b**) Gated THP-1 cells are then displayed on a 1D-histogram representing the distribution of EtBr fluorescence among the THP-1 cell population analyzed. A marker (Region B) is set so that approximately 5 % of the THP-1 cells incubated with no plasma or with plasma samples from malaria-naïve individuals (*green histogram*) are positive for EtBr fluorescence. THP-1 cells incubated with IE opsonized with plasma from malaria-exposed individuals (*red histogram*) display higher percentage of EtBr-positive THP-1 cells

of EtBr+ THP1-cells in the test sample, and expressed relative to the positive control (*see* **Note 15**). The percentage of THP-1 cells that phagocytosed IEs opsonized with positive control plasma samples is usually in the range of 30–45 % (after adjusting for negative controls). If this value is below 30 %, the assay is considered unsuccessful and should be repeated. For the rabbit anti-human IgG antibody positive control, the percentage of EtBr-positive THP-1 cells is in the range 50–65 % (after adjusting for negative controls). If this value is below 50 %, the assay is considered unsuccessful and should be repeated. There are several reasons for unsuccessful assays, which include uneven heat and/or gas distribution during phagocytosis and ineffective THP-1 cells cultured in expired THP-1 medium (THP-1 medium lifespan is approximately 3 months).

5. Results can be analyzed using the Kaluza® software (Beckman Coulter) and Hyperview® Analysis software (IntelliCyt) or similar programs. Typical readouts are shown in Fig. 1.

4 Notes

1. Perform all steps under sterile conditions.
2. U-bottom 96-well plates are coated with 170 μl NCS for at least 1 h, 2 days before an experiment. Plates are washed twice with 200 μl PBS, wrapped in cling wrap and stored at 4 °C. NCS can be reused up to five times.
3. Test samples can also be acquired using other flow cytometers with an autosampler attached, for example a FACSCantoII flow cytometer (BD Biosciences).
4. THP-1 cells are maintained at a density of 2×10^5 cells/ml. From 2 days prior to experiment day, THP-1 cells are kept at a density of 5×10^5 cells/ml. The cells can be passaged for up to 10 cycles. Cell density should be checked every 3 days to avoid high cell density (e.g., 1×10^7 cells/ml), which may lead to differentiation of THP-1 cells.
5. Aliquot patient plasma or sera and heat-inactivate at 57 °C for 45 min to remove complement factors and store at −80 °C. Patient samples should be plated on the day of the experiment. If this is not possible, plate 1 day before and wrap the plate in cling-wrap and store at −80 °C.
6. Thirty microliter of purified IEs at a density of 5×10^5 cells is required per test sample. Approximately 125 ml of parasite culture at 5–8 % parasitemia, 4 % hematocrit will be sufficient to test up to 300–350 test samples in a single experiment.
7. The volume of the polypropylene tube needed depends on the volume of purified IEs to be collected. In this example approximately 10 ml of IEs were collected.

8. If parasitemia is <85 % repurify using MACS separation column. Repurifying using Percoll is futile.
9. Account for 30 % loss of IEs.
10. THP-1 cells stained blue are nonviable cells. Do not include in calculation.
11. For efficient phagocytosis, plates should be well spread out in the humidified CO_2 incubator to ensure the heat and gas are evenly distributed.
12. HyperCyt® Autosampler is an attachment that may work differently with different flow cytometers.
13. Ethidium Bromide excitation spectrum peaks at ~510 nm and its fluorescence emission spectrum peaks at ~600 nm. Use the appropriate laser and detection filter to ensure optimal excitation and detection of EtBr fluorescence.
14. By microscopy, approximately 5 % of the THP-1 cells exposed to IEs with negative controls have taken up IEs.
15. Samples with an adjusted mean variance of >20 % and a replicate mean difference of more than 10 percentage points between duplicates are rerun [10]. A typical readout from a run is shown in Table 1 and details whether samples will need to be run again.

Table 1
To determine whether samples are required for retesting

	Replicate values	Replicate mean	Corrected % of EtBr positive THP-1 cells	Phagocytosis index relative to positive control	Replicate mean difference	Adjusted mean variance	Repeat
No plasma control	5.2 5.6	5.4	0	0	0.2	(0.2/5.4)×100=3.7	No
Malaria-naïve control	5.3 5.7	5.5	0.1	0	0.2	(0.2/5.5)×100=3.6	No
Positive control	45.1 46.1	45.6	40.2	100.0	0.5	(0.5/45.6)×100=1.1	No
Sample 1	15.5 19.5	17.5	12.1	30.1	−2.0	(−2.0/17.5)×100=11.4	No
Sample 2	26.1 60.1	43.1	37.7	93.8	−17.0	(−17.0/43.1)×100=39.4	Yes

The replicate mean difference is calculated. The replicate mean difference value is then divided by the mean replicate and multiplied by 100 to obtain a percentage point. Samples with an adjusted mean variance of >20 percentage points and a replicate mean difference of >10 percentage points between duplicates are rerun

References

1. Sherman IW, Eda S, Winograd E (2003) Cytoadherence and sequestration in Plasmodium falciparum: defining the ties that bind. Microbes Infect 5(10):897–909
2. Beeson JG et al (2001) Parasite adhesion and immune evasion in placental malaria. Trends Parasitol 17(7):331–337
3. Baird JK et al (1991) Age-dependent acquired protection against Plasmodium falciparum in people having two years exposure to hyperendemic malaria. Am J Trop Med Hyg 45(1):65–76
4. Fried M et al (1998) Maternal antibodies block malaria. Nature 395(6705):851–852
5. Boeuf P et al (2011) Relevant assay to study the adhesion of Plasmodium falciparum-infected erythrocytes to the placental epithelium. PLoS One 6(6), e21126
6. Ataíde R et al (2010) Using an improved phagocytosis assay to evaluate the effect of HIV on specific antibodies to pregnancy-associated malaria. PLoS One 5(5), e10807
7. Tsuchiya S et al (1980) Establishment and characterization of a human acute monocytic leukemia cell line (THP-1). Int J Cancer 26(2): 171–176
8. Trager W, Jensen J (1976) Human malaria parasites in continuous culture. Science 193(4254):673–675
9. Ribaut C et al (2008) Concentration and purification by magnetic separation of the erythrocytic stages of all human Plasmodium species. Malar J 7:45
10. Aitken EH et al (2010) Antibodies to chondroitin sulfate A-binding infected erythrocytes: dynamics and protection during pregnancy in women receiving intermittent preventive treatment. J Infect Dis 201(9): 1316–1325

Chapter 13

Miniaturized Growth Inhibition Assay to Assess the Anti-blood Stage Activity of Antibodies

Elizabeth H. Duncan and Elke S. Bergmann-Leitner

Abstract

While no immune correlate for blood-stage specific immunity against *Plasmodium falciparum* malaria has been identified, there is strong evidence that antibodies directed to various malarial antigens play a crucial role. In an effort to evaluate the role of antibodies in inhibiting growth and/or invasion of erythrocytic stages of the malaria parasite it will be necessary to test large sample sets from Phase 2a/b trials as well as epidemiological studies. The major constraints for such analyses are (1) availability of sufficient sample quantities (especially from infants and small children) and (2) the throughput of standard growth inhibition assays. The method described here assesses growth- and invasion inhibition by measuring the metabolic activity and viability of the parasite (by using a parasite lactate dehydrogenase-specific substrate) in a 384-microtiter plate format. This culture method can be extended beyond the described detection system to accommodate other techniques commonly used for growth/invasion-inhibition.

Key words *Plasmodium*, Antibodies, Growth inhibition, High-throughput, Functional assay

1 Introduction

Antibodies are the main adaptive immune defense mechanisms against blood stages of *Plasmodium*. Depending on the antigen and epitope specificity, antibodies can prevent the rupture of mature parasitized red blood cells (pRBC), block the dispersal of merozoites, block invasion of new erythrocytes or bind to the merozoites and subsequently inhibit parasite development in the newly invaded erythrocyte. The quantitative assessment of antibody titers/concentrations often does not correlate with biological/clinical responses. Therefore, functional assays such as growth inhibition assays have been more indicative of biological activities in sera from immunized or malaria-exposed individuals. There is evidence from epidemiological and vaccination studies that growth inhibition correlates with reduced parasitemia [1–4]. In an effort to reveal the role of growth inhibitory antibodies in protection from disease or reduction of morbidity, high-throughput assays are

Ashley M. Vaughan (ed.), *Malaria Vaccines: Methods and Protocols*, Methods in Molecular Biology, vol. 1325,
DOI 10.1007/978-1-4939-2815-6_13, © Springer Science+Business Media New York 2015

needed to test large numbers of clinical samples. The readout method described in this chapter is the measurement of parasite metabolic activity, which has been shown to be more sensitive than other methods that (a) measure changes in the DNA content of pRBC (e.g., SybrGreen or Syto-16) or (b) evaluate blood smears (methods compared in ref. 5). The Plasmodium lactate dehydrogenase (pLDH)-based method quantitates both invasion and growth inhibition and therefore minimizes the risk of false negative results. The assay setup described in this chapter was developed out of a need to test large numbers of field samples with very limiting volumes. The protocol allows for the testing of 180 samples, four negative controls and four positive controls all in triplicate. The controls are run on each side of the plate to control for intra-plate variation. Depending on the number of subjects per study cohort, it is possible to decrease the number of replicates to either duplicates or singulars. However, we strongly recommend consulting a statistician to determine whether replicates are needed.

The assay volume in this method assumes 20 μl, but can be reduced to 10 μl. The samples can be either whole serum or purified immunoglobulins. In cases where the samples are derived from subjects living in malaria-endemic areas, dialysis is strongly recommended in order to remove any pharmacological agents (including folk medicine) that can interfere with parasite activity and thus increase the chance of false positive results regarding the biological activity of antibodies in such individuals.

The ability to employ a high-throughput growth inhibition assay that captures a wide range of anti-parasite activities will be the key to uncovering the role of antibodies induced by either vaccine and/or natural exposure in protection against disease.

2 Materials

Prepare all solutions under sterile (tissue culture) conditions or sterile filter prior to use.

2.1 Culture Medium

1. Ultrapure water (tissue culture grade, endotoxin free).
2. Human O+ serum from a commercial source or blood bank (*see* **Note 1**).
3. RPMI Medium 1640 powder. RMPI 1640 powder is custom formulated to contain 5940 mg/L HEPES, 1.36 mg/L hypoxanthine, 50 mg/L L-isoleucine, 1 mg/L phenol red, 300 mg/L L-glutamine, no para-aminobenzoic acid and no sodium bicarbonate. Reconstitute powder appropriately and sterile filter using a 0.2 μm filter receiver in a biological hood and store at 4 °C until complete medium is needed. Use within 4 weeks of preparation.

4. Sodium Bicarbonate ($NaHCO_3$), 7.5 % wt/vol.
5. Complete Medium with Serum (CMS): For 500 ml of CMS combine 50 ml human serum O+, 16 ml of Sodium Bicarbonate ($NaHCO_3$), 7.5 % wt/vol and 434 ml of reconstituted RPMI 1640 powder. Filter using a 0.2 μm 500 ml filter receiver in biological hood. Gas media with 5 % CO_2, 5 % O_2, 90 % N_2 and store at 4 °C (*see* **Note 2**).

2.2 Dialysis in Case of Testing Serum Samples or Purified Immunoglobulins

1. Dialysis medium: Sterile 1× PBS and Sterile RPMI-NaOH. 1× PBS working solution (diluted 10× PBS, Ca, Mg free) and RPMI-NaOH: To 1 L of sterile RPMI 1640 medium add 15.8 ml of sterile 0.6 M NaOH, pH 7.3 for a final concentration of 9.5 mM NaOH, 4.4 ml of sterile 5 M NaCl for a final concentration of 22 mM NaCl and 17.8 ml of sterile tissue culture water. Final volume will be slightly over 1 L. Store at 4 °C.
2. Slide-A-Lyzer MINI Dialysis Units, 10–100 μl capacity, 10,000 MW cutoff, Pierce, Rockford, IL, Cat. No: 69572.
3. Magnetic stir plate.
4. Magnetic stir bar.
5. Two-liter plastic container with lid.
6. NanoDrop 1000 or equivalent (to determine the concentration of purified IgG), Thermo Scientific, Wilmington, DE.

2.3 Plasmodium Parasite Cultures

The method described here uses synchronized parasites; however the assay can be executed using asynchronous cultures that are incubated for one cycle length (*see* **Note 3**).

2.4 GIA Components

1. 384-well plates (Perkin Elmer, PPN 6007650) (*see* **Note 4**).
2. 96-well V-bottom plate.
3. 1.5 ml microcentrifuge tubes.
4. Sterile, individually wrapped multi-channel basins (Thomas Scientific, Cat. No: 7684D10 or equivalent).
5. 12-channel multi-pipettor (5–50 μl range) or equivalent with Rainin LTS tips.
6. Gilson 2 μl, 20 μl, 200 μl, 1,000 μl pipettors or equivalent with sterile tips.
7. Optional: Axypet-16 (16-channel pipettor), Axygen Scientific tips, Axygen Union City, CA.
8. For serum assays: heat block or water bath capable of maintaining 56 °C.
9. Optional: Tube rotator.
10. Optional for accurate measurement of viable parasitemia (*see* **Note 5**):

   (a) Dihydroethidine (HE, Life Technologies/Molecular Probes D-1168, 25 mg): prepare 10 mg/ml stock solution with DMSO and freeze aliquots. Working solution: dilute HE prior to use to 50 μg/ml with 1× PBS.
   (b) Flow cytometer with blue laser (488 nm excitation) and ability to detect 570 nm signal.
11. LDH substrate buffer (prepare 500 ml of buffer in advance and freeze in 25 ml aliquots).
   (a) 50 ml of 1 M Tris–HCl (pH 8.0).
   (b) 450 ml sterile, tissue culture grade water.
   (c) 2.8 g sodium L-lactate.
   (d) 1.25 ml Triton X-100.
   (e) Stir on a magnetic stirrer at RT for at least 30 min, aliquot into 25 ml portions (50 ml tubes), store at −20 °C.
12. Nitro Blue Tetrazolium (NBT) solution.
   (a) Thaw 2 × 25 ml aliquot of LDH buffer, pool, and warm to RT.
   (b) Add one NBT tablet (10 mg, Sigma Cat# N5514) and dissolve (30 min) by gentle mixing, do not shake. Cover with aluminum foil. The prepared solution can be kept at 4 °C up to 3 weeks (covered with aluminum foil).
13. 3-Acetylpyridine Adenine Dinucleotide (APAD) stock solution (10 mg/ml), Sigma Cat# A5251-100 mg.
   (a) Dissolve 100 mg of APAD in 10 ml of tissue culture grade water.
   (b) Store in 50 μl aliquots at −30 °C.
14. Diaphorase stock solution 50 units/ml: Diaphorase from *Clostridium kluyveri*, Sigma, Cat. # D5540-500UN.
   (a) Dissolve 500 units Diaphorase in 10 ml of tissue culture water.
   (b) Store in 200 μl aliquots at −30 °C.
15. Microplate reader, Spectramax 384plus (Molecular Devices, Sunnyvale, CA) or equivalent.
16. Eppendorf 5430R Table Top Microcentrifuge with fixed angle rotor or equivalent.
17. Eppendorf 5810R Table Top Centrifuge with swinging bucket rotor and microtiter plate carriers or equivalent.
18. Titramax-100 platform shaker, Heidolph Instruments (Thomas Scientific Cat#8293X01) or equivalent.

3 Methods

Carry out all procedures under sterile tissue culture conditions. The readout method described here works for any sample format, i.e., serum/defibrinated plasma (heparinized samples cannot be used in a growth inhibition assay since the heparin interferes with parasite invasion; this applies also to the source material for immunoglobulin preparation) and immunoglobulins.

3.1 Sample Types

3.1.1 Preclinical Serum Samples

Depending on the species from which the samples originated either full serum can be tested or purification of immunoglobulins has to be performed:

Sera derived from rabbits and nonhuman primates can be tested without any further manipulation as long as the serum has been collected in specialized serum separator tubes and processed after clotting is complete (45–60 min incubation at room temperature after blood draw). Serum should be aliquoted on the same day and frozen at −20 °C. Repeated thawing and freezing will increase non-specific toxicity.

If purification of immunoglobulins is required (in case of samples that have shown to have toxic effect or in case of mouse serum), the purification method will depend on the species of immunoglobulin (*see* Subheading 3.1.3).

3.1.2 Clinical Serum Samples

The preparation of clinical serum samples for GIA depends on the immune status of the study subjects:

Sera collected from individuals that have either received antimalarial drugs or other medication that may provide antiparasitic activity (including folk medicine) can be prepared for the growth inhibition assay by either (a) purification of immunoglobulins or (b) dialysis to remove potentially active drugs in an effort to preserve the whole spectrum of immunoglobulins and/or complement factors.

Dialysis:

1. Label and insert Slide-A-Lyzer MINI dialysis units into floating racks. To pre-wet membrane, place rack into a container containing at least 1 liter of dialysis buffer (first round of buffer exchange) plus the magnetic stir bar. Transfer sample into unit (making note of the sample start volume), putting sample directly onto the membrane surface and seal with the provided cap for the unit (*see* **Note 6**).
2. Place covered container on stir plate and dialyze for 1 h at 4 °C with constant stirring. Exchange buffer and repeat dialysis to achieve at least three exchanges with PBS and one

exchange with RPMI/NaOH/NaCl (for concentrations, *see* Subheading 2.2, **item 1**).

3. Recover samples after setting dialysis unit into a microcentrifuge tube and conducting a brief centrifugation in a microcentrifuge. Record volume changes (*see* **Note 7**).
4. Calculate a correction factor based on the starting volume that determines which final volume will be used in the assay (*see* **Note 8**).

3.1.3 Purified Immunoglobulins

The species of immunoglobulins, oxidized lipids, antimalarials, and other drugs, or inadequate sample collection/storage condition may require the purification of antibodies from the source material (*see* **Note 9**):

1. Upon purification, immunoglobulins need to be dialyzed as described in Subheading 3.1.2 to remove excess salt and transfer the immunoglobulins into a buffer that is compatible with the growth inhibition assay.
2. Determine the concentration of the immunoglobulins by NanoDrop and dilute the sample with RPMI/NaOH/NaCl to the desired concentration (typically 2× as an equal volume of sample diluted with an equal volume of parasite suspension).

3.2 Sample Preparation

While serum samples are tested at concentrations of up to 20 % (vol/vol) (*see* **Note 10**), immunoglobulins are typically tested at a range from 2 mg/ml to 20 mg/ml. If using serum samples proceed as described below (Subheading 3.2.1), if using immunoglobulins skip to Subheading 3.2.2.

3.2.1 Heat-Inactivation

If the aim of the experiment is the assessment of anti-parasite activity exclusively mediated by antibodies without the contribution of complement factors, proceed with heat inactivation of the sera:

1. Heat-inactivate sera (56 °C, 20 min)
2. Transfer onto ice for 5 min to cool prior to further processing.

3.2.2 Elimination of RBC-reactive antibodies

Pre-absorption with erythrocytes to eliminate any background growth inhibition caused by antibodies that bind to the erythrocytes from the donor.

1. Prepare 50 % hematocrit RBC (leukoreduced and washed; malaria naive O+ donor, ideally same donor as the RBC for the parasite culture)
2. Add RBC to each sample at a 1:20 ratio and incubate at RT for 1 h; resuspend every 20 min by gently vortexing or incubate samples on tumbler
3. Spin samples for 2 min at 13,000 × *g* to pellet RBCs

Order of samples in preparation plate:

	1	2	3	4	5	6	7	8	9	10
Row 1	Ctrl-1	S-1	S-3	S-5	S-7	S-9	S-11	S-13	S-15	Ctrl-1
Row 2	Ctrl-2	S-2	S-4	S-6	S-8	S-10	S-12	S-14	S-16	Ctrl-2

Order of samples in assay plate (384-well plate) after transfer with 12-channel multi-pipettor:

	1	2	3	4	5	6	7	8	9	10	11	12	13	14	15	16	17	18	19	20
Row	Ct1	Ct2	S-1	S-2	S-3	S-4	S-5	S-6	S-7	S-8	S-9	S-10	S-11	S-12	S-13	S-14	S-15	S-16	Ct1	Ct2

Fig. 1 Plate layout in preparation plate and assay plate (*see* **Notes 11** and **12**)

Table 1
Example for dilution scheme for serum samples (*see* Note 13)

Serum concentration in assay (% vol/vol)	Serum sample volume in 96-well preparation plate	Diluent volume in 96-well preparation plate
20	16 μl	24 μl
10	8 μl	32 μl
5	4 μl	36 μl
2.5	2 μl	38 μl

4. Carefully remove supernatant and transfer to 96-well V-bottom plate (preparation plate) or fresh 1.5 ml microcentrifuge tubes

3.2.3 Dilution of Test Samples (Table 1, **Note 11***)*

1. Transfer the appropriate volume of pre-absorbed serum sample needed for the experiment into a sterile V-bottom 96-well plate (preparation plate, *see* Fig. 1). Each well in the 96-well plate will contain the volume needed for one triplicate in the 384-well plate. *See* **Note 13** for an example of a sample dilution.
2. Plate layout should be in a zigzag pattern (as shown in Fig. 1).

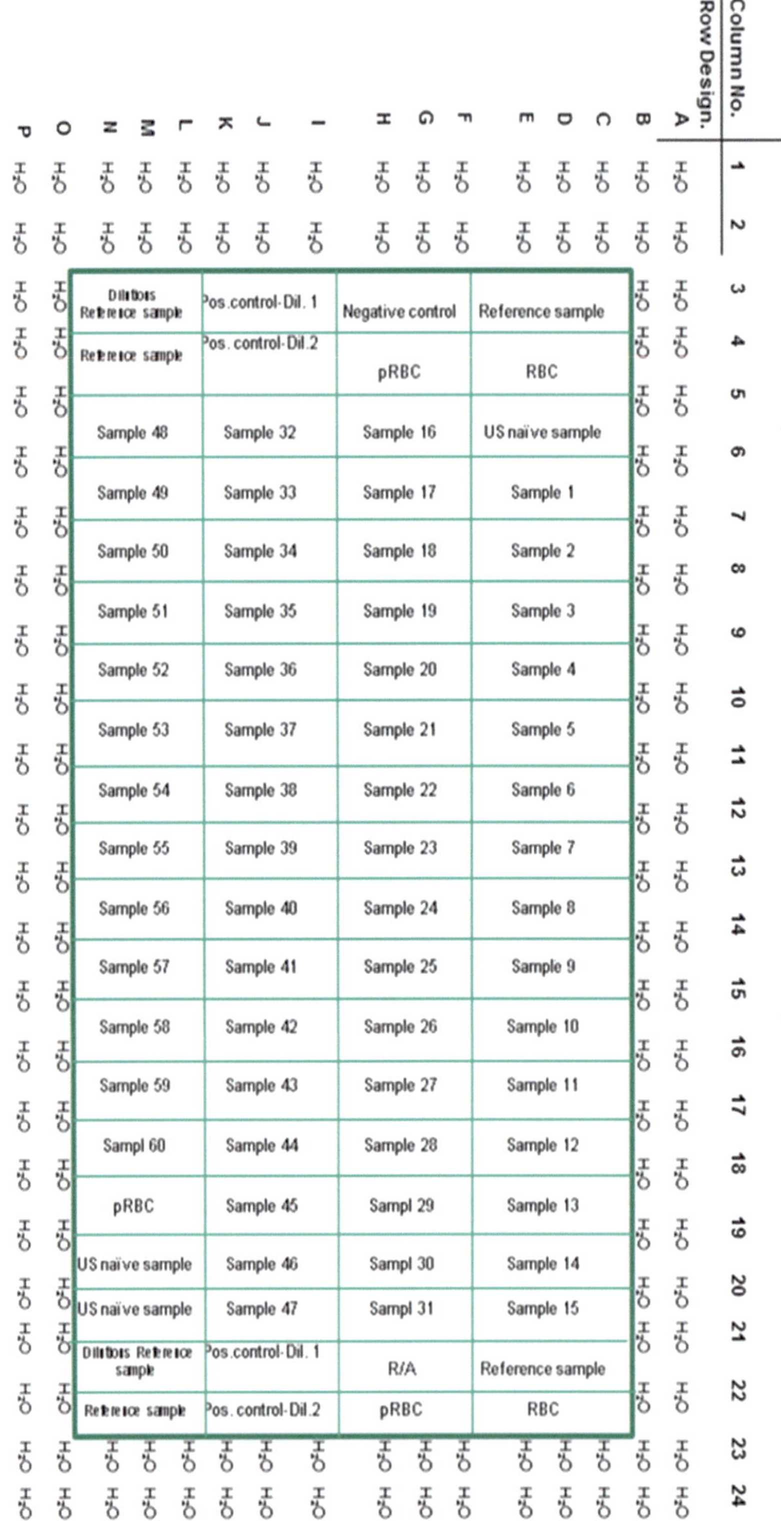

Fig. 2 An example for a final plate layout

3. Dilute serum with CMS as needed (*see* **Note 13**)
4. Mix and dispense 10 μl/replicate well into the assay plate (*see* Fig. 1).
5. The two outer rows and columns are filled with 90 μl of distilled, sterile water to minimize evaporation (*see* Fig. 2 for a final plate layout example)

3.2.4 Preparation of GIA Parasite Suspension

1. Determine parasitemia of synchronized *P. falciparum* late-trophozoite stage/early-schizont stage cultures (*see* **Note 14**) using the dihydroethidine (HE) method prior to processing the samples and committing to assay setup (*see* **Note 15**):
   (a) Stain 50 μl of parasite culture with 500 μl HE
   (b) Incubate samples for 20 min at 37 °C
   (c) Analyze samples by flow cytometry (i.e., the count the number of infected erythrocytes to determine the parasitemia). Acquire at least 100,000 events.
2. Calculate the volume of diluted parasites needed (i.e., 5 ml per 384-well plate). Concentration of parasite dilution prior to adding to assay plates: 0.3 ± 0.1 % parasitemia, 4 % hematocrit. Final hematocrit in the plate will be 2 % (approx. 0.3 % parasitemia)
3. Dilute parasites needed for the entire assay in a 25 cm^2 plug cap flask and subdivide this suspension into individual 25 cm^2 plug cap flasks for each plate (e.g., if the bulk dilution was for 4 plates, then parasites are diluted in 20 ml and then 4 × 5 ml are aliquoted into four 25 cm^2 plug cap flasks).
4. Gas the flasks with 5 % CO_2, 5 % O_2, 90 % N_2 and incubate at 37 °C until ready for dispersion into assay plates.
5. Add 10 μl of parasite suspension to each well using either a 12-channel pipettor or a 16-channel pipettor.
6. Add 10 μl of 4 % hematocrit RBC suspension to the designated control wells for RBC only.
7. Seal assay plates in plastic bag with pre-moistened blotter paper after gassing. Incubate for one cycle length at 37 °C (*see* **Note 3**).

3.2.5 GIA Harvest

1. Remove assay plates from incubator, open bag and add 80 μl of cold 1× PBS to each assay well.
2. Spin plates (e.g., Eppendorf 5810R; microtiter plate carriers) for 10 min at 1,300 × *g* at 4 °C.
3. After centrifugation, remove and discard 80 μl of supernatant from the assay plate without disturbing the cell pellet.
4. Seal plates with a self-adhesive plate sealer before replacing the plate lid
5. Store plates at −20 °C until ready for development. Place plates individually in the freezer (not stacked) to assure even freezing of all plates and wells.

3.2.6 Plate Development

1. Add NBT tablet to thawed LDH buffer, wrap in aluminum foil and bring up to RT (will need 10 ml per plate).
2. Thaw assay plates for 30–40 min at RT with self-adhesive plate sealer in place. Do not stack plates to assure even thawing
3. Prepare complete LDH substrate by adding 50 μl of 3-Acetylpyridine Adenine Dinucleotide (APAD) stock and 200 μl of Diaphorase stock for every 10 ml of NBT solution, mix well and immediately add to assay plates (40 μl per well)
4. Start timer (30 min incubation) as soon as entire plate has received substrate solution
5. Spin the plate for 1 min at 1,800 × *g* to eliminate air bubbles.
6. Cover with foil and place on a flatbed shaker (Titramax-100 shaker use 350 setting) at room temperature
7. Read plates at 650 nm and export data into Excel spreadsheet or other analysis software.

3.2.7 Calculations

- Audit OD values of replicates to assure that:
  - OD values are above 0.15
  - %CV is < 12 %. Any samples with higher %CV need to be repeated.
  - Positive plate controls and reference samples are within historical range
- Calculate Percent Inhibition using absorbance at 650 nm using the formula:

$$\%\,\text{Growth inhibition} = 100 \times \left[1 - \left\{\frac{\text{OD Immune sample} - \text{OD RBC}}{\text{OD pre}\quad\text{immune sample} - \text{OD RBC}}\right\}\right]$$

4 Notes

1. In case malaria-naïve serum is not available, parasite cultures should be adapted to grow in AlbuMAX-supplemented culture medium [6]; AlbuMAX I, Invitrogen/Gibco Cat. No 11020-021.
2. Culture medium should be prewarmed to 37 °C before use.
3. Determine cycle length of parasite lab strain/adapted field isolate-synchronize parasites and culture for various time points at which microscopic slides or DNA-staining with subsequent flow cytometric analysis is performed. Determine the time point at which the parasites have completed one cycle. This will become the incubation time length for the GIA in the future. We determined the cycle length of commonly used lab strains such as 3D7 and 7G8 to be approx. 40 h, FVO to be 48 h and CAMP/FUP to be approx. 44–46 h.

4. Manufacturer of 384-well plates: we have tested various manufacturers of sterile 384-well plates for their ability to support optimal parasite growth (as defined by having the same multiplication rate as in larger culture vessels). The culture conditions described here were established using the various laboratory strains 3D7, FVO (Welcome), CAMP/FUP.
5. Determination of parasitemia can be achieved at a minimum by preparing blood smears from parasite cultures, staining with Giemsa [5] and counting the number of parasites per 2,000 erythrocytes. We have found that setting up cultures based on the percentage of parasitemia determined by methods such as Giemsa-stained blood smears or staining with DNA-dyes such as SybrGreen or Syto-16 leads to large variability in the overall signal of the GIA [7]. This is likely due to the fact that these methods do not allow the discrimination of live/dead parasites; thus, we describe here a method that has been proven to generate the most robust assay results.
6. Slide-A-Lyzer MINI Dialysis Units are ideal for volumes up to 100 μl as they are rated 100 % leak-proof, are made of low-protein binding plastic, and have small membrane surface area, thus reducing sample volume loss.
7. The most common volume change that occurs is an increase in volume (rarely exceeds 20 %).
8. If sample has lost 75 % of its original total volume, this sample has to be excluded from further analysis. Calculate sample volume needed for assay as follows:

$$\text{Test volume} = \text{post - dialysis volume} / \text{pre - dialysis volume} \times \text{volume needed for assay.}$$

9. Methods for immunoglobulin purifications differ significantly in their ability to purify/enrich the different isotypes of antibodies. Also, the species from which the immunoglobulins are derived plays a major role in the efficacy and yield of the various purification assays [8, 9]. We recommend using the Protein A/G or polyethylene glycol method for human and non-human immunoglobulins, caprylic acid/ammonium sulfate for mouse immunoglobulins and Protein A/G for rabbit immunoglobulins.
10. When determining sample volumes needed for the experiment, consider processing an approx. 10 % excess (e.g., 25 μl sample per assay strain if using 20 % serum concentration). The typical sample volume required for a 20 % serum assay is 20 μl of sample per assay strain—*see* **Note 13** for example dilution.
11. Most accurate pipetting has been achieved with the Finnpipette 12-channel multi-pipettor (5–50 μl range) which is versatile as it can be used for the dilution of samples in the V-bottom plate (=preparation plate, Fig. 1) as well as for the loading of the 384-well plate (=assay plate, Fig. 1).

12. The channels of a 12-channel pipettor can load alternating columns into the 384-well plate. Thus, in order to achieve sequential sample line up as shown in the schematic (Fig. 1), the samples are loaded into the preparation plate in a zigzag fashion (Fig. 1).
13. Example of dilution scheme for serum assay for one strain (*see* Table 1). Multiply the volumes listed in Table 1 by the number of assay strains tested.

    The total volume of the diluted samples is 40 μl of which 30 μl will be loaded into the triplicate wells of the assay plate. The excess 10 μl assure that sufficient sample is available in cases of pipetting inaccuracies.
14. Synchronize either with temperature-cycled incubators [10] or by Percoll enrichment. If synchronizing by purifying schizonts by Percoll gradients, perform the synchronization 2 days prior to assay setup (i.e. re-culturing the schizonts for the next cycle before using for the experiment).
15. This step is a go/no go decision—if the culture has a parasitemia <1 % then do not proceed as the health of the culture is in question. This in turn can leave to inflated GIA responses with test and reference samples.

Acknowledgements

The authors would like to thank Dr. Wolfgang Leitner for critical reading of the manuscript.

Disclaimer The opinions or assertions contained herein are the private views of the authors, and are not to be construed as official, or as reflecting true views of the Department of the Army or the Department of Defense.

References

1. Dent AE, Bergmann-Leitner ES, Wilson DW et al (2008) Antibody-mediated growth inhibition of Plasmodium falciparum: relationship to age and protection from parasitemia in Kenyan children and adults. PLoS One 3(10), e3557
2. John CC, Moormann AM, Pregibon DC et al (2005) Correlation of high levels of antibodies to multiple pre-erythrocytic Plasmodium falciparum antigens and protection from infection. Am J Trop Med Hyg 73(1):222–228
3. John CC, O'Donnell, Sumba PD et al (2004) Evidence that invasion-inhibitory antibodies specific for the 19-kDa fragment of the merozoite surface protein-1 (MSP-1_{19}) can play a protective role against Blood-stage Plasmodium falciparum infection in individuals in a malaria endemic area of Africa. J Immunol 173:666–672
4. Thera MA, Doumbo OK, Coulibaly B et al (2010) Safety and immunogenicity of an AMA1 malaria vaccine in Malian children: results of a phase 1 randomized controlled trial. PLoS One 5(2), e9041
5. Bergmann-Leitner ES, Duncan EH, Mullen GE et al (2006) Critical evaluation of different methods for measuring the functional activity of antibodies against malaria blood stage antigens. Am J Trop Med Hyg 75(3):437–442
6. Ringwald P, Meche FS, Bickii J et al (1999) In vitro culture and drug sensitivity assay of

Plasmodium falciparum with nonserum substitute and acute-phase sera. J Clin Microbiol 37(3):700–705

7. Bergmann-Leitner ES, Duncan EH, Burge JR et al (2008) Short report: miniaturization of a high-throughput pLDH-based Plasmodium falciparum growth inhibition assay for small volume samples from preclinical and clinical vaccine trials. Am J Trop Med Hyg 78(3):468–471
8. Bergmann-Leitner ES, Leitner WW (2008) Antibody purification. In: Biological research methodology—a handbook. Taylor&Francis Group Publishers/CRC Press ISBN 9780849376160
9. Bergmann-Leitner ES, Mease RM, Duncan EH et al (2008) Evaluation of immunoglobulin purification methods and their impact on quality and yield of antigen-specific antibodies. Malar J 7(1):129
10. Haynes JD, Moch JK (2002) Automated synchronization of Plasmodium falciparum parasites by culture in a temperature-cycling incubator. Methods Mol Med 72:489–497

Chapter 14

Measuring *Plasmodium falciparum* Erythrocyte Invasion Phenotypes Using Flow Cytometry

Amy Kristine Bei and Manoj T. Duraisingh

Abstract

Having the ability to rapidly, accurately, and robustly measure *Plasmodium falciparum* merozoite invasion is a critical component in effective assessment of a blood stage vaccine's mechanism of action. Being able to measure invasion of erythrocytes accurately, objectively and in a high throughput fashion is of critical importance. Here, we describe a simple and robust flow cytometry method that allows for the measurement of the key invasion parameters of parasite multiplication rate and erythrocyte selectivity—both important determinants of disease severity—from the schizont to the ring stage of the parasite's life-cycle, thus separating invasion from growth of the parasite. Importantly, this method is able to accurately detect low levels of parasitemia and heterogeneity within the population that can be missed by enzymatic methods. Lastly, this method has been successfully adapted and employed in field based research settings for parasitemia measurements in vivo, ex vivo, and in vitro and to measure invasion inhibition by antibodies and the use of alternative pathways for invasion.

Key words Flow cytometry, Plasmodium, Erythrocyte invasion, Merozoite, Malaria, Blood-stage vaccine, Neutralizing antibodies

1 Introduction

The process of erythrocyte invasion is an essential step in the *Plasmodium* parasite's life cycle and a virulence determinant in the disease, in addition to a vaccine target [1]. Recently, there has been a renewed interest in the development of a blood-stage vaccine against malaria [2, 3], and with such interest comes the need for a sensitive, robust, and high-throughput technique to measure invasion and invasion inhibition, of both laboratory adapted strains and parasites from malaria infected patients.

Depending on the specific question and scientific application, there are many aspects to measuring merozoite invasion: (1) measuring parasitemia, PMR, and erythrocyte selectivity; (2) measuring erythrocyte invasion pathways; (3) measuring antibody inhibition of invasion. For some applications, measuring in vivo parasitemia in a high-throughput manner is essential.

Ashley M. Vaughan (ed.), *Malaria Vaccines: Methods and Protocols*, Methods in Molecular Biology, vol. 1325,
DOI 10.1007/978-1-4939-2815-6_14, © Springer Science+Business Media New York 2015

As erythrocyte selectivity has been described as a virulence factor of malaria disease in some [4–7], but not all studies [8], being about to measure erythrocyte selectivity can also be important. Regardless of the specific invasion phenotype of interest, having the ability to rapidly, accurately, and robustly measure essential erythrocyte determinants of *Plasmodium falciparum* merozoite invasion, both in the lab and in the field, is a critical component in evaluating the efficacy of a blood stage malaria vaccine.

Until recently [9], genetic modification of the erythrocyte was not possible and studies of essential erythrocyte determinants of invasion were limited to rare erythrocyte mutants and biochemical methods of removing nonoverlapping sets of erythrocyte receptors by enzymatic cleavage [10–12]. Such biochemical (enzymatic) methods still represent the accepted standard in the field for studying erythrocyte receptor usage—or, invasion pathways—especially as they can be conducted in malaria endemic settings [8, 13–17], and will be described here.

Perhaps most critical in evaluating a blood stage malaria vaccines is the ability to determine the invasion inhibitory potential of vaccine-generated neutralizing antibodies against parasite invasion. There are many methods to measure such inhibition [18–24]; and the method described in this chapter for measuring parasitemia by flow can be easily adapted to any of these methods to detect even very low levels of reinvasion parasitemia, with reproducible accuracy to 0.1–0.2 %.

This chapter will describe methods used to measure ex vivo and in vitro parasitemia, as well as invasion phenotypes related to virulence and/or vaccine efficacy such as erythrocyte selectivity, invasion pathway, multiplication rate, and antibody mediated invasion inhibition. Technically, all of the assays described here are simple and can be easily scaled for high-throughput cytometers (such as those with 96 well-plate capacity). All the experiments described have been performed in the field with a flow cytometer equipped with a blue (488 nm) laser, the default for nearly all, even simple portable flow cytometers.

The key advantages of the method described here are the ability to separate the measurement of invasion from intraerythrocytic growth of the parasite, the ability to accurately measure very low parasitemia at the ring stage (0.1 %), and the ability to measure DNA content, and by extension, erythrocyte selectivity, and the ability to measure not only laboratory adapted strains of parasites but also uncultured isolates directly from infected patients in the field.

2 Materials

2.1 Equipment

1. Tissue culture hood.
2. Incubator: 37 °C.

3. Mixed gas cylinder or gas mixing device [25]: 1 % O_2, 5 % CO_2, N_2 balance.
4. Modular Incubator Chamber (Billups-Rothenberg).
5. Centrifuge that can spin both conical tubes (15–50 mL) and 96 well plates.
6. Flow Cytometer with filters appropriate for detection of common fluorochromes including fluorescein isothiocyanate (FITC): BD FacsCalibur was used for all experiments described, but a BD Accuri has also been shown to be useful for high throughput field-based experiments.
7. Light Microscope: equipped with a 40× objective and 100× oil objective as well as a Miller Reticle.
8. Hemocytometer.
9. Cell Counter.
10. Pipettes: multichannel (p200), single channel (p2, p10, p20, p200, p1,000), and pipette aids for serological pipettes.

2.2 Reagents

1. *P. falciparum* culture adapted isolates or *P. falciparum* uncultured field isolates.
2. Water: Tissue culture grade water, Milli-Q Synthesis or double distilled (ddH_2O).
3. Human blood (O+ erythrocytes).
4. Pooled AB human serum, heat inactivated at 56 °C for 1 h; sterile-transferred to bottles or 50 mL conical tubes and frozen at −20 °C until needed.
5. Unsupplemented RPMI media: made according to the protocol in Subheading 3.1.
6. AlbuMAX: 5 % (w/v) AlbuMAX II (Gibco) is made with unsupplemented RPMI media, sterile filtered and aliquoted into 50 mL conical tubes; freeze at −20 °C until ready for use. Store at 4 °C no longer than 14 days.
7. Sodium bicarbonate: 3.6 % Sodium bicarbonate is made in sterile water, sterile filtered and aliquoted into 50 mL conical tubes; freeze at −20 °C until ready for use. Store at 4 °C no longer than 30 days.
8. Sodium hydroxide: Using a 5 M commercial stock, make a 1 M working solution by diluting 100 mL of 5 M NaOH into 500 mL of water; store in a sealed glass container at room temperature for up to 1 year.
9. Sorbitol: 5 % (w/v) d-sorbitol made in sterile water, sterile filtered. Store at 4 °C no longer than 3 months.
10. Phosphate buffered saline (PBS): 1× PBS, pH 7.4.
11. PBS–BSA: 1× PBS, pH 7.4 with 0.5 % bovine serum albumin (BSA) with 0.02 % sodium azide (*see* **Note 1**).

12. SYBR Green I Buffer: make a 5–10× final stock by adding 0.5–1 μL of SYBR Green I stock (10,000×, Molecular Probes) to 1 mL of PBS (*see* **Note 2**).
13. Fixing solution: 1 % paraformaldehyde (PFA) with 0.0075 % glutaraldehyde in 1× PBS, pH 7.4; made fresh for each experiment or stored at 4 °C no longer than 7 days (*see* **Note 3**).
14. Alsever's solution: Can be purchased commercially or made. To make, dissolve 4.2 g NaCl, 8.0 g Citric Acid ($3Na{\cdot}2H_2O$), 0.55 g Citric Acid·H_2O, 20.5 g d-Glucose in 1 L sterile water, sterile filter and store at 4 °C no longer than 14 days.
15. 1 % PFA/Alsever's solution: 1 % paraformaldehyde in Alsever's Solution, made fresh for each experiment or stored at 4 °C no longer than 14 days.
16. Enzyme sources and stock concentrations:
    (a) Neuraminidase (Nm): 1 U/mL (Sigma).
    (b) Trypsin (T): 3.334 mg/mL (Sigma).
    (c) Chymotrypsin (Chymo): 3.334 mg/mL (Worthington).
17. RNase A: 0.5 mg/mL RNase A (MP Biomedicals) in 1× PBS.
18. Petri dishes or flasks for parasite cultures.
19. 96-well plates flat bottom plates for invasion assays.
20. 96-well flat bottom half-well plates for inhibition assays.
21. Microscopy slides for culture morphology monitoring.

3 Methods

3.1 Preparation of RPMI Media

RPMI media preparation is an essential step for invasion and inhibition assay erythrocyte preparation and for the successful and robust growth of ex vivo or in vitro *P. falciparum* parasite cultures. The unsupplemented media, described here, will serve as the base for preparing uninfected erythrocytes for assays, for resuspending purified IgG for inhibition assays, as well as for final supplementation which is required for parasite culture.

1. To make 1 L of RPMI media for in vitro culture, add 700 mL of sterile water to a 2 L flask and stir constantly with a magnetic stir bar.
2. Add 10.44 g RPMI powder (Sigma) to the flask.
3. Add 5.94 g HEPES to the flask.
4. Add 50 mg of hypoxanthine to 9 mL of sterile water and 500 μL 1 M NaOH. Shake vigorously until all the hypoxanthine has dissolved, and then add to the flask.
5. Add 0.5 mL gentamicin to the flask.
6. Add 250 mL of sterile water to the flask.

7. Adjust the pH to *exactly* 6.75 with 1 M NaOH
8. Sterile filter using 1 L filter units and aliquot as needed (*see* **Note 4**).

3.2 Preparation of Supplemented RPMI Media

1. To 100 mL of unsupplemented RPMI add 5 mL of AlbuMAX
2. Add 5 mL of heat inactivated AB serum
3. Add 5.9 mL of Sodium bicarbonate
4. Store supplemented RPMI media at 4 °C no longer than 14 days.

3.3 Preparation of *P. falciparum* Cultures

1. If ex vivo parasites are used from *P. falciparum* infected patients, the parasites will already be semi-synchronous at the ring stage and no further synchronization is needed. If culture adapted parasites are used, synchronous ring stage cultures should be maintained for at least two reinvasion cycles prior to the assay.
2. To synchronize in vitro parasite cultures, when the parasite stage is mostly early rings (1–8 h post-invasion), transfer culture to a 15 mL conical tube and centrifuge at 800 × *g* to pellet erythrocytes.
3. Remove supernatant and add 5 mL of 5 % d-sorbitol, resuspend well and incubate at 37 °C for 10 min.
4. Centrifuge at 800 × *g* for 5 min, wash twice with 10 mL unsupplemented RPMI media.
5. Centrifuge at 800 × *g* for 5 min, wash once with 10 mL supplemented RPMI media.
6. Centrifuge at 800 × *g* for 5 min, resuspend in 10 mL supplemented RPMI media, plate in a petri dish or flask, gas and replace in the 37 °C incubator.
7. Repeat at next reinvasion cycle when parasites are early rings again.

3.4 Preparation of Acceptor Cells (O+ Cells from the Same Donor)

Acceptor cells serve as the base for erythrocyte invasion assays and inhibition assays. Enzymatic treatment of erythrocytes reveals specific "invasion pathways" by cleaving nonoverlapping sets of receptors. The enzymatic treatment of these erythrocytes is described below.

1. Aliquot 200 μL of packed O+ erythrocytes (100 % hematocrit) into 15 mL conical tubes containing 10 mL PBS for each individual enzyme treatment—final: 2 % hematocrit (*see* **Note 5**).
2. Centrifuge at 800 × *g* for 5 min, wash cells twice with PBS, once with unsupplemented RPMI.
3. Prepare Trypsin and Chymotrypsin enzyme stocks just before treating.

Table 1
Erythrocyte enzyme treatments

Enzyme treatment	Volume of enzyme (stock concentration)	Volume of RPMI	Volume of RBC	Final enzyme concentration
Nm	40 μL Nm	360 μL RPMI	200 μL RBC	66.7 mU/mL Nm
Low T	12 μL T	388 μL RPMI	200 μL RBC	66.7 μg/mL T
High T	180 μL T	220 μL RPMI	200 μL RBC	1.0 mg/mL T
Nm/Low T	40 μL Nm, 12 μL T	348 μL RPMI	200 μL RBC	66.7 mU/mL Nm, 66.7 μg/mL T
Chymo/Low T	180 μL Chymo, 12 μL T	208 μL RPMI	200 μL RBC	1.0 mg/mL Chymo, 66.7 μg/mL T
Chymo	180 μL Chymo	220 μL RPMI	200 μL RBC	1.0 mg/mL Chymo
Nm/T/Chymo	40 μL Nm, 180 μL T, 180 μL Chymo	0 μL RPMI	200 μL RBC	66.7 mU/mL Nm, 1.0 mg/mL T, 1.0 mg/mL Chymo
RPMI	0 μL	400 μL RPMI	200 μL RBC	NA

4. Set up enzyme treatments with unsupplemented RPMI according to the following guidelines (Table 1):
5. Incubate at 37 °C in a rotating incubator for 1 h.
6. Wash cells twice with 10 mL PBS, once with 10 mL incomplete RPMI.
7. Resuspend cells in 10 mL supplemented RPMI media—final: 2 % hematocrit.

3.5 Preparation of Donor Cells (Ex Vivo Parasitized Cells from Patients or In Vitro Cultures)

Enzymatic treatment of the donor parasitized erythrocytes is performed to remove essential erythrocyte receptors and prevent reinvasion into the patients' own cells. This procedure allows the parasites to develop and mature within the donor cells, but when the merozoites emerge, they are only able to invade the acceptor cells, described previously, thus eliminating competition for invasion into two different cell populations: those of the infected donor and those of the acceptor.

1. Transfer culture or parasitized patient blood to a 15 mL conical tube.
2. Centrifuge at 800 × *g* for 5 min, resuspend parasitized cells to 2 % hematocrit (remove 200 μL parasitized RBCs and resuspend in 10 mL RPMI).
3. Dilute parasitemia to 2 % (between 0.75 and 2 % is ideal) with uninfected O+ cells (also at 2 % hematocrit).

4. Wash cells three times as above (800×*g* for 5 min) with unsupplemented RPMI.
5. Treat cells with Nm/T/Chymo and incubate at 37 °C in a rotating incubator for 1 h (*see* **Note 6**).
6. Wash cells 2 times with unsupplemented RPMI, 1 time with supplemented RPMI.
7. Resuspend cells to 2 % hematocrit (200 μL parasitized RBCs in 10 mL supplemented RPMI).

3.6 Plating of Invasion Assays

1. Plate parasitized donor cells and uninfected/enzyme treated acceptor cells 50:50 (v/v) in a 96-well flat bottom plate at a final parasitemia of 1 % (between 0.375 % and 1 % is ideal) and a final hematocrit of 2 % (and generally a final volume of 100 μL). Plate samples in triplicate and plate an additional well with positive control cells (RPMI treated acceptor cells) to monitor assay progression and morphology (this well will not be read by flow cytometry but is useful in determining when the assay reaches completion).
2. For determination of parasite multiplication rate (PMR), initial parasitemia must also be measured by flow analysis. In a U-bottom plate, plate an additional row of triplicate samples with parasitized donor cells and RPMI treated acceptor cells 50:50 (v/v) for each parasite sample. With this plate only, continue directly to Subheading 3.9 for assay harvesting.
3. Incubate assay plates at 37 °C in a candle jar or a gassed incubator or modular incubator chamber gassed with 1 % O_2, 5 % CO_2, nitrogen balance (94 % N_2) until parasite reinvasion (approximately 48 h post-blood draw/plating—monitor parasite growth by microscopy in a control well).

3.7 Preparation of IgG for Inhibition Assays

Many methods exist for purifying IgG for inhibition assays [18, 22, 24, 26], but the unifying criteria are that the antibodies are specific and pure; free from other contaminating serum proteins, which could potentially inhibit invasion. The method below is one such method that has been used to assess antibody-mediated inhibition of invasion.

1. From plasma or serum from pooled or individual exposed donors, purify IgG using Protein G Sepharose columns. (If plasma is used, be sure to collect in EDTA tubes rather than heparin tubes, as heparin can inhibit erythrocyte invasion).
2. Wash IgG extensively using unsupplemented RPMI if proceeding directly to antibody inhibition assay, or PBS if continuing to further purify using specific antigens.
3. If antigen-specific IgG are required, couple the antigen of interest to cyanogen bromide (CNBr)–activated Sepharose

columns and run purified IgG, diluted 1:10 with PBS, over the column.

4. To allow rapid and extensive washing, column chromatography was performed on an AktaFPLC (GE Healthcare).
5. Wash extensively with PBS (at least 20 column volumes, or until the A_{280} (UV absorbance at 280 nm) reaches baseline).
6. Elute antibodies with 100 mM glycine (pH 2.5) in 500 μL fractions into wells containing 50 μL of 1 M Tris–HCl (pH 8.0) to limit the amount of time the antibodies are exposed to low pH.
7. Pool fractions containing peaks, dialyze into unsupplemented RPMI, and concentrate using Amicon Ultra-15 Centrifugal Filter Units. Sterile filter the resulting IgG fraction using Ultrafree-MC Sterile 0.22 μm Centrifugal filter units and adjust the final stock concentration according to the application (*see* **Note 7**), and store antibody stocks at −80 °C until ready for assay plating.

3.8 Plating of Invasion Inhibition Assays (See Note 8)

1. Pellet donor cells by centrifugation 800 × *g* for 5 min (at 2 % hematocrit from Subheading 3.4, **step** 7) and resuspend at 4 % hematocrit (200 μL parasitized RBCs in 5 mL supplemented RPMI).
2. Prepare IgG samples at the desired concentration (*see* **Note** 7), and at 2× final volume, including the appropriate control (*see* **Note 9**).
3. Plate parasitized donor cells, IgG samples and uninfected/enzyme treated acceptor cells 25:25:50 (v/v/v) in a 96-well flat bottom half-well plate for a final parasitemia of 1 % and a final overall hematocrit of 2 % (and generally a final volume of 25–50 μL). Plate samples in triplicate if IgG amounts allow, otherwise plate in duplicate and plate an additional well with positive control cells (RPMI treated acceptor cells) to monitor assay progression and morphology (this well will not be read by flow cytometry but is useful in determining when the assay reaches completion).

3.9 Harvesting Assays and Preparing Samples for Flow Cytometry

1. When parasites have reinvaded and assay is ready for harvesting (fewer than 2 schizonts per 100 infected cells are observed), remove assay plates from the incubator. Re-gas the modular incubator chamber if it contains other assays not yet ready to harvest.
2. Using a p200 multichannel pipette, resuspend cells well and transfer assay wells to a U-bottom plate for ease of centrifugation. Be sure to add an additional well of uninfected erythrocytes at 2 % hematocrit if it is not explicitly included in the assay template. (This well will be used to guide the flow cytometer settings).

Table 2
Flow cytometer settings: voltage and amplifier

Parameter	Detector	Voltage	Amp Gain	Mode
P1	FSC	E00	1.00	Lin
P2	SSC	396	1.00	Lin
P3	FL1	310	1.00	Log

Table 3
Flow cytometer settings: compensation

Parameter	Detector	Voltage
FL1	0 %	FL2
FL2	0 %	FL1
FL2	0 %	FL3
FL3	0 %	FL2

3. Pellet samples by centrifugation (800×*g*, 5 min). If cells are to be stored for up to 2 weeks prior to staining (at 4 °C) and fixation is required, follow alternative fixation protocol, described in **Note 3**.
4. Remove supernatant and wash cells twice with 100 μL of PBS–BSA.
5. Incubate cells with 75 μL of SYBR Green I Buffer for 20 min at 25 °C, with constant agitation.
6. Wash cells twice with 100 μL of PBS–BSA.
7. If cells are to be fixed, resuspend with 100 μL of Fixing solution, incubate at room temperature for 15 min, then wash twice with 100 μL of PBS (*see* **Note 3**). If cells do not need to be fixed, proceed directly to Subheading 3.9, **step 8**.
8. Resuspend in 200 μL of filtered PBS.

3.10 Acquiring Flow Cytometry Data

1. Set the flow cytometer settings according to the following guidelines (Tables 2 and 3), outlined in Subheading 3.10, **steps 1–4** (*see* **Note 10**). The following menu subheadings are based on acquisition using CellQuest Pro software (version 0.3 df3b). Under the "Cytometer" menu, "Detectors/Amps" sub-menu, set the parameters according to Table 2.
2. Under the "Cytometer" menu, "Threshold" sub-menu, set the Primary parameter: FSC, Value: 52.

3. Under the "Cytometer" menu, "Compensation" sub-menu, set all compensation percentages according to Table 3 (no compensation needed).
4. Save settings as a template for future use.
5. Under the "File" menu, open a new acquisition template ("Open new document").
6. Create a dot plot and a histogram plot for acquisition (Fig. 1a, b(ii)). Under the "Plots" menu, "Format histogram" sub-menu, Link the histogram plot to Gate R1 (the erythrocyte gate) of the dot-plot.
7. Under the "Acquire" menu, open the "Parameter description" sub-menu. With the "Setup" option selected, run an uninfected erythrocyte sample. Gate erythrocytes (Gate R1) based on uninfected "pure" erythrocyte population (Fig. 1a).
8. Under instrument settings, adjust FL1 channel so that uninfected erythrocytes fall between 10^0 and 10^1 (Fig. 1b). Re-save instrument settings.
9. Under the "Acquire" menu, "Acquisition & Storage" sub-menu, set the following acquisition parameters: Acquisition Gate: Accept all events; Collection Criteria: Event Count: 100,000 of G1 = R1 (*see* **Note 11**); Storage Gate: Data file will contain ALL events; Resolution: 1,024, Parameters saved to FCS Data file.
10. To set the infected erythrocyte gates, with the "Setup" option selected, Select and run a sample that should represent the positive control and is known to have high reinvasion based on microscopy results (*see* **Note 12**).
11. Make markers for single, double, triple, and quadruple infected peaks (M1, M2, M3, M4) as well as one that includes M1–M4, (M5) (Fig. 1c, ii). M5 represents the total parasitemia; M1–M4 can be used to determine the selectivity index. Re-save acquisition document.
12. Under the "Acquire" menu, open the "Parameter description" sub-menu, determine the file name for the data and the directory to which they will be saved. De-select the "Setup" option and run each sample. Acquisition will stop automatically based on the cell numbers programed into the "Acquisition and storage" sub-menu (*see* Subheading 3.10, **step 9** and **Note 11**).

3.11 Analyzing Flow Cytometry Data

1. Remove FCS files from acquisition computer and open with analysis software of choice. The analysis procedure described here will be using FlowJo analysis software (version 9.5.3).
2. Recreate the gates as defined for data acquisition, both the erythrocyte gated dot plot (Fig. 1a) and the FL1 histogram with markers M1–M5 (Fig. 1c, ii).

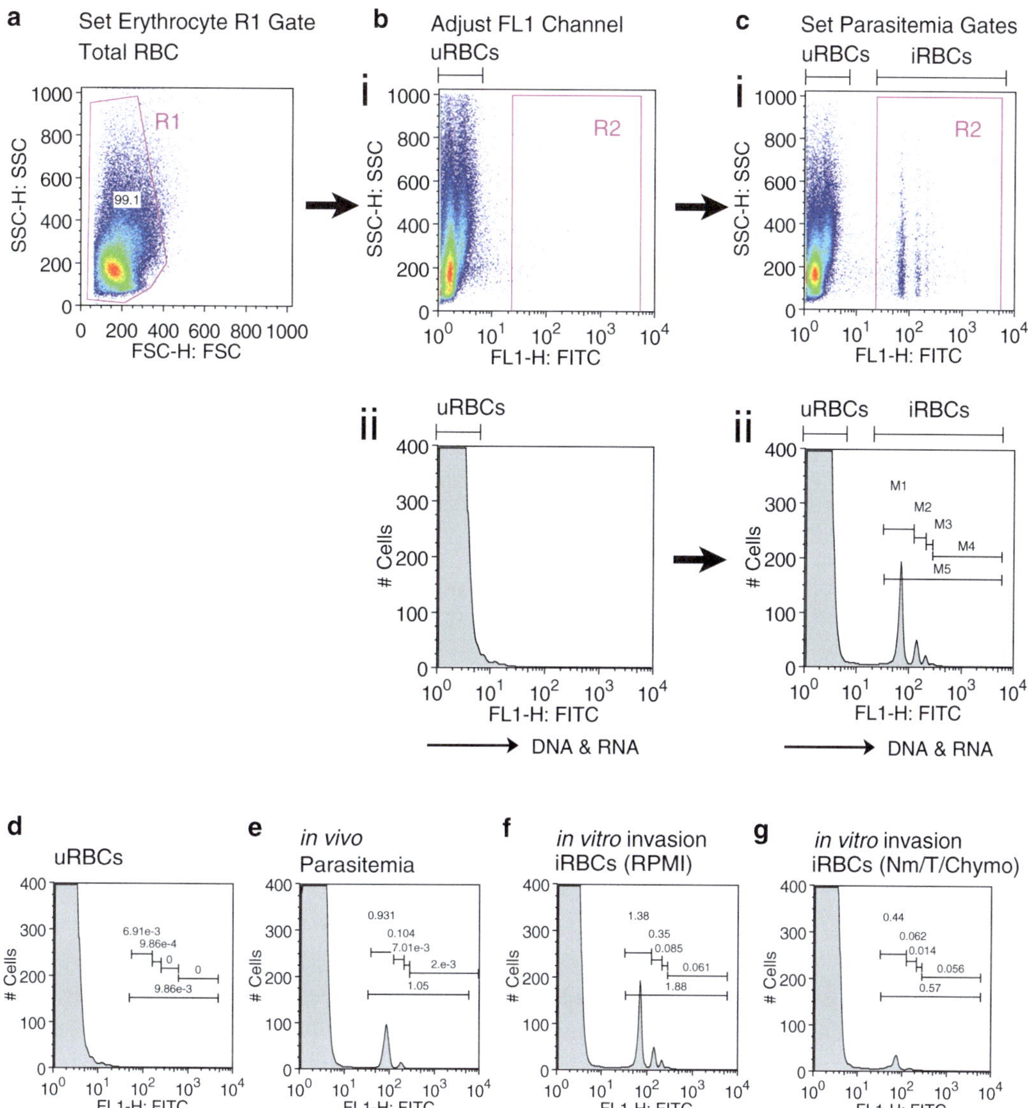

Fig. 1 Gating strategy and examples of data generated by SYBR Green Flow Cytometry. (**a**–**c**) Gating strategy. (**a**) Setting the erythrocyte R1 gate in the forward scatter (FSC) by side scatter (SSC) dot plot. (**b**) Adjusting the FL1 channel to ensure proper reading of infected and uninfected controls. Plots shown represent the FL1 (FITC) by side scatter (SSC) dot plot (i) as well as the FL1 (FITC) histogram (ii). Settings are adjusted so uninfected erythrocytes register between 10^0 and 10^1 on the log scale. (**c**) Setting the parasitemia gates based on infected erythrocytes. Plots shown represent the FL1 (FITC) by side scatter (SSC) dot plot (i) as well as the FL1 (FITC) histogram (ii). Infected erythrocytes are gated as R2 (**c**.i) or M1-M5 (**c**.ii) with M1 representing singly infected, M2 representing doubly, M3 representing triply, M4 representing quadruply infected erythrocytes, and M5 representing total parasitemia. (**d**–**g**) Example parasitemia data generated in the histogram view for uninfected erythrocytes (**d**), ex vivo measured parasitemia (**e**), in vitro measured reinvasion into RPMI treated erythrocytes (*positive control*) (**f**), in vitro measured reinvasion into Nm/T/Chymo treated erythrocytes (*negative control*) (**g**)

3. Validate the gates with uninfected erythrocytes (Fig. 1d) and a positive control sample with high parasitemia (Fig. 1f).
4. Once gates have been set and validated, advance through all samples and export data into Microsoft Excel.

3.12 Analyzing In Vivo and Ex Vivo/In Vitro Parasitemia and Erythrocyte Selectivity

For the purposes of this chapter, "in vivo" is the condition where parasitized blood is analyzed immediately from the patient, "ex vivo" is the condition where parasitized blood is cultured directly from the patient for one cycle of reinvasion, and "in vitro" is the condition where the parasites used have been culture adapted.

1. To calculate in vivo parasitemia, average triplicate measurements for each sample. No subtraction is necessary as there is no appropriate uninfected control matched to the infected patient sample (*see* **Note 13**). The M5 value will represent the total parasitemia and markers M1–M4 will be used to determine in vivo selectivity index (Fig. 1e) [4, 5].
2. To calculate in vivo selectivity index, average triplicate measurements for each marker (M1, M2, M3, M4, M5) for each sample without background subtraction. To calculate ex vivo or in vitro selectivity index (*see* **Note 14**), average triplicate measurements for marker (M1, M2, M3, M4, M5) for each sample (Fig. 1f) and subtract from this value the averaged triplicate values from uninfected erythrocytes (Fig. 1d). Based on DNA content, markers correspond to the following: M1 = single infected erythrocytes, M2 = double infected erythrocytes, M3 = triple infected erythrocytes, M4 = quadruple infected erythrocytes, M5 = total parasitemia.
3. The selectivity index (SI) is a ratio of the total number of observed multiply-infected erythrocytes (O) compared to the total number of expected multiply-infected erythrocytes (E) from a random process, estimated by a Poisson distribution. Expected multiply-infected erythrocytes (E) is calculated as follows: $[P(n)/(1-P(0))] \times$(total number of infected cells considered), where $P(n)$ is the probability of observing "n" parasites per cell [4, 5].

$$\mathrm{SI} = \frac{\left[\text{Total number of observed multiply infected erythrocytes}\,(\mathrm{O})\right]}{\left[\text{Total number of expected multiply infected erythrocytes}\,(\mathrm{E})\right]}$$

$$\mathrm{SI} = \frac{\left[\#\text{ of observed}\,(\text{double}+\text{triple}+\text{quadruple})\text{ multiply infected erythrocytes}\right]}{\left[\#\text{ of expected}\,(\text{double}+\text{triple}+\text{quadruple})\text{ multiply infected erythrocytes}\right]}$$

3.13 Measuring Ex Vivo/In Vitro Invasion Pathway and Multiplication Rate

1. Average M5 parasitemia triplicate measurements for each sample.
2. Subtract M5 background measurements for each sample. Background measurements include uninfected erythrocytes (Fig. 1d) and (Nm/T/Chymo treated cells) (Fig. 1g) (*see* **Note 15**).
3. To determine the % Invasion for each enzyme treated cell population, divide the background-subtracted samples by the parasitemia for the RPMI treated sample and multiply by 100:

$$\text{Invasion}\,(\%) = \frac{[\text{M5 parasitemia into enzyme treated cells}\,(\%)]}{[\text{M5 parasitemia into RPMI treated cells}\,(\%)]} \times 100$$

4. To determine the Parasite Multiplication Rate (PMR), use the following equation (*see* **Note 16**):

$$\text{PMR} = \left(\frac{[\text{Final RPMI parasitemia}\,(\%)]}{[\text{Initial RPMI parasitemia}\,(\%)]}\right) \times 2$$

3.14 Measuring In Vitro Invasion Inhibition by Antibodies

1. To measure invasion inhibition, average M5 parasitemia triplicate (or duplicate) measurements for each sample.
2. Subtract M5 background measurements for each sample. Background measurements include uninfected erythrocytes (Fig. 1d) and (Nm/T/Chymo treated cells) (Fig. 1g) (*see* **Note 15**), if enzyme treated donor cells were used in the assay set up.
3. To determine the Invasion Inhibition percentage for each antibody, use the following equation:

$$\text{Invasion Inhibition}\,(\%) = 100\left(\frac{[\text{M5 parasitemia into antibody containing wells}\,(\%)]}{[\text{M5 parasitemia into control wells}\,(\%)]} \times 100\right)$$

4 Notes

1. Adding 0.02 % sodium azide to the PBS–BSA is optional depending on the duration of storage and the sterile conditions used. PBS–BSA is always filter-sterilized and aliquoted in the tissue culture hood, so sodium azide is often unnecessary. However, adding sodium azide may be preferred if a large amount of buffer is to be stored at 4 °C for extended periods and sterile aliquoting is not performed.
2. Generally, SYBR Green Buffer is made at a final working concentration of 10× (1 μL SYBR/1,000 μL PBS) [27]. However,

to save reagents and cost, it is also possible to use a final working concentration of 5× (0.5 μL SYBR/1,000 μL PBS). As with any dye-based staining procedure, the concentration and the time will affect the intensity of the signal, and hence the flow cytometry settings. The FL1 flow cytometry instrument settings will need to be adjusted accordingly so that uninfected cells fall between the 10^0 and 10^1 region (Fig. 1b). This is done in the "Cytometer" menu, "Instrument settings" sub-menu of CellQuest Pro and should be adjusted prior to acquisition of all data.

3. The decision whether to fix or not fix *Plasmodium* infected cells depends on the biosafety rules of the institution and the particular flow cytometer. Occasionally, even when fixed correctly, fixative reagent batches can cause lysis, which will alter parasitemia measurements. We describe here a very gentle fixing method that is still in agreement with biosafety recommendations, should fixing be absolutely required. Otherwise, we would recommend running samples unfixed, immediately after staining and harvesting (*see* Subheading 3.9, **step** 7). If samples need to be stored prior to harvesting, the following alternative fixation protocol can be used:
   (a) Starting after **step 3** in Subheading 3.9, wash once in 100 μL Alsever's solution.
   (b) Pellet samples by centrifugation (800 × *g*, 5 min).
   (c) Resuspend cells in 1 % PFA/Alsever's solution and fix for 10 min at room temperature.
   (d) Pellet samples by centrifugation (800 × *g*, 5 min).
   (e) Resuspend cells in Alsever's solution. Parafilm around the edges of the 96-well plate and store at 4 °C for up to 14 days.
   (f) When ready to stain and acquire by flow cytometry, return to Methods (Subheading 3.9, **step 4**).
4. When preparing the RPMI media, the final volume will not quite equal 1 L (~960 mL). Do not be tempted to top up the volume to 1 L with water as this will alter the osmolality when the supplements are added.
5. There are two possible methods for measuring and adjusting hematocrit. The first is to carefully and accurately count cells using a hemocytometer and adjust final hematocrits to the same cell numbers/mL (with the approximation that 100 % hematocrit is the same as 1×10^{10} cells/mL). Therefore to make a 2 % hematocrit solution of cells, one would adjust the cells to 2×10^8 cells/mL The second is to adjust by volume assuming that well-packed erythrocytes (centrifuged at 800 × *g* for 5 min) represent 100 % hematocrit. Therefore to make a

2 % hematocrit solution of cells, one would add 200 μL of packed erythrocytes (100 % hematocrit) to 10 mL of buffer. Either method is reasonable but one should be selected and used consistently throughout the protocol.

6. For assessment of invasion pathway usage, treatment of parasitized donor cells with Nm/T/Chymo is one method of preventing reinvasion into donor cells and measuring invasion specifically into the enzyme treated cells of interest. Another method of specifically measuring acceptor cell invasion that does not require enzymatically treating parasitized donor cells is by distinguishing acceptor cells from donor cells by fluorescent staining prior to parasite invasion [17, 28]. Each method has its own challenges: enzyme treatment, as described here, involves more manipulation; whereas, dual-staining methods can result in merozoite invasion competition between untreated donor cells and enzymatically treated acceptor cells, an effect which has been quantified in optimization experiments [28].

7. Final IgG concentrations can vary depending on many factors such as whether affinity purified IgG or total IgG is used, the specific affinity purified target, whether a gradient of concentrations or single concentrations are to be tested, and whether the goal is to obtain maximum inhibition and an IC_{50} or attempt to replicate a specific range of physiological IgG concentrations (naturally occurring or post-vaccination) [18–24]. For these reasons, we will not state a specific concentration for IgG.

8. There are many different ways to perform invasion inhibition assays in the presence of IgG. No matter what plating method is used [18, 22, 24], all can be harvested by flow cytometry if desired. We have found that flow cytometry harvesting can increase the sensitivity normally detected by enzymatic assays such that rather than a limit of detection of 0.6 % (data not shown), we are able to accurately measure between 0.1 % and 0.2 % parasitemia [27]. Depending on the reinvasion rates of the strains of interest (this is a much more relevant concern for ex vivo or short term in vitro adapted field lines than robust laboratory adapted lines), this may or may not be a concern and a reason to harvest by flow cytometry.

9. Another important consideration for inhibition assays is the specific control comparator for the experiment such that the appearance of nonspecific inhibition (or enhancement) is minimized. Some studies use supplemented media alone whereas others use an equivalent concentration of isotype control antibody from unexposed individuals or populations. However, as this chapter is largely concerned with the measurement of the resulting parasitemia by flow cytometry, specifics of invasion inhibition assay design will not be discussed in depth.

10. Exact flow cytometer settings will vary from machine to machine, so these are merely guidelines. But if Fig. 1 is used as a guide, the appropriate settings for the individual user's machine can be obtained and saved. Note that the settings may need slight adjustment each time a new experiment is run (for each independent staining procedure) as the time of staining and the time to acquisition by flow can slightly affect the FL1 intensity. Follow the FL1 channel adjustment guidelines (Subheading 3.10, **step 8**) with uninfected cells before acquiring all sample data.

11. If the primary downstream analysis will be calculating ex vivo or in vitro selectivity index, the acquisition settings can be changed to require the same number of infected cells be acquired per sample. For example, under the "Acquire" menu, "Acquisition and Storage" sub-menu, specify the "Collection Criteria": Event Count: 1,000 of gate G2 = R2 (Fig. 1c, i). In this way, for each sample, the same number of infected erythrocytes will be counted. If multiple analyses (PMR, parasitemia, etc.) are to be performed on the same sample, either two separate acquisitions can be run and saved (one as described in **step 9** in Subheading 3.10 for parasitemia with 100,000 erythrocytes counted (G1 = R1) and one as described here with 1,000 parasitized erythrocytes counted (G2 = R2)), or the selectivity index can be calculated taking into account the specific number of infected erythrocytes counted for each sample, which will vary based on the parasitemia. Both acquisition schemes will save all events, but the difference is whether or not the total erythrocytes or the infected erythrocytes are the defining cell count criteria for stopping the acquisition.

12. While infected erythrocyte markers are needed during the analysis stage, they are not essential during the acquisition stage. However, should the user want to have an idea of the parasitemia as the samples are being run, they can be added to the acquisition template. Also, should the user be using CellQuest Pro as their analysis platform, the markers are useful to save into the acquisition template as they can be converted to the analysis template after all samples are collected.

13. We and others have found a very high correlation between SYBR Green measured parasitemia and microscopy measured parasitemia in in vitro parasite cultures [27, 28]. When measuring in vivo parasitemia, there are 3 potential sources of background when measuring with SYBR Green: (a) RNA-containing reticulocytes, (b) Gametocytes, and (c) Nonviable parasites. One of the advantages of SYBR Green is that is has at least an 11-fold greater sensitivity for DNA than for RNA [29]. However, should this still prove insufficient and if background levels are high due to increased reticulocytes, samples can first

be treated with RNase A prior to SYBR Green staining [28]. Briefly, this involves centrifuging cells just prior to SYBR Green Staining (Subheading 3.9, **step 3**), washing once with PBS, incubating with 100 μL of RNase A for 1 h at 37 °C, followed by two washes with PBS prior to continuing the staining procedure at **step 4** in Subheading 3.9. (Background due to human white blood cells is not an issue as these cells are much larger and more granular than erythrocytes and also have a much higher DNA content, so they are gated out of the analysis.) Gametocytemia of infected patients will be incorporated into total parasitemia by this method as gametocytes contain twice the DNA content of a single genome [30] and would resemble double infected ring-stage parasites or trophozoites. However, it has been proposed that DNA and RNA specific staining, which allows for careful separating of parasite asexual stages [31], could also be applied to separate gametocytes based on their unique DNA and RNA content combinations [32]. Lastly, while less likely to be an issue due to the clearance of dead parasites by the spleen in vivo, if one was monitoring parasitemia over time with drug treatment or in vitro culture parasitemia over multiple cycles without sub-culture (for example), nonviable parasites clearly identifiable by microscopy would not be distinguished from viable parasites by SYBR Green flow cytometry. Dyes measuring mitochondrial membrane potential as a marker for parasite viability have been used for this purpose [33], albeit measuring the ring stage, which is most prevalent in in vivo samples, is more difficult. This source of background emphasizes the need for occasional microscopy spot checks of morphology prior to harvesting certain kinds of assays.

14. When calculating in vitro selectivity index, it is important to consider and record whether the assay was conducted under static or shaking conditions, as shaking, similar to in vivo conditions under physiologic flow, can decrease the number of multiply infected cells [34, 35] (although this effect is greater in petri dishes and flasks than in 96-well plates).
15. While we have found the parasitemia measurements performed by flow to correlate extremely well with microscopy for all enzyme treatments used in invasion assays, the exception can sometimes lie with the background calculation. The flow measurements of Nm/T/Chymo treated cells occasionally do not correlate with microscopy. We have found this problem more often with ex vivo field strains rather than laboratory adapted lines. We speculate that the most likely source of the lack or correlation is that often (especially at high parasitemia), when all cells are treated with Nm/T/Chymo and reinvasion is completely inhibited, schizont material (specifically merozoites)

can attach to the outside of enzyme treated cells but do not invade. These stuck merozoites are counted as "infected" cells by flow cytometry as the cellular unit contains a FITC-positive stuck merozoite, but flow does not distinguish whether the merozoite is inside or outside the erythrocyte. By microscopy it is clear that the cells are uninfected, and hence the disconnect between the flow and the microscopy for the Nm/T/Chymo treated cells. For this reason, it is up to the user how to deal with this disconnect, and there are a few possibilities. Firstly, many in the invasion field do not perform this negative control subtraction and instead measure just the enzyme treatments [17]. Another possibility is to qualitatively assess the Nm/T/Chymo treated cells by microscopy to verify that there is no background in the assay (and the enzyme treatments have been successful) rather than measure them by flow and subtract. A third possibility is to set a stringent cut-off criterion for a successful assay: PMR must be greater than 1 and the RPMI reinvasion parasitemia must be at least twice the Nm/T/Chymo background level. The downside of the third option is that it may result in excluding data that is still accurate and informative. It is important to note that this caveat only affects measuring invasion pathway by flow and considering the Nm/T/Chymo population. For all other applications not involving enzyme treatments, it is irrelevant.

16. For PMR calculations in which Nm/T/Chymo treated parasitized donor cells are mixed 50:50 (v/v) with acceptor cells, multiplying by a factor of 2 accounts for the fact that only ½ of the cells in the well can be invaded [16]. If PMR is calculated using a non-enzyme treated culture (for example, if parasitized erythrocytes are directly cultured and parasitemia is measured at each reinvasion cycle) the factor of 2 is not used.

Acknowledgements

The authors would like to acknowledge Dr. Jeffrey Dvorin for critical reading of the manuscript.

References

1. Wright GJ, Rayner JC (2014) Plasmodium falciparum erythrocyte invasion: combining function with immune evasion. PLoS Pathog 10(3), e1003943
2. Crabb BS, Beeson JG (2005) Promising functional readouts of immunity in a blood-stage malaria vaccine trial. PLoS Med 2(11), e380
3. Richards JS, Beeson JG (2009) The future for blood-stage vaccines against malaria. Immunol Cell Biol 87(5):377–390
4. Simpson JA, Silamut K, Chotivanich K, Pukrittayakamee S, White NJ (1999) Red cell selectivity in malaria: a study of multiple-infected erythrocytes. Trans R Soc Trop Med Hyg 93(2):165–168
5. Chotivanich K, Udomsangpetch R, Simpson JA, Newton P, Pukrittayakamee S, Looareesuwan S, White NJ (2000) Parasite multiplication potential and the severity of Falciparum malaria. J Infect Dis 181(3):1206–1209

6. Walliker D, Sanderson A, Yoeli M, Hargreaves BJ (1976) A genetic investigation of virulence in a rodent malaria parasite. Parasitology 72(2): 183–194
7. Bungener W (1985) Virulence of plasmodium yoelii line YM is caused by altered preference for parasitized and unparasitized immature and mature erythrocytes. Trop Med Parasitol 36(1):43–45
8. Deans A-M, Nery S, Conway DJ, Kai O, Marsh K, Rowe JA (2007) Invasion pathways and malaria severity in Kenyan Plasmodium falciparum clinical isolates. Infect Immun 75(6): 3014–3020
9. Bei AK, Brugnara C, Duraisingh MT (2010) In vitro genetic analysis of an erythrocyte determinant of malaria infection. J Infect Dis 202:1722–1727
10. Reed MB, Caruana SR, Batchelor AH, Thompson JK, Crabb BS, Cowman AF (2000) Targeted disruption of an erythrocyte binding antigen in Plasmodium falciparum is associated with a switch toward a sialic acid-independent pathway of invasion. Proc Natl Acad Sci U S A 97(13):7509–7514
11. Duraisingh MT, Maier AG, Triglia T, Cowman AF (2003) Erythrocyte-binding antigen 175 mediates invasion in Plasmodium falciparum utilizing sialic acid-dependent and -independent pathways. Proc Natl Acad Sci U S A 100(8):4796–4801
12. Duraisingh MT, Triglia T, Ralph SA, Rayner JC, Barnwell JW, McFadden GI, Cowman AF (2003) Phenotypic variation of Plasmodium falciparum merozoite proteins directs receptor targeting for invasion of human erythrocytes. EMBO J 22(5):1047–1057
13. Baum J, Pinder M, Conway DJ (2003) Erythrocyte invasion phenotypes of Plasmodium falciparum in The Gambia. Infect Immun 71(4):1856–1863
14. Bei AK, Membi CD, Rayner JC, Mubi M, Ngasala B, Sultan AA, Premji Z, Duraisingh MT (2007) Variant merozoite protein expression is associated with erythrocyte invasion phenotypes in Plasmodium falciparum isolates from Tanzania. Mol Biochem Parasitol 153(1): 66–71
15. Jennings CV, Ahouidi AD, Zilversmit M, Bei AK, Rayner J, Sarr O, Ndir O, Wirth DF, Mboup S, Duraisingh MT (2007) Molecular analysis of erythrocyte invasion in Plasmodium falciparum isolates from Senegal. Infect Immun 75(7):3531–3538
16. Lantos PM, Ahouidi AD, Bei AK, Jennings CV, Sarr O, Ndir O, Wirth DF, Mboup S, Duraisingh MT (2009) Erythrocyte invasion profiles are associated with a common invasion ligand polymorphism in Senegalese isolates of Plasmodium falciparum. Parasitology 136(1):1–9
17. Gomez-Escobar N, Amambua-Ngwa A, Walther M, Okebe J, Ebonyi A, Conway DJ (2010) Erythrocyte invasion and merozoite ligand gene expression in severe and mild Plasmodium falciparum malaria. J Infect Dis 201(3):444–452
18. Persson KEM, McCallum FJ, Reiling L, Lister NA, Stubbs J, Cowman AF, Marsh K, Beeson JG (2008) Variation in use of erythrocyte invasion pathways by Plasmodium falciparum mediates evasion of human inhibitory antibodies. J Clin Invest 118(1):342–351
19. Egan AF, Burghaus P, Druilhe P, Holder AA, Riley EM (1999) Human antibodies to the 19 kDa C-terminal fragment of Plasmodium falciparum merozoite surface protein 1 inhibit parasite growth in vitro. Parasite Immunol 21(3):133–139
20. Douglas AD, Williams AR, Illingworth JJ, Kamuyu G, Biswas S, Goodman AL, Wyllie DH, Crosnier C, Miura K, Wright GJ, Long CA, Osier FH, Marsh K, Turner AV, Hill AV, Draper SJ (2011) The blood-stage malaria antigen PfRH5 is susceptible to vaccine-inducible cross-strain neutralizing antibody. Nat Commun 2:601
21. Rayner JC, Vargas-Serrato E, Huber CS, Galinski MR, Barnwell JW (2001) A Plasmodium falciparum homologue of Plasmodium vivax reticulocyte binding protein (PvRBP1) defines a trypsin-resistant erythrocyte invasion pathway. J Exp Med 194(11):1571–1581
22. Miura K, Zhou H, Moretz SE, Diouf A, Thera MA, Dolo A, Doumbo O, Malkin E, Diemert D, Miller LH, Mullen GED, Long CA (2008) Comparison of biological activity of human anti-apical membrane antigen-1 antibodies induced by natural infection and vaccination. J Immunol 181(12):8776–8783
23. Crosnier C, Bustamante LY, Bartholdson SJ, Bei AK, Theron M, Uchikawa M, Mboup S, Ndir O, Kwiatkowski DP, Duraisingh MT, Rayner JC, Wright GJ (2011) Basigin is a receptor essential for erythrocyte invasion by Plasmodium falciparum. Nature 480:534–537
24. Patel SD, Ahouidi AD, Bei AK, Dieye TN, Mboup S, Harrison SC, Duraisingh MT (2013) Plasmodium falciparum merozoite surface antigen, PfRH5, elicits detectable levels of invasion-inhibiting antibodies in humans. J Infect Dis 208(10):1679–1687
25. Bei AK, Patel SD, Volkman SK, Ahouidi AD, Ndiaye D, Mboup S, Wirth DF (2014) An adjustable gas-mixing device to increase feasibility of in vitro culture of Plasmodium falciparum parasites in the field. PLoS One 9(3), e90928

26. Malkin EME, Diemert DJD, McArthur JHJ, Perreault JRJ, Miles APA, Giersing BKB, Mullen GEG, Orcutt AA, Muratova OO, Awkal MM, Zhou HH, Wang JJ, Stowers AA, Long CAC, Mahanty SS, Miller LHL, Saul AA, Durbin APA (2005) Phase 1 clinical trial of apical membrane antigen 1: an asexual blood-stage vaccine for Plasmodium falciparum malaria. Infect Immun 73(6):3677–3685
27. Bei AK, Desimone TM, Badiane AS, Ahouidi AD, Dieye T, Ndiaye D, Sarr O, Ndir O, Mboup S, Duraisingh MT (2010) A flow cytometry-based assay for measuring invasion of red blood cells by Plasmodium falciparum. Am J Hematol 85(4):234–237
28. Theron M, Hesketh RL, Subramanian S, Rayner JC (2010) An adaptable two-color flow cytometric assay to quantitate the invasion of erythrocytes by Plasmodium falciparum parasites. Cytometry A 77(11):1067–1074
29. Zipper H, Brunner H, Bernhagen J, Vitzthum F (2004) Investigations on DNA intercalation and surface binding by SYBR Green I, its structure determination and methodological implications. Nucleic Acids Res 32(12), e103
30. Janse CJ, Ponnudurai T, Lensen AH, Meuwissen JH, Ramesar J, Van der Ploeg M, Overdulve JP (1988) DNA synthesis in gametocytes of Plasmodium falciparum. Parasitology 96(Pt 1):1–7
31. Grimberg BT, Erickson JJ, Sramkoski RM, Jacobberger JW, Zimmerman PA (2008) Monitoring Plasmodium falciparum growth and development by UV flow cytometry using an optimized Hoechst-thiazole orange staining strategy. Cytometry A 73(6): 546–554
32. Shapiro HM, Apte SH, Chojnowski GM, Hanscheid T, Rebelo M, Grimberg BT (2013) Cytometry in malaria—a practical replacement for microscopy? Curr Protoc Cytom Chapter 11:Unit 11.20
33. Jogdand PS, Singh SK, Christiansen M, Dziegiel MH, Singh S, Theisen M (2012) Flow cytometric readout based on Mitotracker Red CMXRos staining of live asexual blood stage malarial parasites reliably assesses antibody dependent cellular inhibition. Malar J 11:235
34. Ribacke U, Moll K, Albrecht L, Ahmed Ismail H, Normark J, Flaberg E, Szekely L, Hultenby K, Persson KE, Egwang TG, Wahlgren M (2013) Improved in vitro culture of Plasmodium falciparum permits establishment of clinical isolates with preserved multiplication, invasion and rosetting phenotypes. PLoS One 8(7), e69781
35. Allen RJ, Kirk K (2010) Plasmodium falciparum culture: the benefits of shaking. Mol Biochem Parasitol 169(1):63–65

Chapter 15

The In Vitro Invasion Inhibition Assay (IIA) for *Plasmodium vivax*

Wanlapa Roobsoong

Abstract

Plasmodium vivax is considered as the most widely distributed human malaria parasite outside Africa. Studies of *P. vivax* malaria have always been limited due to the lack of continuously in vitro-propagated parasite lines. Due to this limitation, studies on *P. vivax* have lagged behind that of *P. falciparum*, which is routinely maintained in in vitro blood-stage culture. This method allows for the short-term ex vivo culture of *P. vivax* blood stages and as such offers a wealth of opportunities to study the biology of the blood stages of the parasite. In this chapter we describe the in vitro erythrocyte invasion inhibition assay (IIA) for *P. vivax*, which can be used as a powerful tool for blood-stage vaccine screening. The major challenges of this assay are the purification of schizont-stage parasites and host reticulocytes. The purification methods for both *P. vivax* schizont-stage parasites and reticulocytes as detailed here have been developed and simplified. The protocols in this chapter have been optimized to ensure that IIA becomes a more feasible and reliable assay.

Key words *Plasmodium vivax*, Invasion inhibition assay, Schizont, Reticulocyte

1 Introduction

Plasmodium vivax malaria has often been described as benign, although recent studies have clearly shown the severe morbidity and mortality associated with *P. vivax* malaria. *P. vivax* malaria studies have always been limited since it is extremely difficult to culture the blood stages of the parasite in vitro. Due to this limitation, study on *P. vivax* has lagged behind that of *P. falciparum, which* can routinely be maintained in in vitro blood-stage culture. Thus, in order to work with *P. vivax*, one must have access to either fresh isolate parasites from patients or monkeys, or have access to cryopreserved blood-stage parasites. The availability of short-term ex vivo culture of *P. vivax* [1–3] offers a wealth of opportunities to study the biology of the blood stages of the parasite, including transcriptomics, proteomics, and metabolomics as well as drug and vaccine screening. In this chapter, we describe the

Ashley M. Vaughan (ed.), *Malaria Vaccines: Methods and Protocols*, Methods in Molecular Biology, vol. 1325,
DOI 10.1007/978-1-4939-2815-6_15,

in vitro erythrocyte invasion inhibition assay (IIA) for *P. vivax*, which can be used as a powerful tool for blood-stage vaccine screening. There are two major factors that contribute to the success of this assay. (1) parasite factors: the synchronous schizont stage is suitable for the invasion inhibition assay. *P. vivax*-infected patients however, typically present with asynchronous stages of parasites and thus, using parasites directly without short-term culture and schizont enrichment normally makes the interpretation of results very difficult. (2) host cell factors: *P. vivax* preferentially invades young erythrocytes [4]; the reticulocytes. Thus, the availability of reticulocytes in an in vitro culture is the key to the success of the invasion assay, as too many or too few target cells can affect the invasion efficiency and cost of running the assay. The protocols in this chapter have been optimized to ensure that IIA becomes a more feasible and reliable assay.

2 Materials

2.1 Equipment

1. 37 °C incubator.
2. Hypoxic chamber (Fig. 1a) or candle jar.
3. Mixed gas (5 % O_2, 5 % CO_2, and 90 % N_2).
4. 25 and 75 cm^2 tissue culture flasks, 6-well and 96-well culture plates.
5. Tabletop centrifuge.
6. 15 and 50 ml centrifuge tubes.
7. 1.5 ml microcentrifuge tubes.
8. 15 ml, 10 ml and 25 ml serological pipettes.
9. 3 ml plastic transfer pipettes.
10. 10 μl, 200 μl, and 1 ml pipette tips and pipettors.
11. Hemocytometer.
12. Compound light microscope.
13. Plasmodipur filters (Euro-Diagnostica).
14. Leukocyte reduction filters (Purecell® RC, PALL Corporation) (Fig. 1b).
15. 0.2 μm bottle top filter (Nalgene).
16. 30 ml Luer Lock Tip Syringe.
17. BD Accuri C6 flow cytometer (BD bioscience) or equivalent.
18. SYBR Green (Invitrogen) or equivalent.

2.2 Culture Components

1. McCoy's 5A incomplete culture medium: 11.9 g McCoy's 5A, 5.94 g HEPES, 2.0 g $NaHCO_3$, 4 g D-glucose, 4 ml 10 mg/ml Gentamicin. Add 900 ml deionized water. Adjust pH to 7.4.

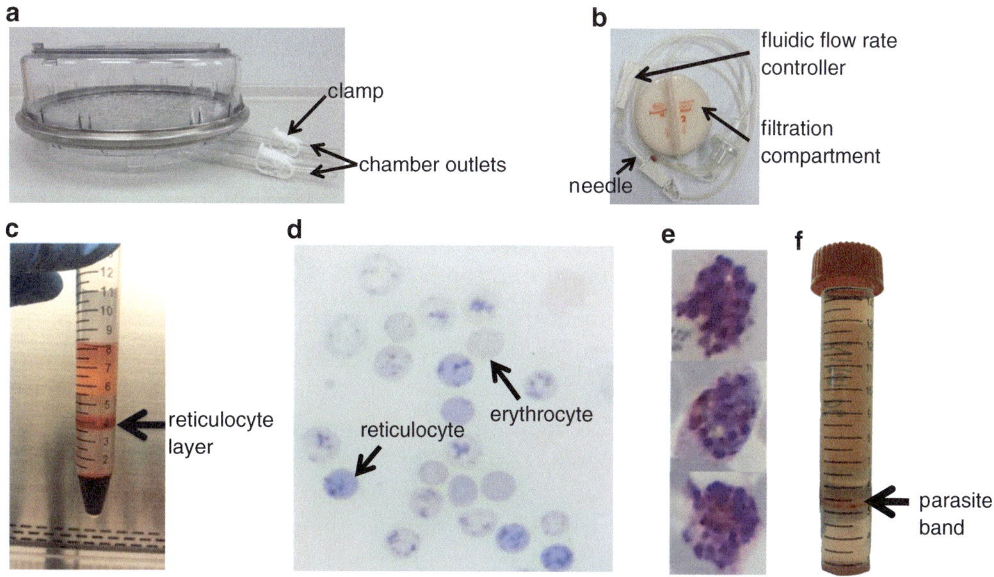

Fig. 1 Parasite culturing, reticulocyte enrichment, and schizont purification. (**a**) Hypoxic chamber. The chamber composing of two outlets in which the gas tube can be inserted for gassing. Once the gassing process has been done, close the outlets with the clamps. (**b**) Leukocyte reduction filter: the filter can be used for 1 unit of blood (250–450 ml). To operate the blood filtration, close the fluidic flow rate controller and then insert the needle to the blood bag. Hang the blood bag with the hanger in the direction following the *arrowhead* on the filtration compartment. Loosen the fluidic flow rate controller and let the blood flow by gravity. Collect the leukocyte-depleted blood in 50 ml tubes. (**c**) Reticulocyte layer: overlayer the leukocyte-depleted blood diluted to 20 % hematocrit in RPMI 1640 incomplete medium on the 19 % Nycodenz and centrifuge at $3000 \times g$ for 30 min. The reticulocyte fraction appears at the RPMI 1640/Nycodenz interface. (**d**) Blue reticulin-stained reticulocytes: the purified reticulocytes are stained with new methylene blue for 15 min before preparing the thin smear. Reticulocytes are defined as cells containing a blue reticulum network. Mature erythrocytes do not stain. (**e**) Giemsa-stained mature schizont stage of *P. vivax* from the ex-vivo short-term culture. Parasites are cultured in McCoy's 5A medium supplemented with 25 % heat-inactivated human AB serum for 18–24 h at 37 °C under hypoxic condition (5 %O_2, 5 % CO_2, 90 % N_2). To check the maturation of the parasites, thick and thin blood smears are prepared. The thin smear is fixed with absolute methanol for 30 s and the thick smear is not fixed. Smears are stained with 10 % Giemsa solution for 15 min before observation with a light microscope. (**f**) Purified schizont fraction: mature-stage parasites from short-term culture are purified using 45 % Percoll. The parasite culture is diluted to 20 % hematocrit with RPMI 1640 incomplete medium before layering on 45 % Percoll and centrifuged at $1200 \times g$ for 20 min. The parasite band appears at the RPMI 1640/Percoll interface

Adjust volume to 1 l. Filter-sterilize through a 0.2 μm bottle top filter. Store at 4 °C.

2. RPMI 1640 incomplete medium: 10.4 g RPMI 1640, 5.94 g HEPES, 2.0 g $NaHCO_3$, 2 g D-glucose, 4 ml 10 mg/ml Gentamicin. Add 900 ml deionized water. Adjust pH to 7.4. Adjust the volume to 1 l. Filter-sterilize through a 0.2 μm bottle top filter. Store at 4 °C.
3. Human AB serum: We obtain human AB serum from the Interstate Blood Bank. As *P. vivax* preferentially invades

Duffy-positive erythrocytes, serum from Duffy negative donors cannot be used in this protocol since it may contain antibodies to the Duffy antigen, resulting in an inhibition of invasion.

(a) Sera are pooled in a sterile bottle.

(b) Sera is heat-inactivated by incubation at 56 °C for 30 min.

(c) The heat-inactivated serum is filter-sterilized through a 0.2 μm bottle top filter.

(d) The heat-inactivated sera is then aliquoted in 50 ml tubes (25 ml aliquots) and stored at −20 °C until required.

4. McCoy's 5A complete culture medium: To McCoy's 5A incomplete medium, add heat-inactivated human AB serum to a final concentration of 25 % serum (*see* **Note 1**). Store at 4 °C.

2.3 Purification Components

1. 45 % Percoll: Mix 40.5 ml Percoll with 4.5 ml sterile 10× phosphate buffered saline (PBS), pH 7.4. Add 55 ml sterile of 1× PBS, pH 7.4. Store at 4 °C.
2. KCl buffer: 8.5734 g KCl 4.7662 g HEPES, 0.095 g $MgCl_2$, 0.138 g $NaH_2PO_4{*}H_2O$, 1.8016 g D-glucose, 0.2342 g EGTA, 8.5734 g KCl, 0.7013 g NaCl. Add 900 ml deionized water. Adjust pH to 7.4. Adjust the volume to 1 l and filter-sterilize. Store at 4 °C.
3. 19 % Nycodenz-KCl: Mix 31.67 ml of 60 % Nycodenz (Nycoprep Universal, Axis Shield) with 68.33 ml of KCl buffer (*see* **Note 2**).
4. 10 % Giemsa: Dilute Giemsa solution to 10 % with 1× PBS, pH 7.4. Prepare Giemsa solution fresh (not more than 30 min) before staining.

2.4 Flow Cytometry Analysis Components

1. 0.05 % glutaraldehyde (fixing solution): Mix 5 μl of 50 % glutaraldehyde stock solution (Sigma Aldrich) with 4.95 ml of 1× PBS, pH 7.4.
2. SYBR Green staining solution: Dilute 2 μl of 10,000 × SYBR Green (Invitrogen) with 20 ml of 1× PBS, pH 7.4.

3 Methods

The in vitro invasion inhibition assay (IIA) is composed of four parts; reticulocyte purification (Subheading 3.1), short-term ex vivo culture of *P. vivax* (Subheading 3.2), schizont purification (Subheading 3.3), and the IIA itself (Subheading 3.4). The source of reticulocytes depends on the availability in each laboratory. The reticulocyte purification protocol (Subheading 3.1) presented here works well for both peripheral blood and cord blood. Purification of reticulocytes can be achieved at any time prior to the IIA and purified reticulocytes can be kept at 4 °C (but not longer than 2 weeks from blood collection date) after purified. While the purification of reticulocytes is not challenging, purification of schizont-stage parasite (Subheading 3.2) is more delicate procedure; immature schizonts will fail to egress as merozoites and conversely, if the schizonts are too mature, they may rupture during the purification process which will have adverse effects on the IIA.

3.1 Reticulocyte Purification

1. Leukocyte depletion from whole blood. We obtain bags of whole peripheral blood from The Red Cross blood bank unit.
   (a) Leukocytes are removed using a leukocyte reduction filter. Insert filter set spike to the blood bag using a twisting motion and then hang on a drip stand.
   (b) Let the blood pass through the filter set by gravity flow. Collect the leukocyte-depleted blood in 50 ml tubes and keep at 4 °C until the reticulocyte purification step.
2. Purification of reticulocytes.
   (a) Centrifuge leukocyte-depleted blood at 1000 × *g* for 10 min and discard the plasma supernatant.
   (b) Wash packed blood twice with 20 ml RPMI 1640 incomplete medium, centrifuge at 1000 × *g* for 10 min and discard supernatant after each wash.
   (c) Dilute packed blood to 20 % hematocrit with RPMI 1640 incomplete medium.
   (d) Transfer 4 ml of room temperature 19 % Nycodenz to 15 ml tubes.
      - Gently layer 4 ml of cold 20 % hematocrit blood on top of 19 % Nycodenz. Centrifuge at 3000 × *g* for 30 min with no brake (*see* **Note 3**).
      - Collect the reticulocytes at the interface (Fig. 1c) in 50 ml tubes using a 3 ml plastic transfer pipette. Sometimes an additional second minor band of reticulocytes may be present which can also be collected.
      - Add at least 2 volumes of RPMI 1640 incomplete medium. Centrifuge at 1000 × *g* for 10 min and discard supernatant. Wash the purified reticulocytes twice more with 30 ml of RPMI 1640 incomplete medium.
      - Determine the volume of packed purified reticulocytes. Add an equal volume of McCoy's 5A incomplete medium to create a 50 % hematocrit. Keep the purified reticulocytes at 4 °C for not more than 2 weeks after the blood drawing date.

- Determine the purity of the reticulocytes by mixing 5 μl of 50 % hematocrit of purified reticulocytes with 5 μl of New Methylene Blue (Retic Chex, Stirek) and incubate for 15 min before making a thin smear. Determine the percentage of reticulocytes (blue staining cells) present in at least 5000 cells (Fig. 1d).

3.2 Short-Term Ex Vivo Culture of *P. vivax*

There are two types of *P. vivax* infected blood that can be used for IIA; fresh isolates (either from patients or monkeys) and cryopreserved parasites. The protocol presented here works well with both types of parasites. For researchers carrying out experiments using cryopreserved parasites, the leukocyte removal part can be omitted. The thawing protocol for cryopreserved parasites is available elsewhere [5].

1. Fresh parasite-infected blood should be drawn into sterile, heparinized tubes. The infected blood can be kept at 37 °C for up to 4 h if immediate blood processing is not possible.
2. Centrifuge the infected blood at 800 × *g* for 10 min. The plasma supernatant can be kept as aliquots at −20 °C for other studies. Wash packed infected blood once with 20 ml RPMI 1640 incomplete medium at 37 °C, centrifuge at 800 × *g* for 10 min and discard supernatant.
3. Dilute the infected blood to 50 % hematocrit with RPMI 1640 incomplete medium at 37 °C. Pass the diluted blood through a Plasmodipur filter pre-wet with 5 ml RPMI 1640 incomplete medium. Collect the filtrate into 50 ml tube. The maximum capacity of the Plasmodipur filter is 25 ml of ≤50 % hematocrit blood. Centrifuge at 800 × *g* for 10 min and discard the supernatant.
4. Dilute the leukocyte-depleted packed infected blood to 5 % hematocrit with warm McCoy's 5A complete medium and transfer to a 6-well plate or 25-cm^2 flask for a small culture volume or 75-cm^2 flasks for a large culture volume.
5. Transfer the culture flasks to a hypoxic chamber (Fig. 1a). Flush the mix gas (5 % O_2, 5 % CO_2, and 90 % N_2) through the outlet for 1 min. Close the chamber outlets and incubate the parasite cultures at 37 °C. The incubation period depends on the stage of the parasites at the blood collection time point. Younger parasite stages take longer time to mature to the schizont stage but typically maturation takes 18–24 h.
6. Monitor parasite maturation by preparing thick and thin smears from the culture. Fix the thin smear with absolute methanol for 30 s while leaving thick smears unfixed before staining with 10 % Giemsa for 15 min. Observe the maturation of parasites under a light microscope with a 10× eyepiece and 100× objective. The suitable schizont for performing the IIA is a segmented schizont (Fig. 1e).

3.3 Schizont Purification (Segmented Schizonts Are Required for IIA)

1. Transfer parasite cultures to 50 ml tubes. Centrifuge at 800 × *g* for 10 min and discard the culture supernatant.
2. Wash the packed infected blood with 30 ml RPMI 1640 incomplete medium at 37 °C. Centrifuge at 800 × *g* for 10 min and discard supernatant. Dilute packed infected blood to 20 % hematocrit with RPMI 1640 incomplete medium at 37 °C.
3. Transfer 4 ml of room temperature 45 % Percoll to 15 ml tubes. Gently layer 4 ml of 20 % hematocrit infected blood onto the Percoll. Centrifuge at 1200 × *g* for 20 min with no brake.
4. Use a 3 ml plastic transfer pipette to collect the purified schizont at the interface into 15 ml tubes (Fig. 1f).
5. Add 2 volume of RPMI 1640 incomplete medium at 37 °C. Centrifuge at 500 × *g* for 10 min and discard the supernatant.
6. Wash the parasite pellet twice with 10 ml RPMI 1640 incomplete medium at 37 °C. Centrifuge at 500 × *g* for 5 min and discard supernatant after washing (*see* **Note 4**).
7. Dilute the parasite pellet with 1 ml RPMI 1640 incomplete medium. Mix 10 μl of diluted parasite with 90 μl of 0.1 % Trypan blue and then transfer 10 μl to a hemocytometer in order to determine the total number of cells.
8. Take 1 μl of the schizont preparation and prepare a thin smear for Giemsa staining. Let the smear dry and fix with methanol for 30 s. Stain with 10 % Giemsa for 10 min. Determine the percentage purity by counting the number of schizonts in the total of at least 500 counted cells.
9. Determine the number of schizonts present in the sample: Total schizont number = (total number of cells × % purity)/100.

3.4 In Vitro Invasion Inhibition Assay (IIA)

In the utilization of this protocol, reticulocytes from both peripheral blood and cord blood can be used and we obtain similar invasion efficiencies. The assay has been optimized for a 96-well plate, with 200 μl culture volume per well at 3 % hematocrit and 0.1 % schizont parasitemia. In testing the ability of antibody samples or alternative interventions to prevent invasion, each condition is carried out in triplicate. After incubation, parasite DNA content is quantified with SYBR Green staining followed by flow cytometry. A successful intervention will lead to a statistically significant decrease in DNA content due to inhibition of invasion and subsequent growth.

1. Prepare the host reticulocytes: We have optimized the reticulocyte percentage for the assay to 4 % reticulocytes and 96 % autonomous packed blood cells.

   For example, suppose that after purification, a sample contains 40 % reticulocytes and the final reticulocyte percentage in each well must equal 4 %.

The hematocrit in each well must equal 3 % and thus each well containing 200 μl culture volume must contain $(200 \times 0.03) = 6$ μl of packed blood.

In the above example, the final volume of reticulocytes required would be $(4\ \%/40\ \%) \times 6$ μl = 0.6 μl reticulocytes and 5.4 μl packed cells from autonomous blood are obtained after purification, the final % reticulocytes in each well is 4 % and the total packed cell is 6 μl/well.

2. There are two types of control that need to be carried out in each assay. The first is a negative control into which only reticulocytes and culture medium are added without schizonts. The "negative control" wells will be used for gating purposes for the SYBR Green staining procedure in the flow cytometry analysis. The second is an "invasion control" where no antibody or other intervention is added.
3. Add 40 μl of warm McCoy's 5A complete medium containing 6 μl of 4 % reticulocyte-enriched blood to each culture well required for the assay.
4. Add 160 μl of warm McCoy's 5A complete medium to the "negative control" wells and 100 μl to the "invasion control" wells. For experimental wells, add 100 μl of 2× antibody sample or other intervention diluted in warm McCoy's 5A complete medium.
5. Dilute the purified schizont preparation to 1×10^6 cells/ml with warm McCoy's 5A complete medium. Transfer 60 μl of the diluted schizont to all wells apart from the "negative control" wells. This will give a final 0.1 % schizont parasitemia. The total volume in each well is now 200 μl.
6. Place the plate in an hypoxic chamber (Fig. 1a). Flush mixed gas (5 % O_2, 5 % CO_2, and 90 % N_2) for 1 min and then close the chamber outlets. Incubate at 37 °C for 18 h.
7. Determine parasite content in each well using SYBR Green staining of parasite DNA followed by flow cytometry. Thin smears are also prepared from each culture wells for further confirmation of experimental success. A thin smear of the "invasion control" must show an increase in parasitemia to at least 0.2 %. This demonstrates parasite viability and the subsequent ability of the intervention to inhibit invasion.
8. For SYBR Green staining, centrifuge the culture plate at $500 \times g$ for 5 min and discard the culture medium. Wash the culture wells once with 200 μl PBS. Add 100 μl of 0.05 % glutaraldehyde and incubate at room temperature for 10 min to fix the parasites. Centrifuge the culture plate at $500 \times g$ for 5 min and discard the supernatant. After washing once with

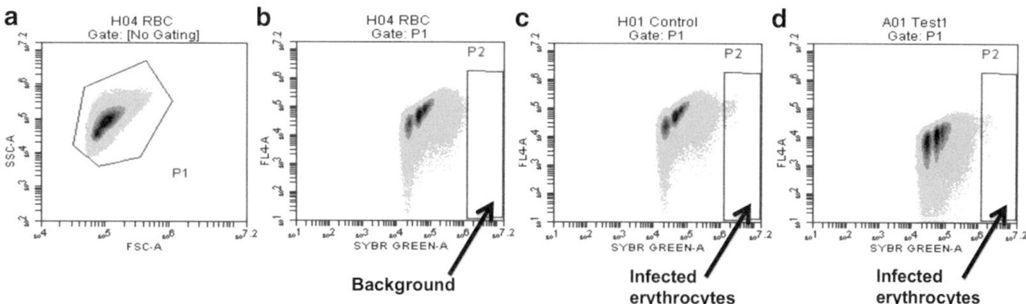

Fig. 2 Flow cytometry for the measurement of infected reticulocytes. Gating ensures that only SYBR green-bound parasites are detected. (**a**) The events are viewed in the FSC-A/SSC-A plot and the population in gate P1 is selected to be viewed on the SYBR Green-A/FL4-A plot. (**b**) The purified reticulocytes alone are stained with SYBR Green and used to observe background staining (gate P2) and with this gating, purified reticulocytes generate almost no background. (**c**) The infected erythrocytes appear in gate P2 of the control sample in which intervention has not been added. (**d**) Test samples with successful interventions lead to a drop in the number of parasite-infected reticulocytes

200 μl PBS, add 100 μl of SYBR Green in PBS (1:10,000 dilution) and incubate at room temperature for 10 min in the dark. Centrifuge the culture plate at 500 × *g* for 5 min and discard supernatant. Add 200 μl of PBS to each well and process for flow cytometry.

9. We perform flow cytometry in a BD AccuriC6 flow cytometer. A total of 500,000 events are acquired for each well and erythrocytes are gated (Fig. 2a). Uninfected reticulocytes in the negative control wells stained with SYBR green are used to define cell populations with background staining and almost no reticulocytes are stained with SYBR green under these conditions (gate P2, Fig. 2b). Positive events of control parasite-infected and test-intervention wells are then captured in gate P2 (Fig. 2c, d), which shows the numbers of parasite-infected erythrocytes. To determine invasion inhibition, we use the following equation.

$$\% \text{ inhibition} = 100 - \left(100 * \left[\left(\text{T} - \text{N}\right) / \left(\text{P} - \text{N}\right)\right]\right)$$

where:

N = SYBR Green positive cells (%) of normal erythrocytes without parasite and interventions (negative control wells) (% of the cells in gate P2 in Fig. 2b).

P = parasitemia (%) of infected erythrocyte in control parasite-infected wells (% of the cells in gate P2 in Fig. 2c).

T = parasitemia (%) of infected erythrocytes in test-intervention wells (% of the cells in gate P2 in Fig. 2d).

4 Notes

1. McCoy's 5A complete medium should be used within 1 week of preparation. Repeat warming of the medium at 37 °C is not recommended.
2. 19 % Nycodenz-KCl should be prepared fresh and used at room temperature when performing the gradient centrifugation of reticulocytes.
3. In our hands, performing the reticulocytes enrichment in 15 ml tube work best. The total volume in each tube should be between 7 and 9 ml, 8 ml is the optimum total volume. When layering the diluted blood on the 19 % Nycodenz-KCl, one can use either a 3 ml transfer pipette or a 10 ml serological pipette.
4. Percoll residue can be removed by centrifuging at 500 × *g* for 5 min.

References

1. Borlon C et al (2012) Cryopreserved *Plasmodium vivax* and cord blood reticulocytes can be used for invasion and short term culture. Int J Parasitol 42(2):155–160
2. Chotivanich K et al (2001) Ex-vivo short-term culture and developmental assessment of *Plasmodium vivax*. Trans R Soc Trop Med Hyg 95(6):677–680
3. Udomsangpetch R et al (2007) Short-term in vitro culture of field isolates of *Plasmodium vivax* using umbilical cord blood. Parasitol Int 56(1):65–69
4. Mons B (1990) Preferential invasion of malarial merozoites into young red blood cells. Blood Cells 16(2–3):299–312
5. Blomqvist K (2008) Thawing of glycerolyte-frozen parasites with NaCl. In: Moll K et al (eds) Methods in malaria research. MR4, Manassas, VA, p 15

Chapter 16

The Ex Vivo IFN-γ Enzyme-Linked Immunospot (ELISpot) Assay

Martha Sedegah

Abstract

The quantification of single cell interferon-gamma (IFN-γ) release for assessing cellular immune responses using the Enzyme-linked immunospot (ELISPOT) assay is an invaluable technique in immunology. Peripheral blood mononuclear cells (PBMC) are stimulated in vitro with recombinant proteins, peptides and recently whole malaria organisms. Stimulation may be short term (20–36 h) or long term (cultured ELISpot, up to 7 days). ELISpot is also able to quantify other cytokines secreted by antigen-specific T-cells, such as interleukin-2, interleukin-5, and other interleukins. ELISpot is playing an important role especially in vaccine research studies.

Key words ELISPOT, Peripheral blood mononuclear cells, PBMC, Interferon-gamma, IFN-γ, Cytokines, T cells

1 Introduction

The Enzyme-linked immunospot (ELISpot) assay is an adaptation of the enzyme-linked immunosorbent assay (ELISA) and was initially used for antibody-secreting B cells [1, 2]. This was adapted to measure the release of interferon-gamma (IFN-γ) from mitogen-stimulated human peripheral blood lymphocytes (PBMC), measured by alkaline phosphatase as spots surrounding IFN-γ producing cells and allows microscopic enumeration of these spot-forming cells. Thus, ELISpot differs from intracellular cytokine stain (ICS) methodologies that uses flow cytometry to detect the phenotype of individual cells and the cytokines they produce within antigen-specific cells. Both methodologies are widely used in a many different research and clinical settings, and each offer specific advantages depending on the desired outcomes. A major concern

Ashley M. Vaughan (ed.), *Malaria Vaccines: Methods and Protocols*, Methods in Molecular Biology, vol. 1325,
DOI 10.1007/978-1-4939-2815-6_16,

was the need to obtain repeatable outcomes that would allow comparison of results from different laboratories [3–6], and led to efforts standardize assays and harmonize standing operating procedures (SOPs) [5, 7, 8–10], compliance with good laboratory practice and the Code for Federal Regulations [9].

In this laboratory, the ELISpot method uses PBMC cells, freshly isolated, or previously cryopreserved, which have been stimulated with antigen (in the form of synthetic peptides [11–16], recombinant proteins [4, 17], or whole organism) in vitro. The cells are then incubated in nitrocellulose-lined microtiter wells that have been pre-coated with anti-cytokine antibody. After incubation (for 18–36 h), the local production of cytokines around "producing cells" can be visualized by adding a second antibody that is labeled with the enzyme alkaline phosphatase or horseradish peroxidase, and then adding a substrate that is enzymatically converted into an insoluble colored product. Cytokine producing cells can then be visualized as "spots." The basic methodologies based on synthetic peptides used in this laboratory have been previously published [11]. More recently, whole malaria parasites, purified and cryopreserved sporozoites, have been used [18, 19].

2 Materials

All solutions should be prepared using ultrapure (Type 1) Millipore® water and analytical-grade reagents, and are prepared at room temperature. Culture media are prepared at 4 °C but warmed to room temperature prior to use.

2.1 Cell Culture Media

1. *R10 Medium*: 10 % Fetal Bovine Serum (Sigma Cat#F4135), 100 U/mL Penicillin, 100 μg/mL Streptomycin (Life Technologies Cat#15140-122), 2 mM L-Glutamine (Life Technologies Cat#25030-081), in RPMI medium (Life Technologies Cat#22400-105). Filter through a 0.22 μm filter unit.
2. *R2 Medium*: 2 % Fetal Bovine Serum, 100 U/mL Penicillin, 100 μg/mL Streptomycin, 2 mM L-Glutamine, 96 % RPMI. Filter through a 0.22 μm filter unit.
3. *HR10 media*: 10 % Human AB Serum (Sigma Cat#H4522), 100 U/mL Penicillin, 100 μg/mL Streptomycin, 2 mM L-Glutamine, 1 % 100× MEM-non-essential amino acids (Life Technologies Cat#11140-050), 87 % RPMI-1640. Filter through 0.22 μm filter unit, then through 0.08 μm filter unit and store at 4 °C until used. For example, 500 mL HR10:

50 mL Human AB Serum, 5 mL Penicillin-Streptomycin, 5 mL L-Glutamine, 5 mL 100× MEM Non-essential, 435 mL RPMI-1640.

2.2 Chemicals and Reagents

1. *Coating buffer*: 0.1 M bicarbonate buffer, pH = 9.6. Combine 250 mL of double-distilled water with 0.398 g Na_2CO_3 and 0.733 g $NaHCO_3$ in a glass beaker. Mix coating buffer solution on the stir plate with a magnetic stir bar. After the reagents have been dissolved into solution, measure pH to pH 9.6. Filter coating buffer solution prior to use.
2. *0.5 % fetal bovine serum (FBS) in 1× PBS pH = 7.4*: buffer to prepare biotinylated anti-human IFN-γ monoclonal antibody (mAb) 7-B6-1 and Streptavidin-Alkaline Phosphatase solution.
3. *Washing buffer*: 1× PBS with 0.05 % Tween 20. Tween 20® (Sigma Cat#1379) is a commercial brand name for polyoxyethylene sorbitol monolaurate. Depending on the volume of washing buffer to be prepared, 0.05 % of Tween 20® is directly added to 1× PBS solution (e.g. 2 L washing buffer = 200 mL 10× PBS, 1799 mL Millipore® ultrapure water and 1 mL Tween 20®).
4. *Streptavidin-Alkaline Phosphatase solution*: Streptavidin-Alkaline Phosphatase conjugate 1:1000 dilution in 1× PBS pH = 7.4 with 0.5 % Fetal Calf Serum. Calculate required volume of 1:1000 dilution of Streptavidin-ALP (Mabtech Cat. #3310-8) with 0.5 % of Fetal Calf Serum to be prepared (e.g. 10 mL total solution requires 0.01 mL of Streptavidin-ALP, 0.05 mL of Fetal Calf Serum and 9.94 mL 1× PBS).
5. *Chromogenic-alkaline phosphatase substrate solution*: chromogenic-alkaline phosphatase substrate (AP conjugate substrate kit, Bio-Rad Cat. #170-6432) is used at 1:25 dilution in double-distilled water. Calculate required volume of 1:25 dilution Chromogenic Alkaline Phosphatase Substrate Solution (e.g. 10 mL total solution requires 0.4 mL 25× AP Color Development Buffer added to 9.6 mL room temperature double-distilled water). Add 0.1 mL AP color reagent A and 0.1 mL AP color reagent B immediately before use. Incubate at RT for 15 min. Stop development by washing in Millipore® ultrapure water and then air-dry.

2.3 Isolation of Peripheral Blood Mononuclear Cells (PBMC)

2.3.1 Materials and Reagents

- Ficoll-Paque: (GE Health Care Cat# 17-1440-03).
- R10 Medium.
- R2 Medium.
- Polypropylene Conical Tubes, 50 mL.
- Freezing medium: 90 % Fetal Bovine Serum and 10 % dimethyl. Filter through a 0.22 μm filter.

2.3.2 Procedure

1. Aliquot the blood evenly into each 50 mL tube containing R10 medium to create a 2:1 blood/media ratio (e.g. Place 10 mL R10 and 20 mL anticoagulant-treated blood for a final volume of 30 mL). Mix by drawing the blood and medium in and out with Pasteur pipette.
2. Carefully underlay the diluted blood with 12 mL Ficoll-Paque.
3. Centrifuge at 360 × *g* for 25 min at room temperature with no brake. Observe separation of blood into three layers:
   (a) Packed red blood cells at the bottom.
   (b) Middle ring band of mononuclear cells.
   (c) Upper most diluted plasma layer: Collect upper plasma layer into labeled 50 mL tubes and store at −80 °C. Gently pipette up the lymphocyte layer by placing the pipette tip right above the cell layer and aspirating all the cells. Be careful not to disturb the RBC layer. Transfer cells into designated tubes containing R2. Tap up to 45 mL using R2. Centrifuge at 470 × *g* for 15 min at room temperature (First wash).
4. Pour out the supernatant, and resuspend the cell pellet in R2 using a 10 mL pipette. Tap up tube to 45 mL using R2. Carefully remove any debris using a 10 mL pipette. Mix well. Centrifuge at 470 × *g* for 12 min at room temperature (second wash).
5. Pour out supernatant, and resuspend the cell pellet in R2 using a 10 mL pipette. Using R2, make sure the tube contains exactly 50 mL. Sample is ready for counting (count#1).
6. Take the amount of cells needed for the ELISPOT assay, centrifuge the cell suspension at 470 × *g* for 12 min at room temperature and resuspend the cell pellet in HR10 medium at the cell concentration required for use in ELISPOT assay (e.g. rest at 5×10^6 cells/mL for an assay that requires 4×10^6 cells/mL typically used to test malaria peptides) and allow to rest for 1 h at 37 °C, 5 % CO_2 incubator.
7. Centrifuge the remainder of the cell suspension at 470 × *g* for 12 min and resuspend in filtered cold freezing medium at a designated concentration (for example 20×10^6 cells/mL) for cryopreservation.
8. After 1 h of rest, prepare the cells for count#2 and adjust final concentration to 4×10^6 cells/mL in R10 medium for a final count#3 to confirm cell concentration.

2.4 Antigens and Mitogens

1. *Antigens*: (a) Synthetic 15mer peptides: either single 15mer peptides or pools of 15mer peptides that usually overlap by 11 amino acids. (b) Synthetic 9-10mer HLA-defined epitopes predicted by algorithms such as NetMHC [20] or SYPEITHI [21].

2. *Whole organisms*: this laboratory uses *Plasmodium falciparum* sporozoites [19]: Cryopreserved sporozoites are stored in a liquid nitrogen freezer and thawed on the day of the assay to be used as antigens. Sporozoites are thawed in a 37 °C water bath by gentle shaking of vials just immediately prior to plate set-up. Dilute sporozoites to 250,000/mL using HR10 media.
3. *Mitogens as positive controls*: Concanavalin A (ConA) that induces mitogenic activity of T cells (Con A, *Conavalia ensiformis*, Sigma-Aldrich cat. #C5275); CEF MHC class I control peptide pool "plus" for detecting CD8+ T cell IFN-γ activities in human PBMC (CTL cat. #CTL-CEF-002); phytohemagglutinin lectin (PHA-L) to induce PBMC replication (PHA-L lectin from *Phaseolus vulgaris*) (Sigma-Aldrich cat. #L4144).

2.5 Antibodies

- Anti-human IFNγ mAb-1-D1K (Mabtech cat. #3420-3-1000).
- Biotinylated Anti-human IFN-γ mAb 7-B6-1 (Mabtech cat. #3420-6-1000). Calculate required volume at concentration of 1 μg/mL prepared in 1× PBS pH 7.4 with 0.5 % FCS (for example 10 mL total solution requires 0.01 mL biotinylated antibody, 0.05 mL FCS and 9.94 mL 1× PBS pH 7.4).

2.6 Plastic and Glass Ware

- Sterile, clear 96-well filter plate with 0.45 μm pore size hydrophobic Polyvinylidene Difluoride (PVDF) membrane.
- Filter System: 500 mL, 200 mL, 150 mL, 0.22 μm and 0.8 μm Nalgene© Rapid Flow™ Filter Units and bottle top filter.

3 Methods

3.1 Cellular Procedure: Sterile

1. To prepare antibody solution: calculate required volume needed and add 15 μg/mL of the 1 mg/mL mAb anti-IFN-γ in 0.1 M bicarbonate buffer pH 9.6, and filter through 0.22 μm filter unit. For example: mix 0.1 mL mAb 1-D1k and 9.9 mL 0.1 M bicarbonate buffer, total volume 10 mL. Coat 96-well PVDF-backed plates with anti-IFN-γ mAb1-D1k at 15 μg/mL diluted with Sodium bicarbonate buffer at pH 9.6, 100 μL/well, overnight at 4 °C and wrapped in aluminum foil to protect from light.
2. Wash the pre-coated plates with plain RPMI-1640 medium six times in a biological hood, patting the plates dry on sterile gauze pads between washes.
3. Add 200 μL/well of HR10 medium, wrap plates in aluminum foil to protect from light and incubate for 2–3 days at 4 °C.
4. On day of assay, retrieve plates from 4 °C fridge and bring in biological hood. Remove previous HR10 media by flicking to

small basin and tapping onto sterile gauze. Block with 200 μL/well of blocking HR10media. Do this at least 1 h prior to plate set-up to allow plates to reach room temperature.

5. According to the ELISpot plate layout template, using triplicate or quadruplicate replicates, add 100 μL/well (except for supplementary HR10 media) of the following stimulants in this order (if applicable).
6. Supplementary HR10 media: the volume to be added (either 50 μL or 75 μL) is determined by the cells to be plated on the well, to bring the total culture volume to 200 μL/well.
7. Positive Controls: CEF concentration 4 μg/mL; ConA concentration 1.25 μg/mL; PHA concentration 1.25 μg/mL all prepared in medium HR10.
8. Peptides: Prepare peptide pool, for instance Cp1-9, Ap1-12, PfSSP2, PfLSA1, PfAg2, PfMSP1 (3D7) [13, 22] at working concentration of 2.5 μg/mL for a final concentration of 1.25 μg/mL. For individual peptide pools (PfCSP pool 1 to pool 9 and PfAMA1 pool 1 to pool 12), working concentration is 20 μg/mL for a final concentration of 10 μg/mL. We plate 100 μL of working concentration per well and add 100 μL of the PBMCs to end up with final concentration per well that is one half of the working concentration.
   - Proteins: prepared at the same concentrations as peptide.
   - Whole organism (sporozoites): Varying concentrations of *P. falciparum* sporozoites ranging from 10,000 to 150,000 per well were tested and the optimum concentration established prior to actual assay. To use in the assay as stimulant, take needed number of vials of sporozoites from liquid nitrogen storage and gently place in water bath set to 37 °C. Do not shake vials. Allow to thaw approximately 30 s. Once thawed, place in 50 mL tube and add calculated volume of HR10 media to obtain desired sporozoite concentration to be plated in 100 μL per well.
9. After either thawing PBMCs or isolating fresh PBMCs by density gradient, adjust PBMCs to 4×10^6/mL in HR10 media and add either 100 μL or 50 μL of cell suspension (400,000 or 200,000) to designated wells for a total of 200 μL per well. Note: volume of cells to be added could be different based on the corresponding stimulants; for example CEF and ConA uses 100,000 cells or 25 μL of cells at 4×10^6/mL as these stimulants often induce responses that are much higher than malaria peptides, and therefore smaller numbers of cells are used (*see* **Note 1**).
10. Incubate plates at 37 °C, 5 % CO_2 for 36–40 h. Once plates are in the incubator, do not disturb their location/orientation, and minimize opening/closing of incubator.

3.2 ELISpot Development: Non-sterile

1. After completion of incubation time, remove the cells from plates by tapping on paper towels and wash six times with washing buffer (Subheading 2.2, **item 3**) using an ELISA washer (Dynex Ultrawash Plus®).

   Add 100 μL/well of filtered biotinylated anti-IFN-γ mAb 7-B6-1 mAb at 1 μg/mL in 0.5 % FBS-1× PBS pH = 7.4. Incubate plates for 3 h at room temperature, and then wash six times with washing buffer.
2. Add 100 μL/well of streptavidin-alkaline phosphatase conjugate diluted 1:1000 with 0.5%FCS-1× PBS pH 7.4. Incubate plates at room temperature for 1 h, then wash six times with washing buffer and three times with 1× PBS only.
3. Add 100 μL/well of chromogenic alkaline phosphatase substrate solution at 1:25 dilution using double-distilled water. Incubate for 15 min at room temperature. Terminate the colorimetric reaction by soaking the plates in Millipore water followed by washing each plate with tap water and allowing to air-dry overnight. Enumerate the IFN-γ SFC (Spot Forming Cells) using the AID ELISpot Reader System ELR02 (AID; Advanced Imaging Devices, Autoimmun Diagnostika GMBH, Germany) or similar.

3.3 Reading the Spots

ELISpot image acquisition is executed through an automated reader using the AID ELISpot Reader system (Manufacturer: Cell Technology, Inc. for Advanced Imaging Devices (AID) Model ELR02). The reader must be well-maintained and properly calibrated and is to be operated only by trained personnel with camera settings previously established. The count settings to properly identify a spot should have been previously established and all parameters set to decrease variability.

3.4 Calculation of Positive Activities

Outliers are values from either quadruplicates or triplicates experiments that contribute more than 50 % of Standard Deviation and are 3× higher or lower than the mean of the remaining three of the quadruplicates (or two in triplicates) points. These outliers are removed from analysis and are not included in the calculation of spot forming cells/million. For each CSP and AMA1 peptide pool tested against any given bleed, a positive response is defined as (1) a statistically significant difference ($p = 0.05$) between the average of the number of spot forming cells in triplicate or quadruplicate test wells and the average of triplicate or quadruplicate negative control wells (Student's two tailed t-test), plus (2) at least a doubling of spot forming cells in test wells relative to negative control wells, plus (3) a difference of at least ten spots between test and negative control wells. Volunteer samples are designated as responders when positive against at least one of the pools tested at any post immunization sampling [11] (*see* **Note 2**).

4 Notes

1. Typically, malaria peptides and control stimulants such as CEF or ConA differ in the activities each induces. If a standard cell number is used, there is a risk that a strong stimulant such as CEF or ConA may induce responses that cannot be counted. To overcome this problem, different numbers of PBMC's are used with malaria peptides and with CEF or ConA. For malaria peptides, add either 100 μL or 50 μL of cell suspension (400,000 or 200,000) to designated wells for a total of 200 μL per well. But for CEF and ConA the number of cells is reduced and 100,000 cells or 25 μL of cells at 4×10^6/mL are added to each well.
2. Example of calculation and identification of positive and negative outcomes (Table 1): in this example, the assay was performed in triplicates, the mean is then calculated, corrected for the medium only controls, and the statistical analysis performed. Here, two peptides were used to stimulate PBMC (400,000/well) and activities were determined to be positive (Peptide 1) or negative (Peptide 2).

Table 1
Example of calculation and identification of positive and negative outcomes

Plate #1	Well	Peptide	Peptide
400K cells/well	A	49	23
	B	55	10
	C	38	14
	Mean	47	17
Subtract medium	A	40	14
	B	46	1
	C	29	5
	SFC/m	96	17
	t test	0.007	0.226
	SI	5.3	1.7
	Difference	38	7
	Result	POSITIVE	NEGATIVE

Acknowledgments

The following have made major contributions to the development and use of this assay: Harini Ganeshan, Maria Belmonte, Jun Huang, Esteban Abot, and Arnel Belmonte, and helped write this chapter with Michael R. Hollingdale.

References

1. Czerkinsky CC et al (1983) A solid-phase enzyme-linked immunospot (ELISPOT) assay for enumeration of specific antibody-secreting cells. J Immunol Methods 65(1–2): 109–121
2. Sedgwick JD, Holt PG (1983) A solid-phase immunoenzymatic technique for the enumeration of specific antibody-secreting cells. J Immunol Methods 57(1–3):301–309
3. Janetzki S et al (2004) Evaluation of Elispot assays: influence of method and operator on variability of results. J Immunol Methods 291(1–2):175–183
4. Janetzki S et al (2005) Standardization and validation issues of the ELISPOT assay. Methods Mol Biol 302:51–86
5. Cox JH et al (2002) Accomplishing cellular immune assays for evaluation of vaccine efficacy in developing countries. In: Rose NR, Hamilton RG, Detrick B (eds) Manual clinical laboratory immunology. ASM Press, Washington, DC, pp 301–315
6. Scheibenbogen C et al (2000) Quantitation of antigen-reactive T cells in peripheral blood by IFNgamma-ELISPOT assay and chromium-release assay: a four-centre comparative trial. J Immunol Methods 244(1–2):81–89
7. Janetzki S, Britten CM (2012) The impact of harmonization on ELISPOT assay performance. Methods Mol Biol 792:25–36
8. Slota M et al (2011) ELISpot for measuring human immune responses to vaccines. Expert Rev Vaccines 10(3):299–306
9. Zhang W, Lehmann PV (2012) Objective, user-independent ELISPOT data analysis based on scientifically validated principles. Methods Mol Biol 792:155–171
10. Lehmann PV, Zhang W (2012) Unique strengths of ELISPOT for T cell diagnostics. Methods Mol Biol 792:3–23
11. Sedegah M et al (2011) Adenovirus 5-vectored P. falciparum vaccine expressing CSP and AMA1. Part A: safety and immunogenicity in seronegative adults. PLoS One 6(10):e24586
12. Sedegah M et al (2011) Identification and localization of minimal MHC-restricted CD8+ T cell epitopes within the Plasmodium falciparum AMA1 protein. Malar J 9:241
13. Dodoo D et al (2011) Measuring naturally acquired immune responses to candidate malaria vaccine antigens in Ghanaian adults. Malar J 10:168
14. Tamminga C et al (2011) Adenovirus-5-vectored P. falciparum vaccine expressing CSP and AMA1. Part B: safety, immunogenicity and protective efficacy of the CSP component. PLoS One 6(10):e25868
15. Chuang I et al (2013) DNA prime/adenovirus boost malaria vaccine encoding P. falciparum CSP and AMA1 induces sterile protection associated with cell-mediated immunity. PLoS One 8(2):1371
16. Sedegah M et al (2013) Identification of minimal human MHC-restricted CD8+ T-cell epitopes within the Plasmodium falciparum circumsporozoite protein (CSP). Malar J 12:185
17. Rosenberg ES et al (1999) Characterization of HIV-1-specific T-helper cells in acute and chronic infection. Immunol Lett 66(1–3): 89–93
18. Epstein JE et al (2011) Live attenuated malaria vaccine designed to protect through hepatic CD8+ T Cell immunity. Science 334:475–480
19. Seder RA et al (2013) Protection against malaria by intravenous immunization with a nonreplicating sporozoite vaccine. Science 341(6152):1359–1365
20. Nielsen M et al (2003) Reliable prediction of T-cell epitopes using neural networks with novel sequence representations. Protein Sci 12(5):1007–1017
21. Rammensee H et al (1999) SYFPEITHI: database for MHC ligands and peptide motifs. Immunogenetics 50(3–4):213–219
22. Dodoo D et al (2008) Cohort study of the association of antibody levels to AMA1, MSP119, MSP3 and GLURP with protection from clinical malaria in Ghanaian children. Malar J 7:142

Chapter 17

Evaluating IgG Antibody to Variant Surface Antigens Expressed on *Plasmodium falciparum* Infected Erythrocytes Using Flow Cytometry

Andrew Teo, Wina Hasang, and Stephen Rogerson

Abstract

Constant exposure to *Plasmodium falciparum* leads to acquisition of malarial antibodies that can protect against the clinical consequences of infection. One important target of such antibodies is against the parasite-infected erythrocyte (IEs). Current established assays to test the efficacy of antibodies in preventing parasite growth include direct parasite growth inhibition, the agglutination of IEs, and the inhibition of adhesion of IEs (to quantify antibody that inhibits adhesion to purified receptors or cells).

However, many of these assays are labor-intensive and low-output which limits study sizes to small cohorts. Here we present an alternative assay that measures the levels of protective antibodies to variant surface antigens (VSA) of IEs. This assay can be performed using a microtitre plate and requires only a small volume of test serum sample. Serum samples are incubated with IEs and are then analyzed using a semi-automated autosampler attached to a flow cytometer. The assay is accurate, quick, and reproducible. Ultimately this assay could be used on large population-based studies, which could increase the statistical power of clinical studies.

Key words Variant surface antigens, Assay, High throughput, IgG antibody, Malaria, Statistical power

1 Introduction

Among all *Plasmodium* species, *Plasmodium falciparum* infection remains the most deadly. *P. falciparum* infected erythrocytes (IEs) express a unique member of a variant surface antigen (VSA) family, termed *P. falciparum* erythrocyte membrane protein 1 (PfEMP1), that mediates the cytoadherence to endothelial receptors such as cluster of differentiation 36 (CD36) and intercellular adhesion molecule-1 (ICAM-1), and to a placental receptor, chondroitin sulfate A (CSA) [1] . This cytoadherence contributes to immune evasion and parasite survival. Recent studies have demonstrated that PfEMP1 is the major VSA recognized by human immunoglobulin G (IgG) antibodies from patients with acquired immunity to malaria, and that antibody to PfEMP1 is associated with

Ashley M. Vaughan (ed.), *Malaria Vaccines: Methods and Protocols*, Methods in Molecular Biology, vol. 1325,
DOI 10.1007/978-1-4939-2815-6_17, © Springer Science+Business Media New York 2015

protective immunity [2]. Current established assays to quantitate antibody responses to IEs are often time-consuming and thus not conducive for large-scale studies. Here, we present a high-throughput flow cytometry assay, which measures IgG antibody titres against IEs using small amounts of a patient's plasma or serum. Test samples are incubated with IEs, secondary antibody, and fluorophore-conjugated tertiary antibody. Parasite DNA is stained with ethidium bromide. Samples are then analyzed using an autosampler attached to a flow cytometer. This is a reliable and efficient way to screen antibody responses against IEs in clinical studies of correlates of protection in the sero-epidemiology of malaria.

2 Materials

2.1 Equipment

1. Polypropylene 15 ml and 50 ml tubes.
2. Multichannel pipettor.
3. Centrifuge with a microtiter plate holder.
4. HyperCyt® Autosampler (IntelliCyt, NM, USA) attached to a CyAnADP analyzer (Beckman Coulter) (*see* **Note 1**).

2.2 Reagents

1. Cultures of mid-to late-stage *P. falciparum* trophozoite-infected erythrocytes, approximately 4–8 % parasitemia. *P. falciparum* is cultured as previously described [3].
2. Heat-inactivated newborn calf serum (NCS).
3. Casein blocking buffer (Thermo Scientific).
4. Ethidium bromide (EtBr) 1 mg/ml.
5. Secondary antibody: Polyclonal rabbit anti-human IgG (Dako).
6. Tertiary antibody: Alexa Fluor 647 conjugated donkey anti-rabbit (Invitrogen).
7. U-bottom 96-well plates (BD Biosciences).
8. Sterile phosphate-buffered saline (PBS) at pH 7.4.
9. Paraformaldehyde (PFA) at 2 % in PBS, filtered and kept at 4 °C.
10. Washing Solution: PBS with either 1 % NCS or 0.1 % casein added.

3 Methods

3.1 Antibody Binding to IEs

1. Pre-coat the microtitre plate with 170 μl of undiluted NCS for >1 h and wash twice with PBS. The NCS-coated 96-well plates can be wrapped with cling wrap and stored at 4 °C (*see* **Note 2**). Alternatively to NCS, the microtitre plate can be coated

with 170 μl 0.1 % casein for 1 h and used on the day of the experiment.

2. All incubations, washes, and dilutions can be done using PBS with either 1 % NCS or 0.1 % casein.
3. Synchronize in vitro IEs culture to 4–8 % parasitemia at mid-late stage trophozoites. Resuspend and wash cells thrice prior to assay, using washing solution.
4. To NCS-coated U-bottom 96-well plates, aliquot 2.5 μl of test sera samples per well in duplicate on the experiment day. If not possible, aliquot the previous day and store at −80 °C (*see* **Note 3**). Each test plate also contains pooled sera as a positive control (for example, pooled sera from 40 individuals previously demonstrated to have recognition of IEs, can be validated using this assay), and negative controls (sera from six malaria-naive donors) (*see* **Note 4**).
5. Resuspend IEs at 0.2 % hematocrit with wash solution and dispense 47.5 μl of suspension into each well (to give a 1:20 dilution of sera or plasma samples) containing test samples and controls (*see* **Note 5**). Gently tap the sides of the plate to agitate contents, then incubate for 30 min at room temperature (RT) and wash thrice at 350 × *g* for 3 min with wash solution, removing the supernatant after each wash.
6. Add 25 μl of secondary antibody (1:100 dilution), agitate by gently tapping the sides of the plate, followed by incubation for 30 min at RT and wash as above (*see* **Note 6**).
7. Add 25 μl of tertiary antibody (1:500 dilution) with 10 μg/ml of EtBr, agitate by gently tapping the sides of the plate, incubate for 30 min at RT in the dark and wash as above.
8. Resuspend cells in 100 μl of chilled 2 % PFA and store plate at 4 °C for at least 2 h in dark before acquisition. Final density is approximately 5×10^6 cells/ml.

3.2 FACS Acquisition

1. Calibrate the flow cytometer using calibration beads sourced from the manufacturer to ensure reproducibility of experiment.
2. Gate the population of red blood cells (RBC) with its forward scatter (FSC) and side scatter (SSC) characteristics using the no serum control, *see* Fig. 1a.
3. After gating for the RBC population, create a new 2-D histogram and set the *x*-axis to detect $EtBr^+$ fluorescence and set the *y*-axis to detect Alexa Fluor 647^+ fluorescence, Fig. 1b (*see* **Note 7**).
4. Using the no serum control, adjust the photomultiplier (PMT) voltage on the log fluorescence channels so negative population of cells and IEs are optimized geometrically in the first and

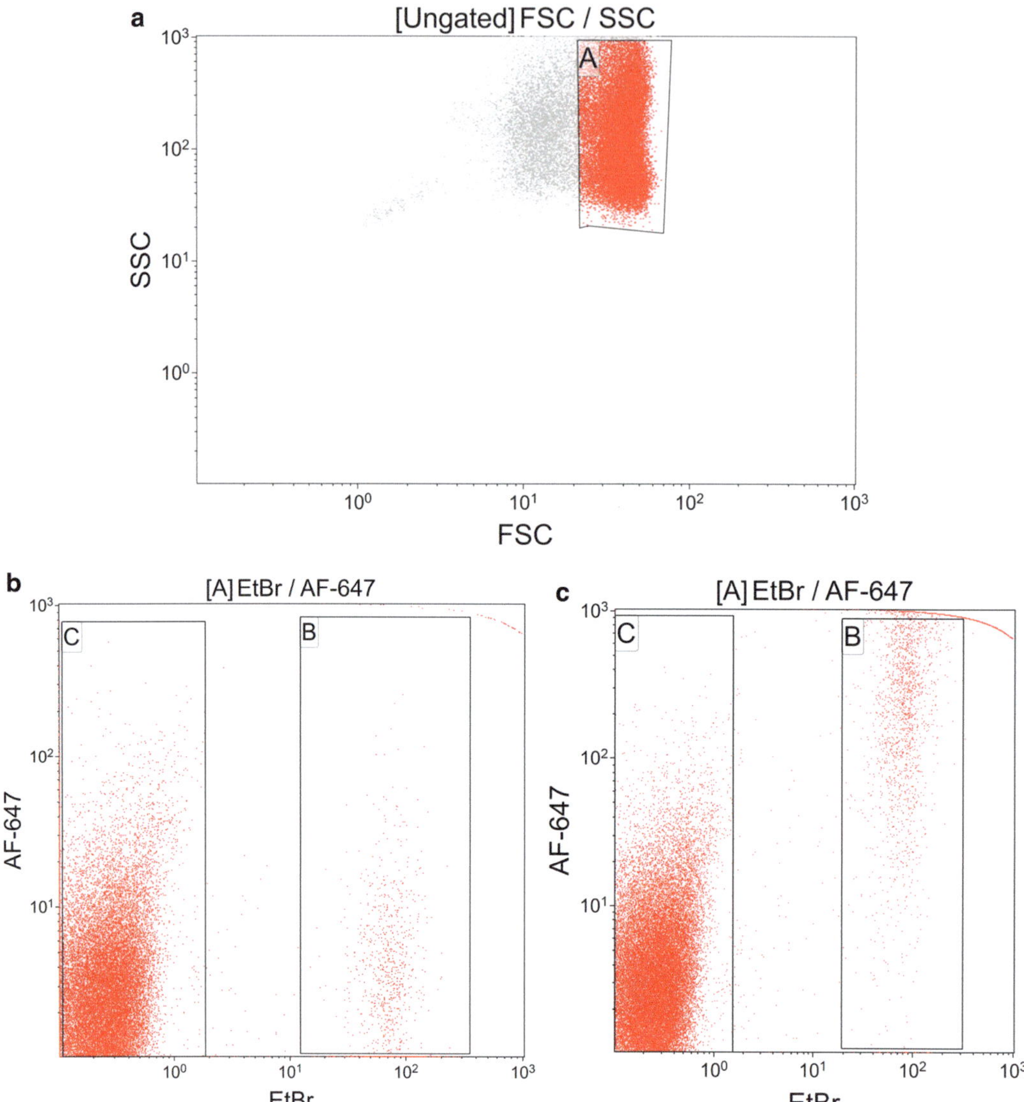

Fig. 1 FACS gating and analysis strategy. (**a**) Typical cytogram of IEs incubated with rabbit anti-human IgG (secondary) and Alexa Fluor 647 donkey-anti rabbit IgG (tertiary) antibody with ethidium bromide. Acquired events are plotted according to their side scatter (SS) and forward scatter (FS) characteristics. Gate A separates both infected and uninfected erythrocytes from cellular debris. (**b**) Gated infected and uninfected erythrocytes are then displayed on a 2D-histogram separating IEs from uninfected erythrocytes. In the region gated (B) are EtBr$^+$ IEs that are Alexa Fluor 647 low. In the region gated (C) are EtBr$^-$ and Alexa Fluor 647$^-$ uninfected erythrocytes. (**c**) Typical 2-D histogram of IEs incubated with malaria-infected patient's plasma. In the region gated (B) are EtBr$^+$ and Alexa Fluor 647 high IEs. In the region gated (C) are EtBr$^-$ and Alexa Fluor 647$^-$ uninfected erythrocytes. The geometric mean fluorescence intensity for gate B indicates the relative amount of antibody bound to IEs in this sample

second decade on the cytogram, *see* Fig. 1b (*see* **Note 8**). Once set, proceed with FACS acquisition.

5. Resuspend cells with multichannel pipettor prior to FACS acquisition. Load the plate onto a Hypercyt® Autosampler

attachment for a CyAnADP flow cytometer, and acquire samples for 15–20 s, at approximately 6000 events/s (*see* **Note 9**).

6. For users without an autosampler, ensure that the flow rate and acquisition time are sufficient to acquire a minimum of 2000 EtBr positive cells for each test sample.
7. Determine the geometric mean fluorescence intensity (MFI) for Alexa Fluor 647 of the $EtBr^+$ IEs, *see* Fig. 1c.
8. Antibody recognition can be expressed as geometric MFI. Determine the MFI for Alexa Fluor 647 in the $EtBr^+$ population. From this, subtract the auto-fluorescence (of the $EtBr^-$ population), to determine the relative amount of antibody bound to IEs (*see* **Note 10**). From this, subtract the mean MFI of the six negative control samples tested, giving the absolute difference (*see* **Note 11**).
9. Evaluate the amount of variation between duplicates and rerun samples with unacceptable variation (*see* **Note 12**).
10. Results are analyzed using software Kaluza® software (Beckman-Coulter) or similar programs.
11. The replicate mean difference is calculated by taking the MFI of one sample replicate and subtracting the uncorrected geometric MFI.
12. Samples with a mean readout of greater than the mean plus three standard deviations of the negative control are considered as positive for IgG against VSA of IEs.
13. The experiment is considered unsuccessful when 70 % of the test samples have a geometric MFI above the pooled positive controls.
14. Reasons for an unsuccessful assay includes the fact that too many cells were lost during the washes or the parasites were not synchronized to mid-late stage trophozoites.

4 Notes

1. Test samples can also be acquired using other flow cytometer attached with an autosampler, for example a BD FACSCantoII flow cytometer; BD Biosciences.
2. U-bottom 96-well plates are coated with 170 µl NCS for at least 1 h, 2 days before an experiment. Plates are washed twice with 200 µl PBS, wrapped in cling wrap, and stored at 4 °C. NCS can be reused up to five times.
3. Aliquot patient plasma or sera and heat-inactivate at 57 °C for 45 min to remove complement factors and then store at −80 °C. Patient samples should be coated on the day of experiment, if this is not possible, coat 1 day before, wrap in cling-wrap, and store at −80 °C.

4. Include in the first test plate a no serum control, which is incubated with only secondary and tertiary antibody with EtBr. This control is to ensure reproducibility of assay.
5. IEs resuspended at 0.2 % hematocrit can also be incubated with test sample at 1:10 dilution. This is preferable when the majority of test samples in the cohort has low levels of detectable antibody, for example cohorts from low or unstable malaria transmission settings.
6. When using secondary or tertiary antibody from a different supplier, perform titration to obtain optimum concentrations.
7. Ethidium Bromide excitation spectrum peaks at ~510 nm and its fluorescence emission spectrum peaks at ~600 nm. Alexa-Fluor 647 excitation spectrum peaks at ~650 nm and its fluorescence emission spectrum peaks at ~660 nm. Use the appropriate laser and detection filter to ensure optimal excitation and detection of EtBr and Alexa-Fluor 647 fluorescence.
8. In our set up, the PMT voltage for ethidium bromide fluorescence is set at 690 V while the Alexa-Fluor 647 fluorescence is in the range between 500 and 550 V.
9. Hypercyt® Autosampler is an attachment and may work differently with different flow cytometers.

Table 1
Determination of whether samples require re-testing

	Replicate MFI	Auto-fluorescence	Corrected average MFI	% relative MFI	Replicate mean difference (*see* Note 12)	Adjusted mean variance	Repeat
Positive control	988.1 968.4	25.2 22.2	954.5	100	9.9	(9.9/978.3) × 100 = 1.0	No
Malaria-naïve control	26.2 27.6	11.4 11.2	15.6	0	0.7	(0.7/26.9) × 100 = 2.6	No
Sample 1	212.6 195.4	6.4 8.3	196.6	(196.6 − 15.6)/(954.5 − 15.6) × 100 = 19.3	8.6	(8.6/204) × 100 = 4.2	No
Sample 2	302.5 126.1	5.5 3.9	209.6	(209.6 − 15.6)/(954.5 − 15.6) × 100 = 20.6	88.2	(88.2/214.3) × 100 = 41.2	Yes

The replicate mean difference is calculated. The replicate mean difference value is then divided by the mean replicate and multiplied by 100 to obtain a percentage point. Samples with an adjusted mean variance of >20 % points and a replicate mean difference of >10 % points between duplicates should be rerun

10. Geometric mean fluorescence intensity acquired for Alexa-Fluor 647 population in gated population (B) is subtracted with gated population (C) to eliminate auto-fluorescence of Alexa-Fluor 647 in uninfected erythrocytes, Fig. 1c.
11. The relative antibody in sample can be expressed as a relative MFI using the positive and negative controls from each plate. Relative antibody: (average of duplicates subtract average of negative controls) divided by (average of positive controls subtract average of negative controls) multiply by 100. A final result on a scale of 0–100 is generated.
12. Samples with an adjusted mean variance of >20 % and a replicate mean difference of >10 % points between duplicates are rerun [4]. An example run is included (Table 1).

References

1. Smith JD, Gamain B, Baruch DI, Kyes S (2001) Decoding the language of var genes and *Plasmodium falciparum* sequestration. Trends Parasitol 17:538–545
2. Chan JA, Howell KB, Reiling L et al (2012) Targets of antibodies against *Plasmodium falciparum-infected* erythrocytes in malaria immunity. J Clin Invest 122:3227–3238
3. Trager W, Jensen J (1976) Human malaria parasites in continuous culture. Science 193:673–675
4. Aitken EH, Mbewe B, Luntamo M et al (2010) Antibodies to chondroitin sulfate A-binding infected erythrocytes: dynamics and protection during pregnancy in women receiving intermittent preventive treatment. J Infect Dis 201: 1316–1325

Chapter 18

Inhibition of Infected Red Blood Cell Binding to the Vascular Endothelium

Marion Avril

Abstract

Plasmodium falciparum-infected red blood cells (IRBC) adhere to the endothelium via receptors expressed on the surface of vascular endothelial cells (EC) and sequester in the microvasculature of several organs. Sequestration is the primary step leading to complications related to the severity of malaria. In order to study this cytoadhesion phenomenon, IRBC in vitro binding assays have been developed using a monolayer of primary or transformed endothelial cells. Here we describe the methodology of an assay to inhibit the binding of IRBC on vascular endothelial cells under static adhesion conditions. Similar techniques could be used for conducting a binding inhibition assay under flow assay conditions using an appropriate device.

Key words Malaria, *Plasmodium*, Cytoadhesion, Microvasculature, Endothelium, Binding assays

1 Introduction

Most human malaria deaths are caused by blood-stage *Plasmodium falciparum* parasites.

Severe malaria is a multifactorial phenomenon involving the microvascular obstruction (sequestration) of *P. falciparum*-infected red blood cells (IRBC) in deep vascular endothelium [1], metabolic disturbances, such as acidosis [2] and the production of inflammatory cytokines, such as TNF-α and IFN-γ [3].

The ability of IRBC to bind to microvascular endothelial cells (cytoadhesion) and become sequestered from the peripheral blood was described in postmortem studies of patients who died from falciparum malaria in the 1890s [4]. IRBC sequestration is not limited to a specific tissue or organ, it is found in many microvascular tissues of the human body, including gut, lung, dermis, heart, and brain [5, 6]. In cerebral malaria, one of the most life-threatening complication of the disease, IRBC accumulate in the microvasculature of the brain [5, 7] leading to acidosis, hypoxia, and harmful inflammatory cytokines in the brain [8].

Ashley M. Vaughan (ed.), *Malaria Vaccines: Methods and Protocols*, Methods in Molecular Biology, vol. 1325, DOI 10.1007/978-1-4939-2815-6_18, © Springer Science+Business Media New York 2015

IRBC adhere directly to various host endothelial receptors, including CD36 [9], intracellular adhesion molecule-1 (ICAM-1) [10], vascular cellular adhesion molecule-1 (VCAM-1), E-selectin (formerly known as ELAM-1) [11], P-selectin, thrombospodin-1 (TSP) [12], chondroitin sulfate-A (CSA) [13, 14], and endothelial protein C receptor (EPCR) [15]. A subset of IRBCs also forms clumps or agglutinates to other IRBC [16] or forms rosettes by adhering to non-infected erythrocytes [17]. In addition to direct parasite adhesion to host receptors, platelets can act as a bridge between IRBC and endothelial cells, providing additional CD36 receptors for cytoadhesion [18]. IRBC adhesion is mediated by the *P. falciparum* erythrocyte membrane protein 1 (PfEMP1) family [19–21]. PfEMP1 proteins encode distinct adhesion properties. Clonal antigenic variation of PfEMP1 variants modifies IRBC binding specificity and enables evasion of host immunity. Field studies have suggested that the ability to bind to CD36 is shared by most wild strains of *P. falciparum*, although levels of adhesion are variable [22, 23]. Other adhesion traits also vary between PfEMP1 proteins and it is likely that additional host receptors involved in this IRBC sequestration remain to be identified. Overall, cytoadhesion is thought to be a major factor in the virulence of *P. falciparum* malaria because of its likely contribution to ischemic pathology, and because it may represent a strategy developed by the parasite to avoid the host's normal splenic clearance mechanisms that remove aged or damaged erythrocytes [24–26]. Even though the mechanism by which IRBC attach to the blood microvasculature is not fully understood, there is considerable interest in elucidating the molecular mechanisms of this adhesion process through in vitro "sequestration models."

The roles and relative importance of the different host receptors in vivo remain ambiguous, and they have been barely studied in adhesion models that mimic circulatory conditions. Furthermore, it is very challenging to test anti-adhesion therapies in an animal model that truly reflects the pathophysiology of severe falciparum malaria in humans. Even though some attempts have been made to develop animal models of sequestration [27] their relevance to human disease mechanisms remain unverified. None of the primate or rodent malaria species develops clinical and pathological features similar to those in humans and *P. falciparum* has co-evolved to recognize human plasma membrane receptors. A few studies using human vasculature grafted onto immunodeficient mice have been used successfully to investigate sequestration and anti-adhesion drugs [28, 29]. Further research in this area would clearly be of benefit, and the development of humanized animal models [30, 31] and transgenic parasites to enable the study of specific human: *P. falciparum* receptor–ligand interactions might be one way forward.

All of the findings mentioned above illustrate the complexity of studying the cytoadhesion interactions between *P. falciparum*

IRBC and host human cell. However, they open up the possibility of developing therapeutic interventions aimed at blocking or reversing parasite adhesion. Knowledge of the molecular mechanisms of parasite adhesion could be used to design vaccines aimed at raising antibodies to block adhesion and prevent sequestration. In the case of a blood stage vaccine for example, the spleen would then be able to remove non-sequestered mature IRBC, and so the build-up of high parasite burdens of avidly sequestering parasites could be avoided and severe malaria prevented. However, the vaccine approach is challenging because of the variability of the parasite adhesion ligand PfEMP1 which is highly polymorphic. For this reason, anti-PfEMP1 vaccines will need to target crossreactive antibody epitopes against a range of different isolates. The in vitro endothelial binding models also open up the opportunity to investigate disease mechanisms. A detailed understanding of disease processes may suggest novel interventions to treat host–pathogen mechanisms. Overall, an in vitro "sequestration model" to vascular endothelium is needed to study the molecular interaction between the IRBC and host receptors, as well as the effect of putative anti-cytoadherence drugs or potential vaccine candidates.

1.1 Basic Experimental Design

IRBC cytoadhesion had been often examined using ex vivo or in in situ model systems in an attempt to simulate the interaction between IRBC and the endothelium, but none is a perfect model of the circulation in every respect. Ex vivo assays usually use either a cross-species mixture of parasite and host animal, or examine non-human malaria parasites. On the other hand, few in vitro assays have been developed using human endothelial cells with laboratory-adapted *P. falciparum* strains. For example, the immortalized Human Brain microvascular Endothelial Cell line (HBEC-5i) has been used as an in vitro model of the blood–brain barrier to study cerebral endothelial vasculature [32]. Endothelial cells lines representing the microvasculature are very useful for the investigation of static assays related to the cytoadhesion of suspensions of IRBC, which could settle onto the sub-confluent monolayers of cultured cells. After a period of incubation (typically 30–60 min) the non-adherent IRBC are removed by a standardized washing procedure. Adherent cells are then counted, most commonly by direct microscopic observation of Giemsa-stained cells.

This type of assay is technically easy and relatively inexpensive, and allows a relatively large number of assays to be carried out simultaneously. However, the assay is performed in a static environment that ignores the shear forces exerted on adherent cells by circulating blood which might be considered in any attempt to assess the pathological importance of cytoadhesion.

For the binding assay of IRBC to vascular endothelium techniques described below, the endothelial cells are grown on a multi-chamber slide, which consists of a removable polystyrene media chamber attached to a specially treated standard glass microscope slide (25×75 mm). The multi-chambered design presents an optimal surface for attachment and growth of cells and allows for parallel studies of multiple conditions. Individual wells are separated by a slightly raised hydrophobic border to prevent cross-contamination between wells. This system is compatible with all imaging equipment and makes the microscopic examination very convenient. The slide may then be fixed, stained and cover-slipped for long term storage.

2 Materials

2.1 Preparing the Endothelial Cell Slides

1. Serological pipettes.
2. Pipettor and hand pipettes.
3. Unplugged glass Pasteur pipettes.
4. 15 ml conical tubes.
5. 37 °C water bath.
6. Multi-chamber 1, 2, 4, or 8-well slides either unmodified or precoated.
   (a) Slide precoated with collagen (BD Biocoat #354557).
   (b) Slide precoated with fibronectin (BD Biocoat # 354630).
   (c) Slide precoated with polylysine (Thermo Scientific Nunc™ Lab-Tek™ II Chamber Slide™ System).
   (d) Unmodified polystyrene slide (Falcon# 354118).
   (e) Slide Biocompatible adhesive (Thermo Scientific Nunc™ Lab-Tek™ II Chamber Slide™ System).
7. Separation device for the multi-chamber slide supplied by the manufacturer.
8. Sterile petri dish.
9. Hemocytometer.
10. PBS 1× without calcium and magnesium.
11. Distilled water.
12. Tissue culture flask (unmodified or pre-coated).
13. 0.25 % Trypsin–EDTA 1× solution.
14. 37 °C incubator supplied with 5 % CO_2 and 95 % relative humidity.
15. Phase contrast microscope with a 40× objective.
16. Tabletop centrifuge.
17. Biological safety cabinet with vacuum line.

2.2 Setting Up for the Binding Assay Experiment

1. Glass slide container.
2. Pre-warmed RPMI-BSA (RPMI-1640 binding medium containing 0.5 % BSA, pH 6.8–7.2).
3. 0.7 % pork gelatin solution (liquefies at 37 °C).

2.3 For the Binding Assay

1. Serological pipettes.
2. Pipettor and hand pipettes.
3. Unplugged glass Pasteur pipettes.
4. 15 ml conical tubes.
5. 37 °C water bath.
6. Mineral oil.
7. Glass microscope slides.
8. Glass coverslips.
9. Giemsa stain.
10. Distilled water.
11. 100 % methanol.
12. Light microscope with 100× objective and 10× eyepiece.
13. Parafilm.
14. Microcentrifuge tubes.
15. 10 μl hand pipettes.
16. Eukitt Mounting media (E.M.S, Catalog #15320–15322).
17. Prolong mounting medium (Life Technologies, P7481).

3 Methods

3.1 Seeding the Monolayer of Endothelial Cells (3–4 Days Before the Assay)

1. Grow the endothelial cells to 80–90 % confluency in a 37 °C incubator supplied with 5 % CO_2 (*see* **Note 1**).
2. The monolayer can be treated with 1× trypsin-EDTA to detach and disperse the cells.
3. Aspirate media from the tissue culture flask using a sterile glass Pasteur pipette.
4. Wash the flask with 5 ml of PBS 1× twice in order to remove serum.
5. Detach the cells from a 25-cm^2 flask by incubating the cells with 2 ml of 1× trypsin-EDTA solution. You can examine the cells under the microscope to ensure that the cell layer is dispersed and detached from the substratum (usually within 5–10 min) (*see* **Note 2**).
6. Add 5–10 ml of growth media and aspirate the cells by gently pipetting.

7. Transfer to cell suspension to a 15 ml tube and centrifuge at $200 \times g$ for 5 min.
8. Discard the supernatant and suspend the pellet with 1 ml of growth media by pipetting gently.
9. Take appropriate aliquot of the cell suspension and transfer it to a new culture flask containing growth media to seed cells. Label the flask with the cell line, passage number and date. Incubate cultures in a 37 °C incubator supplied with 5 % CO_2 and 95 % relative humidity.
10. Determinate the current cell concentration using the hemocytometer.
11. Seed the multi-chamber slide by diluting the cells down to 20–30 % confluency (visual and subjective estimation), then to allow them to grow back for 3–4 days to reach 100 % confluency on the day of the binding assay (*see* **Note 3**).
12. Add the appropriate amount of growth media to the 1 ml cell suspension and distribute the correct volume of cells per well (2.5 ml, 1.2 ml, 0.5 ml, or 0.3 ml for 1, 2, 4, or 8-well chamber slides respectively).
13. Once seeded, place the slide within a sterile petri dish inside the 37 °C incubator supplied with 5 % CO_2 and 95 % relative humidity (*see* **Note 4**).
14. Allow the cells to grow for 3–4 days to achieve 100 % confluency on the day of the binding assay.
15. Change cell culture media in each well every 48 h.

3.2 On the Day of Assay, Prior to Starting the Binding Assay Experiment

1. Pre-warm RPMI-BSA binding medium in a 37 °C water bath.
2. Once cells are confluent (*see* **Note 5**), aspirate the cell media with low vacuum and add 3 ml, 1.5 ml, 0.5 ml, or 0.2 ml of pre-warmed RPMI-BSA binding media per well for 1, 2, 4, or 8-well chamber slides respectively, to block unspecific background of binding.
3. Let the slide pre-incubate in the 37 °C incubator supplied with 5 % CO_2 for no more than 30 min (*see* **Note 6**).
4. Pre-warm 0.7 % pork gelatin solution in a 37 °C water bath.
5. Fill a glass slide container with RPMI-BSA binding medium and reserve it in a 37 °C water bath until the washing step.

3.3 IRBC Gelatin Enrichment

1. Gelatin enrichment of the IRBC is preferred over a MACS column purification in order to preserve the integrity of the RBC membrane surrounding the parasite (*see* **Note 7**). For this, grow IRBC in 5 % hematocrit culture to a parasitemia of 4–8 % synchronized trophozoites.

2. Pellet the IRBC culture by centrifugation for 5 min at 600 × *g*.
3. Discard the supernatant and resuspend the pellet with ten times the pellet volume with pre-warmed 0.7 % pork gelatin solution and transfer into a 15 ml tube. Mix well without creating air bubbles.
4. Incubate upright in a 37 °C water bath for 1 h (*see* **Note 8**).
5. During the gelatin enrichment incubation time, proceed to the pre-incubation of the endothelial cells with the molecules of interest if required (Subheading 3.5).

3.4 Preparing the IRBC Suspension

1. After 1 h incubation at 37 °C, take the gelatin tube out of the water bath.
2. You should see a gradient including a top clear layer followed by a cloudier layer and a dark blood pellet. Mature stage knob positive IRBC are among the top two layers, whereas the non-infected red blood cells or knob negative IRBC are in the pellet.
3. Transfer the top two layers into a new 15 ml tube and add 5 ml of pre-warmed RPMI-BSA media for a wash.
4. Pellet down the enriched IRBC culture by centrifugation 5 min at 600 × *g*.
5. Aspirate with low vacuum and discard the supernatant.
6. Repeat the wash step once.
7. Aspirate with low vacuum and discard the supernatant. Add 20 μl of pre-warmed RPMI-BSA on top of the tiny blood pellet.
8. Take a few microliters (2–3 μl) from the enriched IRBC pellet to make a small smear on a glass microscopic slide. Dry the smear, fix it with 100 % methanol and stain it with 10 % Giemsa for 5 min.
9. In the meantime, resuspend the pellet with 1 ml of pre-warmed RPMI-BSA and calculate the number of RBC present in 1 ml using the hemocytometer. For this, perform a 100× dilution by mixing 10 μl of the IRBC suspension into an Eppendorf tube containing 1 ml of RPMI.
10. Once the Giemsa staining is done, rinse the slide with water, dry and determine parasitemia. Count at least three fields with approximately 200 red blood cells (RBC) per field using the light microscope. The percentage parasitemia = (the number of IRBC/total number of RBC) × 100.
11. Finally, calculate the total number of IRBC/ml = number of RBC/ml × percentage parasitemia (IRBC/RBC).
12. Resuspend the IRBC suspension to a final concentration of 1×10^7 IRBC/ml in pre-warmed RPMI-BSA binding medium.

3.5 Binding Assays of IRBC on a Monolayer of Endothelial Cells

There are two ways to set up a binding assay experiment that allow one to investigate the capability of molecules or reagents to inhibit IRBC binding. The molecule or reagent under investigation could be polyclonal anti-serum, monoclonal antibodies, a recombinant protein, or chemical reagents. A corresponding control should be used such as pre-immune anti-serum, irrelevant monoclonal antibodies, negative control recombinant protein or minimally RPMI-BSA binding media if nothing else is applicable.

Option1, when the molecule or reagent to test is directed against the parasite ligand, it needs to be pre-incubated with the IRBC suspension prior to adding to the vascular endothelial cells.

Option 2, when the molecule or reagent is specific for the receptors or proteins expressed on the surface of the vascular endothelium, it needs to be added to the cell monolayer prior to the IRBC suspension.

In both cases, pre-incubation steps are important and need to be done for 30 min to 1 h prior to adding the IRBC suspension on top of the endothelial cells.

Option 1: Pre-incubation of IRBC and molecule or reagent prior to binding assay experiment on vascular endothelial cells

1. In a microcentrifuge tube, prepare a 50:50 (volume/volume) mixture including the molecule or reagent at 2× final concentration + the IRBC suspension at 1×10^7 IRBC/ml. Use the RPMI-BSA binding medium for all dilutions if needed. Mix well by pipetting. Use volumes appropriate for the well size as detailed above (*see* **Note 9**).
2. Incubate for 30 min at room temperature or in a 37 °C water bath.
3. In the meantime, leave the cell monolayer in RPMI-BSA binding medium inside the 37 °C CO_2 incubator.
4. After a 30 min pre-incubation, remove the slide from the incubator and aspirate (with low vacuum) the RPMI-BSA binding media from each well.
5. Add the IBRC + molecule mixture into the appropriate wells.
6. Replace the slide inside the 37 °C CO_2 incubator and incubate for 1–2 h.
7. You can check under the microscope after the first 10 min that IRBC have settled down nicely on the monolayer of cells (*see* **Note 10**).
8. At the end of the incubation time, proceed to the washing step.

Option 2: Pre-incubation of molecule or reagent on vascular endothelial cells before IRBC binding assay experiment

1. Each molecule or reagent to test and the corresponding control solution should be diluted in pre-warmed RPMI-BSA binding media at the final concentration desired.

2. Aspirate culture medium with low vacuum and add 1.5 ml, 0.75 ml, 0.25 ml, or 0.1 ml (respectively) of the appropriate molecule or test reagent in pre-warmed BSA binging media to the 1, 2, 4, or 8 well chamber slide.
3. Incubate in the 37 °C CO_2 incubator for 30 min. Note: plan to have the gelatin enrichment of the IRBC suspension ready by the end of this 30 min period (so this step should be done while the gelatin is ongoing).
4. Remove the slide from the incubator.
5. Without removing any solution previously added, add (per well) the same volume of the IRBC suspension at 1×10^7 IRBC/ml (i.e., 1.5 ml, 0.75 ml, 0.25 ml, or 0.1 ml for the 2, 4, or 8 wells chamber slide, respectively).
6. Gently pipet the IRBC suspension on the side of the well to insure even across each well. The final concentration of the molecule or reagent will be 1× and the IRBC at 5×10^6 IRBC/ml.
7. Replace the slide inside the 37 °C CO_2 incubator and let it incubate for 1–2 h.
8. Check under the microscope after the first 10 min to verify that IRBC have completely settled on the monolayer of cells (*see* **Note 10**).
9. At the end of the incubation time, proceed to the washing step.

3.6 Washing Steps of the Binding Assay

1. After the 1 h or 2 h incubation time, remove the reserved glass slide washing container (prefilled with RPMI-BSA binding medium) from the 37 °C water bath, and remove the slides from the incubator.
2. Aspirate (with low vacuum) the solution from each well (place the glass Pasteur pipette by the side of the well, without touching the bottom of the well where the IRBC should be settled).
3. Remove the upper chamber wells and the inert silicone gasket using the black and white separation device supplied (*see* **Note 11**) (*see* Fig. 1).
4. Peel off the upper chamber and the silicone gasket from the slide. This step needs to be done as quickly as possible in order to prevent the cells from drying out.
5. Remove the slide from the separation device.
6. Transfer the glass slide into a washing container; place it vertically between two supporting racks (*see* **Note 12**).
7. Quickly attach a sheet of Parafilm on the top of the container and incline the slide container at a 70–90° angle. The slides are now flipped horizontally and upside down, allowing the unbound IRBC to fall off by gravity for 10 min (*see* Fig. 2).

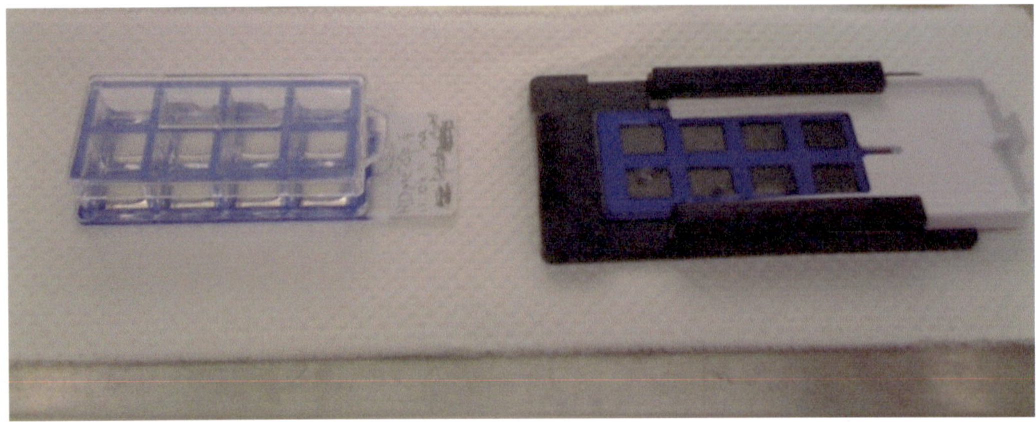

Fig. 1 On the *left* is an 8-well chamber slide and on the *right* is the same slide after removing the upper chamber wells and the inert silicone gasket using the black and white separation device

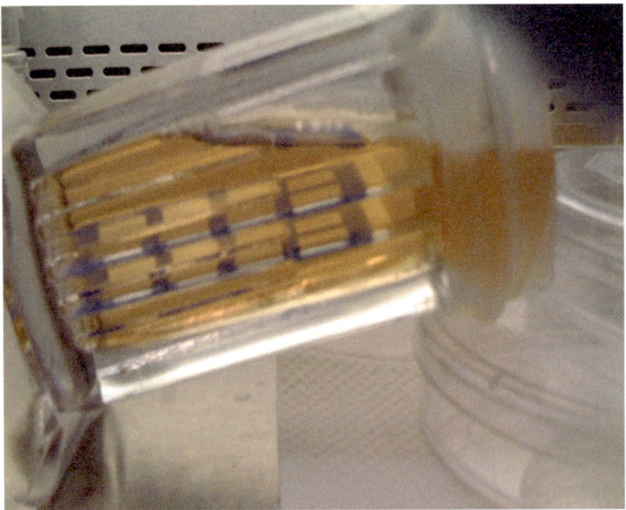

Fig. 2 The slide is placed between 2 supporting racks within the washing container with a sheet of Parafilm on the top of the container. Then the container is inclined at a 70–90° angle allowing the unbound IRBC to fall off by gravity

8. After 10 min, bring the glass container upright, remove and discard the Parafilm and take the slide out of the container.
9. Wipe the back of the slide and place it inside a plastic petri dish.
10. Observe the slide using the phase contrast microscope (with 40× objective) to determine if this washing step was sufficient to remove all unbound IRBC.
11. If so, continue to the preservation/fixation of the slide. If not, proceed to another wash step as described below in **step 12**.
12. Using the same glass slide container in an upright position, gently dunk the slide in and out of the washing medium in a

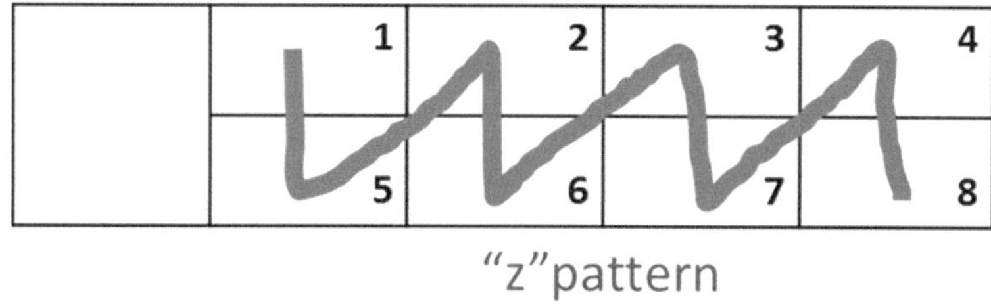

Fig. 3 Representation of the continuous "z" pattern when the mounting solution is added to the surface of the slide

vertical orientation twice, making sure to completely immerse the slide each time.

13. Take the slide out from the container, wipe the back and repeat **step 9**. If floating or unbound IRBC are still visible (*see* **Note 13**), proceed to the next washing step, otherwise continue to the preservation/fixation of the slide.
14. If another wash is needed, re-submerge the slide within the glass container. While holding it straight and firmly (and with the slide completely submerged), do the movement back and forth twice (the idea is to create some shear stress forces to wash in the opposite way relative to the previous step).
15. Remove the slide out from the container, wipe the back and put it back on the petri dish to check for remaining unbound IRBC using the phase contrast microscope (with the 40× objective) .
16. If unbound IRBC remain, alternate the washing steps (dunk up and down and back and forth) until no floating or non-adherent IRBCs are visible.

3.7 Preserve the Slide

3.7.1 For Giemsa Stained Slides

1. Fix the slide by submerging it with 1 % glutaraldehyde for 30 min at room temperature.
2. Rinse off the glutaraldehyde with PBS and air-dry the slide.
3. Fix with 100 % methanol and stain it with 10 % Giemsa for 5 min.
4. Rinse the Giemsa stained slide with water and air-dry it.
5. Under the fume hood, mount a long coverslip on the slide using the Eukitt Mounting solution. In order to avoid introducing air bubbles, use a 1 ml disposable transfer pipette to withdraw mounting solution, and then add to the surface in a continuous z-pattern over all of the wells (*see* Fig. 3). Then, add the cover-slip.
6. Allow to air-dry for 24 h under the fume hood.
7. The slide is then ready for quantification.

3.7.2 For Fluorescent Viewing (If Applicable)

1. Fix the slide in 2 % paraformaldehyde for 10 min (note: paraformaldehyde creates much less fluorescent background then glutaraldehyde).
2. Air-dry the slide.
3. Mount the slide (use a long coverslip) with the Prolong reagent (Life technologies, P7481). Add 32 drops of room-temperature mounting medium to one tube of powdered Prolong anti-fade reagent and mix gently with the 1 ml pipette (with the tip cut to expand the opening which avoids creating air bubbles).
4. Add anti-fade solution in a continuous z-pattern over the wells, apply a coverslip, and allow to dry 24 h at room temperature or 4 °C while protected from light.

3.8 Quantification of IRBC Binding

The binding of IRBC to the vascular endothelial cells can be qualified as either the number of IRBC adherent per mm^2 of confluent endothelial cells or as the number of IRBC adherent per 100 endothelial cells. For a statistical analysis of binding assays, independent biological replicates should be performed at least in triplicate on different days.

1. Count IRBC adherent per mm^2 endothelial cells:
   (a) Choosing randomly in each well, select 4 representative fields of confluent endothelial cells.
   (b) Count the number of adherent IRBC on each of those 4 fields per well under a light microscope with the 40× objective and 10× eyepiece (400× magnification).
   (c) Calculate the number of IRBC/mm^2 = number of IRBC counted/surface area of the counted field (*see* **Note 14**).
2. Count IRBC adherent per 100 endothelial cells:
   (a) Choosing randomly in each well, select four representative fields of confluent endothelial cells.
   (b) Count the number of adherent IRBC on each of those four fields per well under a light microscope with 40× objective and 10× eyepiece (400× magnification).
   (c) Count the number of endothelial cells present in each of those fields.
   (d) Calculate the number of IRBC/100 endothelial cells = (number of IRBC counted × 100)/number of endothelial cells counted.
3. Taking pictures of the binding assays
   (a) Pictures of IRBC binding to the vascular endothelial cells can be taken later under a light inverted microscope (objectives 20× or 40×), equipped with an appropriate camera device.

4 Notes

1. Seeding of the endothelial cell type and their growth curves should be followed according to their manufacturers' recommendations. Transformed or primary endothelial cells are seeded on their appropriate adhesion support, which could be a non-coated or pre-coated tissue culture treated glass slide. Multi-chamber slide are available featuring 1, 2, 4, or 8 wells. The culture area for each well is 8.6 cm^2, 4 cm^2, 1.7 cm^2, or 0.7 cm^2, respectively.
2. To avoid clumping do not agitate the cells by hitting or shaking the flask while waiting for the cells to detach. Cells that are difficult to detach may be placed at 37 °C to facilitate dispersal.
3. The optimal density at which to seed cells depends on the cell-type and may vary from 1,000 cells/cm^2 to 10,000 cells/cm^2.
4. Using the petri dish facilitates manipulating with ease the slide to observe microscopic cell growth and during the binding assay experiment and also can prevent contamination from handling.
5. After 3 or 4 days of growth, the vascular endothelial cells should be nearly 100 % confluent. This can be checked using a phase contrast microscope with a 40× objective. If the cells are 100 % confluent, proceed to the binding assay experiment. If not, allow extra days of growth.
6. If incubation is longer than 30 min in presence of incomplete serum-free media such as the RPMI-BSA binding media, cells may start to retract from the slide. So timing and planning each step of the incubation is critical.
7. MACS purification could create "mechanical forces" that lyse the RBC, releasing "free" parasites which will stick to the endothelial cells and create nonspecific binding.
8. The tube containing the gelatin preparation should remain untouched and upright for 1 h in order for the gradient of gelatin to separate appropriately.
9. The final concentration of the molecule or reagent will be 1× and the IRBC at 5×10^6 IRBC/ml.
10. If the IRBC are not evenly distributed, then you can disperse them by gently rocking the slide back and forth between a 12 o'clock and 6 o'clock position and gently tipping the slide (4 times), and then gently rocking back and forth between 3 o'clock and 9 o'clock (4 times). The goal is to gently agitate the solution so the IRBC are dispersed over the slide but avoid rocking too hard, which create swirls and shear stress. However, we do not observe IRBC distribution to be an issue. They settle and stay evenly distributed of the bottom of the well.

11. As described by the manufacturers' recommendations, place the chamber slide on the black support, and insert the white support between the bottom of the slide and the right edge of the chamber. While holding the slide in the black support, gently insert the white support between the chamber and the slide to lift the chamber walls off of the slide.
12. The washing container can fit up to four glass slides vertically between the supporting racks.
13. The unattached IRBCs or RBCs can be detected by gently lifting and dropping the petri dish on the microscope stand. Adherent IRBCs will not move.
14. The surface area of the field could be calculated using a precise stage micrometer calibration slide (used to calibrate your microscope). It comes with 1 mm total length that is subdivided into 100 divisions, that is, each division is 0.01 mm.

References

1. Udeinya IJ, Graves PM, Carter R, Aikawa M, Miller LH (1983) *Plasmodium falciparum*: effect of time in continuous culture on binding to human endothelial cells and amelanotic melanoma cells. Exp Parasitol 56:207–214
2. Planche T, Krishna S (2006) Severe malaria: metabolic complications. Curr Mol Med 6:141–153
3. Schodel F, Wirtz R, Peterson D, Hughes J, Warren R, Sadoff J, Milich D (1994) Immunity to malaria elicited by hybrid hepatitis B virus core particles carrying circumsporozoite protein epitopes. J Exp Med 180:1037–1046
4. Marchiafava E, Bignami A (1884). On summer-autumnal malaria fever. In: Two monographs on malaria and the parasites of malaria fevers. London: The New Sydenham Society 150:1–232
5. MacPherson GG, Warrell MJ, White NJ, Looareesuwan S, Warrell DA (1985) Human cerebral malaria. A quantitative ultrastructural analysis of parasitized erythrocyte sequestration. Am J Pathol 119:385–401
6. Milner DA Jr, Whitten RO, Kamiza S, Carr R, Liomba G, Dzamalala C, Seydel KB, Molyneux ME, Taylor TE (2014) The systemic pathology of cerebral malaria in African children. Front Cell Infect Microbiol 4:104
7. Taylor TE, Fu WJ, Carr RA, Whitten RO, Mueller JS, Fosiko NG, Lewallen S, Liomba NG, Molyneux ME (2004) Differentiating the pathologies of cerebral malaria by postmortem parasite counts. Nat Med 10:143–145
8. van der Heyde HC, Nolan J, Combes V, Gramaglia I, Grau GE (2006) A unified hypothesis for the genesis of cerebral malaria: sequestration, inflammation and hemostasis leading to microcirculatory dysfunction. Trends Parasitol 22:503–508
9. Barnwell JW, Asch AS, Nachman RL, Yamaya M, Aikawa M, Ingravallo P (1989) A human 88-kD membrane glycoprotein (CD36) functions in vitro as a receptor for a cytoadherence ligand on *Plasmodium falciparum*-infected erythrocytes. J Clin Invest 84:765–772
10. Berendt AR, Simmons DL, Tansey J, Newbold CI, Marsh K (1989) Intercellular adhesion molecule-1 is an endothelial cell adhesion receptor for *Plasmodium falciparum*. Nature 341:57–59
11. Ockenhouse CF, Tegoshi T, Maeno Y, Benjamin C, Ho M, Kan KE, Thway Y, Win K, Aikawa M, Lobb RR (1992) Human vascular endothelial cell adhesion receptors for *Plasmodium falciparum*-infected erythrocytes: roles for endothelial leukocyte adhesion molecule 1 and vascular cell adhesion molecule 1. J Exp Med 176:1183–1189
12. Roberts DD, Sherwood JA, Spitalnik SL, Panton LJ, Howard RJ, Dixit VM, Frazier WA, Miller LH, Ginsburg V (1985) Thrombospondin binds falciparum malaria parasitized erythrocytes and may mediate cytoadherence. Nature 318:64–66
13. Rogerson SJ, Chaiyaroj SC, Ng K, Reeder JC, Brown GV (1995) Chondroitin sulfate A is a cell surface receptor for *Plasmodium falciparum-infected* erythrocytes. J Exp Med 182:15–20
14. Fried M, Duffy PE (1996) Adherence of *Plasmodium falciparum* to chondroitin sulfate

A in the human placenta. Science 272: 1502–1504

15. Turner L, Lavstsen T, Berger SS, Wang CW, Petersen JE, Avril M, Brazier AJ, Freeth J, Jespersen JS, Nielsen MA, Magistrado P, Lusingu J, Smith JD, Higgins MK, Theander TG (2013) Severe malaria is associated with parasite binding to endothelial protein C receptor. Nature 498:502–505
16. Pain A, Ferguson DJ, Kai O, Urban BC, Lowe B, Marsh K, Roberts DJ (2001) Platelet-mediated clumping of *Plasmodium falciparum-infected* erythrocytes is a common adhesive phenotype and is associated with severe malaria. Proc Natl Acad Sci U S A 98:1805–1810
17. Wahlgren M, Fernandez V, Scholander C, Carlson J (1994) Rosetting. Parasitol Today 10:73–79
18. Wassmer SC, Lepolard C, Traore B, Pouvelle B, Gysin J, Grau GE (2004) Platelets reorient *Plasmodium falciparum*-infected erythrocyte cytoadhesion to activated endothelial cells. J Infect Dis 189:180–189
19. Baruch DI, Pasloske BL, Singh HB, Bi X, Ma XC, Feldman M, Taraschi TF, Howard RJ (1995) Cloning the *P. falciparum* gene encoding PfEMP1, a malarial variant antigen and adherence receptor on the surface of parasitized human erythrocytes. Cell 82:77–87
20. Smith JD, Chitnis CE, Craig AG, Roberts DJ, Hudson-Taylor DE, Peterson DS, Pinches R, Newbold CI, Miller LH (1995) Switches in expression of *Plasmodium falciparum* var genes correlate with changes in antigenic and cytoadherent phenotypes of infected erythrocytes. Cell 82:101–110
21. Su XZ, Heatwole VM, Wertheimer SP, Guinet F, Herrfeldt JA, Peterson DS, Ravetch JA, Wellems TE (1995) The large diverse gene family var encodes proteins involved in cytoadherence and antigenic variation of *Plasmodium falciparum*-infected erythrocytes. Cell 82: 89–100
22. Marsh K, Marsh VM, Brown J, Whittle HC, Greenwood BM (1988) *Plasmodium falciparum*: the behavior of clinical isolates in an in vitro model of infected red blood cell sequestration. Exp Parasitol 65:202–208
23. Ockenhouse CF, Ho M, Tandon NN, Van Seventer GA, Shaw S, White NJ, Jamieson GA, Chulay JD, Webster HK (1991) Molecular basis of sequestration in severe and uncomplicated *Plasmodium falciparum* malaria: differential adhesion of infected erythrocytes to CD36 and ICAM-1. J Infect Dis 164:163–169
24. David PH, Hommel M, Miller LH, Udeinya IJ, Oligino LD (1983) Parasite sequestration in *Plasmodium falciparum* malaria: spleen and antibody modulation of cytoadherence of infected erythrocytes. Proc Natl Acad Sci U S A 80:5075–5079
25. Berendt AR, Ferguson DJ, Newbold CI (1990) Sequestration in *Plasmodium falciparum* malaria: sticky cells and sticky problems. Parasitol Today 6:247–254
26. Howard RJ (1988) Malarial proteins at the membrane of *Plasmodium falciparum*-infected erythrocytes and their involvement in cytoadherence to endothelial cells. Prog Allergy 41:98–147
27. Willimann K, Matile H, Weiss NA, Imhof BA (1995) In vivo sequestration of *Plasmodium falciparum*-infected human erythrocytes: a severe combined immunodeficiency mouse model for cerebral malaria. J Exp Med 182: 643–653
28. Ho M, Hickey MJ, Murray AG, Andonegui G, Kubes P (2000) Visualization of *Plasmodium falciparum*-endothelium interactions in human microvasculature: mimicry of leukocyte recruitment. J Exp Med 192:1205–1211
29. Yipp BG, Baruch DI, Brady C, Murray AG, Looareesuwan S, Kubes P, Ho M (2003) Recombinant PfEMP1 peptide inhibits and reverses cytoadherence of clinical *Plasmodium falciparum* isolates in vivo. Blood 101: 331–337
30. Arnold L, Tyagi RK, Meija P, Swetman C, Gleeson J, Perignon JL, Druilhe P (2011) Further improvements of the *P. falciparum* humanized mouse model. PLoS One 6:e18045
31. Vaughan AM, Mikolajczak SA, Wilson EM, Grompe M, Kaushansky A, Camargo N, Bial J, Ploss A, Kappe SH (2012) Complete *Plasmodium falciparum* liver stage development in liver-chimeric mice. J Clin Invest 122: 3618–3628
32. Claessens A, Rowe JA (2012) Selection of *Plasmodium falciparum* parasites for cytoadhesion to human brain endothelial cells. J Vis Exp 59:e3122

Chapter 19

Evaluation of Pregnancy Malaria Vaccine Candidates: The Binding Inhibition Assay

Tracy Saveria, Patrick E. Duffy, and Michal Fried

Abstract

The parasite-binding inhibition assay is designed to evaluate the acquisition of naturally acquired functional antibodies that block *Plasmodium falciparum* binding to endothelial or placental receptors. The assay is also used to assess functional activity by antibodies induced by immunization, for example antibodies raised against pregnancy malaria vaccine candidates like VAR2CSA. Here we describe a plate-based assay to measure the levels of adhesion-blocking antibodies. This assay format can be adapted to any lab that is minimally equipped for short-term parasite culture.

Key words Binding inhibition assay, Plate-based assay, IgG purification, CSA

1 Introduction

During pregnancy, *Plasmodium falciparum* parasites sequester in the placenta and adhere to chondroitin sulfate A (CSA) expressed on the surface of the syncytiotrophoblast [1]. Malaria during pregnancy is a major public health problem, associated with severe maternal anemia as well as with low birth weight (LBW) delivery and infant mortality [2, 3]. In areas of stable malaria transmission, the hallmark of pregnancy malaria is parity-dependent susceptibility, whereby women develop resistance over 1–2 pregnancies that controls infection and prevents severe sequelae. This unique epidemiology results from acquisition of immunity to placental parasites, and therefore a vaccine to prevent malaria during pregnancy should mimic naturally acquired immunity acquired by multigravid women.

Currently, an international effort to develop a vaccine to prevent pregnancy malaria focuses on a member of the PfEMP1 variant surface antigen family named VAR2CSA. VAR2CSA is preferentially expressed by placental parasites and parasite isolates selected for binding to CSA [4], and women acquire antibodies to VAR2CSA over successive pregnancies as they develop resistance to placental malaria. VAR2CSA is a large protein of about 350 kDa

Ashley M. Vaughan (ed.), *Malaria Vaccines: Methods and Protocols*, Methods in Molecular Biology, vol. 1325, DOI 10.1007/978-1-4939-2815-6_19,

composed of six extracellular Duffy binding-like (DBL) domains, and is too large to manufacture as an intact molecule. Therefore immunogens are being considered that incorporate one or a combination of VAR2CSA's DBL domains, with or without adjacent interdomain regions.

One of the major challenges in developing a pregnancy malaria vaccine (PMV) is identifying a domain or domain combination that can elicit broadly reactive antibodies. In endemic areas women acquire strain-transcending antibodies that block parasite adhesion to CSA and this property has been an important criterion in selecting candidates. A number of studies have evaluated PMV candidates by assessing the level of inhibition of adhesion by antibodies raised to recombinant forms of VAR2CSA domains or full-length protein.

Several platforms for binding inhibition assays have been described, including a high-throughput assay in 96-well plates of tritium-labeled parasites [5] and a flow-based assay [6]. Here, we focus on the static Petri dish-based assay [7]. This assay format can be adapted to any lab that is minimally equipped for short-term parasite culture, a centrifuge, and a microscope. Therefore, the assay can be used and has been used to analyze anti-adhesion activity on fresh parasite isolates that can thus support the selection of the optimal PMV candidate.

2 Materials

2.1 Reagents

1. Trophozoite-stage parasites at 5–20 % parasitemia, 0.5 % hematocrit (*see* Subheading 3.1).
2. 100 mm × 20 mm polystyrene Petri dishes (Falcon 351029) (*see* **Note 1**).
3. Sterile phosphate-buffered saline (PBS), pH 7.4.
4. Sterile RPMI1640 media.
5. 1 % Gelatin (Sigma G2625) in sterile RPMI 1640 media.
6. Bovine serum albumin (BSA), powder (Sigma A5611 or similar product from other manufacturers).
7. 3 % BSA in sterile PBS.
8. 3 % BSA in sterile RPMI 1640 media.
9. 1.5 % Glutaraldehyde (Sigma G6257) in sterile 1× PBS.
10. 5 % Giemsa (Sigma GS-500) in deionized water or 1 μg/ml 4',6-diamidino-2-phenylindole (DAPI) (Sigma D9542) in deionized water.
11. Chondroitin sulfate A (CSA), sodium salt, from bovine trachea (Sigma C9819-25G).
12. Control and test sera and/or IgG (*see* Subheading 3.3).

2.2 Equipment

1. Tabletop centrifuge (that allows for centrifugation at 1800 × *g*).
2. Microcentrifuge.
3. Laminar flow hood.
4. Incubator at 37 °C.
5. Water bath at 37 °C.
6. Vacuum pump.
7. Rotator (optional).
8. Peristaltic pump (optional).
9. Light or fluorescent microscope.

3 Methods

The binding inhibition assay for CSA-adherent parasites can be used for immuno-epidemiological studies to evaluate acquisition of immunity in exposed populations using human plasma, sera, or IgG. The assay can also evaluate functional activity in animal antisera raised against PMV candidates. For both applications, confirmation of parasite binding to CSA is performed prior to the analysis of anti-adhesion activity to ensure that the parasites are suitable for these measurements.

3.1 Parasite Preparation

Parasite isolates can be from one of the following sources:

1. Laboratory-adapted parasite lines selected for binding to CSA, such as *P. falciparum* CS2 available from MR4 (MRA-96).
2. Fresh isolates obtained from the peripheral blood of pregnant women (*see* **Note 2**).
3. Blood collected from infected placentas (*see* **Note 2**).

Parasites collected from the peripheral blood are commonly at the ring stage and should be allowed to mature in in vitro culture for about 12–20 h until reaching trophozoite/schizont stages, which adhere to endothelial receptors. Placental blood commonly contains mature parasite forms that can be used immediately in the assay. To evaluate anti-adhesion activity, parasites are enriched to a parasitemia of >1 % using a gelatin gradient.

Gelatin enrichment of mature-form parasites:

4. Warm the 1 % gelatin solution in a 37 °C water bath.
5. Pellet the blood at 500 × *g* for 5 min and resuspend with RPMI 1640 to 50 % hematocrit.
6. Add two volumes of gelatin solution and incubate for 30 min in a 37 °C water bath. In the absence of a water bath, an incubator set at 37 °C can be used.

7. Mature parasites remain in the upper layer while uninfected erythrocytes and ring-stage parasites form rouleaux and descend to the bottom layer.
8. Transfer the upper layer to a new tube, pellet the blood containing mature parasites, and wash three times with RPMI 1640 media.
9. Prepare and read a thin blood smear using methanol fixation followed by Giemsa staining: if parasitemia is >20 %, dilute to 20 % with uninfected red blood cells.

3.2 Plate Preparation

1. Using a template, draw circles on the back of a polystyrene Petri dish and label the wells appropriately. To prepare a template, use a circular Petri dish-sized piece of material (e.g., plastic, cardboard, paper) that contains twenty 10 mm circles drawn in 18° increments around the perimeter. Each circle will be able to accommodate approximately 20 μl of liquid (*see* **Note 3**).
2. Apply 15–20 μl of CSA solution at a concentration of 20 μg/ml (in sterile PBS) to the interior surface of the Petri dish within the margins of the marked wells.
3. Allow the CSA to absorb overnight at 4 °C in a humid chamber (e.g., a sealable container with wet paper towels).
4. Alternatively, plates can also be prepared on the same day by incubating for 4 h at 37 °C in a humid chamber.

3.3 IgG Purification of Human and Animal Sera

The method described here is based on using Protein G-coupled GammaBind Sepharose beads (GE Healthcare). Alternatives are available at your own discretion.

3.3.1 Materials

1. IgG Binding Buffer (Thermo Scientific 21019).
2. IgG Elution Buffer (Thermo Scientific 21004).
3. Neutralization buffer (1 M Tris–HCl pH 8.5).
4. Dialysis material for 10 K MWCO (suggest using Thermo Scientific Dialysis Cassettes, 10 K MWCO; requires needles/syringes for application).
5. Centrifuge columns, 0.8 ml (e.g., Pierce PN89868).
6. GammaBind™ Plus Sepharose™ bead slurry (GE Healthcare 17-0886-01).

3.3.2 Procedure

1. Bring all buffers to room temperature.
2. Add 400 μl of bead slurry to the centrifuge column (gently swirl slurry before application to ensure homogenous suspension); twist bottom off column and place in 1.5 ml microcentrifuge tube.

3. Spin for 1 min at 5000 × *g* (all spins are performed for the same time and force).
4. Wash column/beads using 400 μl binding buffer; spin and discard flow through. Repeat one more time.
5. Apply the centrifuge column cork to the bottom of the column.
6. Add 100–450 μl of plasma/serum sample on top of the beads (optimal volume is 150 μl); cap the column (Parafilm® wrap is recommended to prevent leakage).
7. Incubate with gentle rotation end over end, for 20–30 min at 4 °C.
8. Remove cork from column and spin; discard flow through (this can be saved to determine binding efficiency).
9. Wash using 400 μl of binding buffer, inverting the column several times after buffer application. Discard flow through after spin. Repeat wash step twice.
10. Add 25 μl of neutralization buffer to a clean microcentrifuge tube; transfer column to this tube.
11. Add 400 μl of elution buffer to column.
12. Spin; keep flow through containing purified IgG.
13. Repeat **steps 10–12** twice more, using the same column but with fresh microcentrifuge tubes, neutralization buffer and elution buffer.
14. Combine the IgG obtained in the three elutions. Samples are dried prior to dialysis by either lyophilization/freeze-dry or evaporation. Punch a hole on the top of each tube; freeze on dry ice before adding to lyophilizer (run on lyophilizer overnight if necessary) or alternatively, samples can be dried using a SpeedVac™ concentrator.
15. Add 100 μl of water to each tube of dried sample; if samples are aliquoted into multiple tubes combine into one tube.
16. Dialyze against 1 l of 1× PBS for 30–60 min at RT. If using recommended dialysis cassettes, be sure to hydrate the cassette in PBS for 1 min before application.
17. Carefully add sample using needle and syringe; remove all air from the cassette.
18. Float cassette in PBS.
19. Use a magnetic stir bar for gentle stirring of the PBS dialysis medium.
20. Change to fresh 1 l 1× PBS and dialyze for 1–2 h at 4 °C, again with gentle stirring.

21. Change to fresh 1 l of PBS and dialyze overnight at 4 °C, again with gentle stirring (can add an additional PBS change if preparing multiple samples).
22. Remove sample from dialysis membrane and place in fresh microcentrifuge tube.
23. If using dialysis cassette, use needle and syringe to put a small amount of air into cassette before removing sample.
24. Keep sample at 4 °C if planning to use within 48 h; otherwise aliquot and store at −20 °C.
25. Determine the IgG concentration using the BCA assay (Pierce 23225) or similar methodology of your choosing.

3.4 Binding Inhibition Assay: Setup

Binding inhibition assays can be used to test plasma, serum, or IgG from malaria-exposed humans or from animals immunized with vaccine candidates (*see* **Note 4**). These samples are defined as "test sera." The level of binding is compared to the level of binding in the presence of nonimmune serum/plasma or serum/plasma from animals immunized with an irrelevant protein that is expressed and formulated in a similar way as the vaccine candidate (*see* **Note 5**). Inhibition assays are also performed using purified IgG (*see* Subheading 3.3).

1. Incubate parasites at a parasitemia of >1 % and hematocrit of 0.5 % in 3 % BSA/RPMI 1640 media for 30 min at 37 °C or room temperature.
2. Appropriately label microcentrifuge tubes with nomenclature for the serum or IgG being tested. Gently mix the parasite suspension to ensure even distribution and then divide among the labeled microcentrifuge tubes, adding 15–20 μl per tube (use the same volume as the initial receptor volume throughout the assay).
3. Spin for 2 min at 400 × *g* and remove the volume of supernatant equal to the volume of serum to be added. Human serum or plasma is commonly used at a dilution of 1:5–1:10. The appropriate dilution of sera raised against recombinant proteins should be determined.
4. Purified IgG is analyzed at increasing concentrations (0.1 mg/ml thru 1 mg/ml). To maintain an equal concentration of BSA among the samples tested with varying amounts of IgG, remove the volume of supernatant equal to the volume of the highest IgG concentration to be used from all the tubes. Add increasing amounts of IgG and RPMI 1640 media to a final volume of 15–20 μl.
5. Make sure that the parasites are well mixed with the serum/IgG to ensure proper binding of the antibodies to the parasites.
6. Incubate the parasites in serum/IgG for 30 min at 37 °C or room temperature.

7. Block the CSA plates with 3 % BSA/PBS: aspirate the CSA spot and immediately apply 15–20 μl of 3 % BSA/PBS; incubate for at least 30 min at room temperature in a humidified container (e.g., sealable container with moist paper towel, or humidified incubator).
8. Aspirate the BSA/PBS blocking buffer from the wells by suction and immediately add the parasite suspension from step 6. Incubate for 30 min at room temperature in humidified container.

3.5 Binding Inhibition Assay: Washes

3.5.1 Manual Washing

1. To wash the plate, cover the samples with 20 ml of PBS by slowly adding PBS to the center of the Petri dish (*see* **Note 6**).
2. Avoid adding PBS directly to the parasite suspensions.
3. After the wells are covered with PBS, tilt the plate gently to wash off unbound cells. Collect PBS and dislodged cells by suction at the edge of the dish.
4. Repeat the washing process three times.

3.5.2 Automated Washing Station

An automated washing station was designed to allow consistent plate washing to reduce the variation between plates. The system was previously described [8] and includes a rotating platform and a peristaltic pump that regulates the inflow and outflow of the washing solution. The peristaltic pump delivers washing buffer (PBS) through the inlet tubing until the buffer reaches the level of the outlet tubing.

5. Wash in PBS on a rotating platform, by slowly and carefully adding PBS to the center of the plate, and allowing it to gently flow and fill the plate (*see* **Note 6**). When necessary, gently vacuum extra liquid and blood from the center of the plate (*see* **Note 6**). Continue to gently wash until the spots are clear of blood and there is no longer any blood concentrated in the center of the plate.
6. Discontinue PBS addition. Aspirate the remaining PBS using vacuum while the rotating platform is still on—be sure to aspirate in the middle of the plate first, only aspirating from the edges when collecting the final PBS.

3.6 Binding Inhibition Assay: Fixing and Staining

1. Add 10 ml of 1.5 % glutaraldehyde/PBS to the Petri dish and incubate for 10 min at RT.
2. Gently rinse the plate three times with deionized water (gently adding to the center of the plate, not on the spots).
3. Stain with 5 % Giemsa for 5 min or 1 μg/ml DAPI in PBS for 10 min (if using DAPI, cover plates after final rinse and keep away from light).
4. Gently rinse plate three times with deionized water and let the plates dry.

3.7 Binding Inhibition Assay: Counting

3.7.1 Giemsa-Stained Plates

1. Count bound infected red blood cells (iRBCs) stained with Giemsa using a 10× eyepiece and 100× magnifying objective (high-power field). Survey each test site to identify areas with low background (no/few uninfected RBCs).
2. Count 20 fields that contain the highest number of parasites.
3. Follow the same approach (survey for low-background areas and count fields with highest parasite densities) for all the wells.
4. To calculate the level of inhibition, compare the number of bound cells in the presence of test sera (N_{test}) to the number bound in the presence of control sera ($N_{control}$). Calculate the percent inhibition: $100-((N_{test}/N_{control})\times 100)$.

3.7.2 DAPI-Stained Plates

5. Use MetaMorph® or other standard imaging software. Count a minimum of 1000 red blood cells (over several fields of view), using a 10× eyepiece and 40× magnifying objective fluorescent microscope with a UV laser in order to determine the number of DAPI-stained cells, noting both the number of infected and uninfected cells.
6. To calculate the level of inhibition, compare the number of bound cells in the presence of test sera (N_{test}) to the number bound in the presence of control sera ($N_{control}$). Calculate the percent inhibition $100-((N_{test}/N_{control})\times 100)$.

4 Notes

1. The type of Petri dish plate is critical. Falcon 351029 Petri dishes were found to be suitable. Any other plate should be compared to this plate to determine if the plate is suitable for the assay.
2. Informed consent should be obtained from donors before collecting blood or placenta.
3. Throughout the procedure, it is very important to prevent drying of spots. Apply blocking solution or parasite suspension immediately after aspirating liquid from each well.
4. When using human plasma in the inhibition assay, plasma blood type must be matched to parasite blood type to avoid agglutination. It is not necessary to match blood type for long-term cultured parasites adapted to blood type O.
5. Inhibition assays should always include controls. Assays performed with human plasma (or IgG) should include nonimmune sera (e.g., sera collected from malaria-naïve donors) as a negative control, and pooled immune sera from multigravid women as a positive control. Assays of sera (or IgG) from immunized animals should include a negative control

from animals that were immunized with an irrelevant protein produced from the same expression platform and prepared and delivered as immunogen in the same way as the test reagents.

6. Be careful to avoid aspirating parasites directly from wells.

Acknowledgements

P.E.D. and M.F. are supported by the Intramural Research Program of the NIAID-NIH.

References

1. Fried M, Duffy PE (1996) Adherence of *Plasmodium falciparum* to chondroitin sulfate A in the human placenta. Science 272: 1502–1504
2. McGregor IA, Wilson ME, Billewicz WZ (1983) Malaria infection of the placenta in The Gambia, West Africa; its incidence and relationship to stillbirth, birth weight and placental weight. Trans R Soc Trop Med Hyg 77:232–244
3. Desai M, ter Kuile FO, Nosten F, McGready R, Asamoa K et al (2007) Epidemiology and burden of malaria in pregnancy. Lancet Infect Dis 7:93–104
4. Salanti A, Staalsoe T, Lavstsen T, Jensen AT, Sowa MP et al (2003) Selective upregulation of a single distinctly structured var gene in chondroitin sulphate A-adhering *Plasmodium falciparum* involved in pregnancy-associated malaria. Mol Microbiol 49:179–191
5. Nielsen MA, Pinto VV, Resende M, Dahlback M, Ditlev SB et al (2009) Induction of adhesion-inhibitory antibodies against placental *Plasmodium falciparum* parasites by using single domains of VAR2CSA. Infect Immun 77:2482–2487
6. Fernandez P, Petres S, Mecheri S, Gysin J, Scherf A (2010) Strain-transcendent immune response to recombinant Var2CSA DBL5-epsilon domain block *P. falciparum* adhesion to placenta-derived BeWo cells under flow conditions. PLoS One 5, e12558
7. Fried M, Nosten F, Brockman A, Brabin BJ, Duffy PE (1998) Maternal antibodies block malaria. Nature 395:851–852
8. Duffy PE, Fried M (2011) Pregnancy malaria: cryptic disease, apparent solution. Mem Inst Oswaldo Cruz 106(Suppl 1):64–69

Chapter 20

High-Throughput Testing of Antibody-Dependent Binding Inhibition of Placental Malaria Parasites

Morten A. Nielsen and Ali Salanti

Abstract

The particular virulence of *Plasmodium falciparum* manifests in diverse severe malaria syndromes as cerebral malaria, severe anemia and placental malaria. The cause of both the severity and the diversity of infection outcome, is the ability of the infected erythrocyte (IE) to bind a range of different human receptors through *Plasmodium falciparum* erythrocyte membrane protein 1 (PfEMP1) on the surface of the infected cell. As the *var* genes encoding the large PfEMP1 antigens are extensively polymorphic, vaccine development strategies are focused on targeting the functional binding epitopes. This involves identification of recombinant fragments of PfEMP1s that induce antibodies, which hinder the adhesion of the IE to a given receptor or tissue. Different assays to measure the blocking of adhesion have been described in the literature, each with different advantages. This chapter describes a high-throughput assay used in the preclinical and clinical development of a VAR2CSA based vaccine against placental malaria.

Key words Adhesion assay, Placental malaria, Vaccine potency, Antibodies, PfEMP1, VAR2CSA, Binding-inhibition, Clinical development

1 Introduction

The major virulence factor of *Plasmodium falciparum* is the ability of the infected erythrocyte to sequester in the vascular bed, which enable immune evasion and can cause life-threatening complications (reviewed in Smith et al. [1]). Although different gene families coding for adhesins have been described, the key antigen in adhesion is *P. falciparum* erythrocyte membrane protein 1 (PfEMP1). Thus, from a theoretical point of view, these antigens are very promising for malaria vaccine development. Unfortunately, the *var* genes that encode PfEMP1 are highly polymorphic and protection per se is associated with acquisition of a broad repertoire of antibodies against multiple PfEMP1 family members after repeated infections [2–4]. However, protection against severe disease is mediated by humoral responses and appears to be acquired after a few infections [5–7]. Furthermore, recent data suggest that

Ashley M. Vaughan (ed.), *Malaria Vaccines: Methods and Protocols*, Methods in Molecular Biology, vol. 1325, DOI 10.1007/978-1-4939-2815-6_20, © Springer Science+Business Media New York 2015

it is possible to target the binding epitopes of PfEMP1 variants, thereby reducing the risk of escape mutants and targeting of non-protective epitopes of vaccine candidates [8–11]. As the *var* genes are extensively polymorphic the strategy is to develop syndrome specific vaccines. A major breakthrough was the discovery that the conserved PfEMP1 antigen VAR2CSA enables IE to bind to chondroitin sulfate A (CSA) and thereby accumulate in the placenta [12]. Apparently, the tropism for placental CSA of VAR2CSA restricts expression of this molecule to infections of pregnant women, as children and men in malaria endemic areas have very low levels of antibodies to VAR2CSA [13, 14]. The lack of protective antibodies and the tropism for CSA of VAR2CSA hence explains the vulnerability of pregnant women [9].

In the process of PfEMP1 based vaccine development one of the functional assays is, due to difficulties in establishing appropriate animal models, in vitro measurements of antibody-mediated inhibition of infected erythrocyte (IE) binding [15–18]. The antibodies are produced by immunizing animals, often rodents, with recombinant fragments of PfEMP1. As adhesion is occurring to multiple different receptors distinctive binding phenotypes can be recognized: (1) Rossetting, where IEs bind uninfected red blood cells, (2) Clumping, where IEs bind to platelets, (3) Endothelial adhesion, where IEs bind cells lining the vascular endothelium. The distinct phenotype of adhesion determines how to measure the potency of a vaccine in vitro. For parasite binding to the vascular endothelium and placental adhesion in particular several assays are described in the literature, each with different advantages and weaknesses (a non-exhaustive list includes [15, 16, 19–27]) The three most commonly used assays to measure antibody-dependent inhibition of binding are: *The petri dish assay*: Parasite binding is investigated in a petri dish, on which 20 spots are coated with CSA/decorin and blocked with Bovine Serum Albumin (BSA), the latter to prevent nonspecific cell attachment to the plastic dish. Parasite enriched RBCs are pre-incubated with test or control sera and are then added to each spot on the petri dish for 30 min at 37 °C. The dish is washed with phosphate-buffered saline (PBS) either gyrating it by hand or on a gyrating platform, either at a fixed time or until the blood pellets reach the center of the plate. PBS is removed followed by two washes without rotation. The plates are fixed in glutaraldehyde, stained with Giemsa and investigated by microscopy. The counting is performed either manually or is further developed to be more automated using different software options. *The micro capillary method*: A chip with capillary tubes made of material that enable adsorption of protein is coated with CSA/decorin and blocked with BSA. Parasite-infected erythrocytes incubated with either control or test sera are allowed to bind in each capillary tube for 30 min at 37 °C, after which shear wall pressure, similar to a capillary blood vessel, is applied using a peristaltic pump. Parasite binding is assessed by evaluating the number of bound IEs by software and images recorded by a video camera connected to a microscope. *The 96-well assay*: Parasite binding is evaluated in the wells of a 96-well plate, which are all coated with CSA and BSA as described above. After incubation at 37 °C with IEs (treated with tritiated hypoxanthine) in combination with control or test sera, the plate is washed three times with 200 μl of RPMI cell culture media using a pipetting robot that gently resuspend unbound IEs at five different locations in the well using an 8 channel pipette. The washing is repeated three times, after which parasites are counted by liquid scintillation, and the level of tritiated hypoxanthine in the parasite DNA represents the degree of binding.

One of the obvious differences between the three assays is the number of samples that can be processed. In the 96-well assay it is possible to run up to 4 plates or 384 different spots in 1 day, thereby allowing investigation of more sera or/and different dilutions at the same time than in the two other assays. The difference of the conditions during binding is another area where the assays differ considerably. In the petri dish and 96-well assays binding takes place under static conditions to allow maximal interaction between the IEs and the receptor. In the micro-capillary method binding occurs in a way that is imitating physiological conditions in a small blood vessel. Washing is another pivotal step that is different in all assays. In the petri-dish assay washing is performed by adding washing medium to cover the entire bottom of the plate, followed by gentle rotation on a gyro-rotator or by hand, this creates a vortex that gathers unbound cells in the center of the petri dish, from where they can be removed. The problem is that it is not possible to remove the entire volume of washing medium, which increase the risk of contaminating the binding spots during subsequent washing and fixing steps. Furthermore, several of the steps are performed manually, which introduces the risk of inter-person variation. In the micro-capillary assay, washing is inherent to the assay as cells that are inhibited will not adhere to sides of the capillary tube. An issue with this assay is that in most setups one peristaltic pump is managing the flow in chips with multiple channels (often 8 channels). Thus, if there is a small blood clot or excessive adhesion in one channel, the flow-rate is reduced significantly in that channel, which may confer an uneven level of shear flow rates in an adjacent capillaries. In the 96-well assay washing is performed by a pipetting robot or manually with an electronic pipette. The pipetting robot enables removal of unbound cells by pipetting certain volumes of washing medium at five different points in the well and at an exact distance from the bottom of the well. This supports low assay to assay variation and is not influenced by person variation. Assessment of binding is achieved by microscopy in both the petri-dish and the micro-capillary assay. Although software based solutions and automated microscopes have been developed, counting by microscope is often time consuming. In the 96-well assay, parasite binding counting is automated by liquid scintillation based on the incorporation of tritiated hypoxanthine. With regard to implementation costs, the 96-well assay is by far the most expensive to implement, followed by the micro-capillary assay. However, for the petri dish assay, implementation of a semi-automated washing stand as well as an automated microscope for software counting is also expensive. Running costs per test sample are expensive for the micro-capillary method as the chips are costly, followed by the 96-well plate assay.

The choice of assay to use should relate to the binding phenotype of the IE. In the case of placental adhesion the inter-villous space is a low-pressure circuit with a slow flow-rate with blood surrounding protruding villi, which is difficult to mimic. However, the conditions with regard to the flow rates in the placenta are similar to that of a small blood vessel. For all three methods commercially available bovine CSA or decorin is commonly used as a receptor in studies of placental malaria, which may not fully resemble CSA on the syncytiotrophoblast in the placenta. Syncytiotrophoblast or BeWo cells are probably a more biological relevant alternative [28], but they are tedious to work with, as they require optimal conditions to enable stable growth and adherence, which introduce the risk that the washing step also removes the BeWo cell layer. In a clinical development phase of a vaccine multiple occasions of potency testing is required. In addition, in vitro correlates of protection for a disease occurring during pregnancy could come into consideration in order to reduce the length of phase II and III clinical trials. As the inter-assay variation is minimal in the 96-well assay and as it allows for testing many samples simultaneously, we decided to use this assay for screening the potency of multiple different VAR2CSA proteins in our preclinical development phase. The assay is furthermore used in the clinical development of a vaccine against placental malaria. The following is a description of the 96-well assay.

2 Materials

2.1 Parasite Culture

Culture medium: 500 ml RPMI 1640, 25 mM HEPES, 25 mM $NaHCO_3$, 200 mML-glutamine, 25 mg gentamycin (Gibco), 2.5 g AlbuMAX II (*see* **Note 1**), 10 ml normal human serum, 10 mg hypoxanthine (*see* **Note 2**).

Washing medium: 500 ml RPMI 1640, 25 mg gentamycin.

Giemsa stain: 10 % Giemsa in PBS.

Gas mixture: 2 % O_2, 5.5 % CO_2, 92.5 % N_2.

Red blood cells (RBCs): Blood type O Rh^- or Rh^+ RBC in citrate phosphate dextrose adenine (CPDA) buffer without buffy coat (*see* **Note 3**).

2.2 MACS Purification

VarioMACS separator magnet (Miltenyi).

VarioMACS column (Miltenyi).

VarioMACS three-way valve (Miltenyi).

Needle (length: 4 mm, diameter: 0.9 mm).

Ethanol 70 %.

2 % fetal calf serum (FCS) in PBS.

2.3 Binding Assay

Binding medium: 500 ml RPMI 1640, 25 mM HEPES, 25 mM $NaHCO_3$, 200 mML-glutamine, 10 ml FCS.

Incubation medium: 500 ml RPMI 1640, 25 mM HEPES, 25 mM $NaHCO_3$, 200 mML-glutamine, 25 mg gentamycin, 2.5 g AlbuMAX II (*see* **Note 1**).

1 ml of 5 mCi/ml tritiated hypoxanthine diluted in 100 ml PBS (Perkin Elmer) (*see* **Note 2**).

96 well microtiter plates (Falcon 351172).

PBS.

Micro Scint-20 (Sigma).

VarioMACS separator magnet (Miltenyi).

VarioMACS column (Miltenyi).

VarioMACS three-way valve (Miltenyi).

Needle: length 4 mm, diameter 0.9 mm.

96-well Scintillation counter (Perkin Elmer, Topcount MXT).

96-well Filtermate Harvester (Perkin Elmer).

Biomek 2000 pipetting robot (Coulter).

3 Methods

3.1 Parasite Culture

1. Manipulation of parasites is performed in a lamina airflow hood.
2. Suspend RBC at ~4 % hematocrit in prewarmed 37 °C culture medium.
3. Add 5 ml of the RBC suspension to a 50 ml cell culture flask or 25 ml to a 250 ml cell culture flask.
4. Flush 50 ml flasks for ~30 s with gas mixture (250 ml flasks for ~90 s) at 1.5- to 2-bar pressure.
5. Incubate the flasks at 37 °C for 24 h.
6. Remove the culture flask gently from the incubator and remove spent supernatant.
7. Remove 4 μl of RBC to make a Giemsa-stained thin smear.

8. Add new (prewarmed) culture medium to the flask, gas as above, and return the flask to the incubator.
9. Sub-cultivate the parasites by dilution when necessary (*see* **Note 4** below).

3.2 Selection of VAR2CSA Expression

Parasites in continuous culture are routinely selected for VAR2CSA expression by bio-panning on decorin or BeWo cells. Briefly, 3 spots of 20 μl of 5 μl/ml sterile filtered decorin solution are coated on the bottom of a 50 ml culture flask used for adherent cells and left to incubate overnight at 4 °C. The flask is blocked for 1 h by adding 5 ml of parasite culture medium in 37 °C. 200 μl of infected erythrocytes are added, with a 5–10 % primarily late-stage parasitemia. The flask is gassed and incubated on a gyrating table at 37 °C for 1 h. The flask is washed by gently adding 5 ml of washing medium to the side of flask and incubating it for 3 min on the gyration table, after which the medium is removed. This procedure is repeated 3–5 times until the wash no longer contains cells. Binding to the spots can be inspected with an inverted microscope. When washing is complete, 5 ml of parasite medium and 200 μl of uninfected erythrocytes are added; the flask is gassed and incubated for 24 h, thereafter the rings stage culture is transferred to a 50 ml flask. The procedure can also be performed by seeding BeWo cells instead of coating spots of decorin [29, 30].

3.3 MACS Purification of Late Stage Trophozoites and Schizonts from Parasite Culture or Blood Sample

1. Cut off the tip of the plastic needle holster without touching the needle and keep the needle in the holster (*see* **Note 5**).
2. Assemble three-way valve, needle, and column. Apply to the magnet. Apply 2 % FCS in PBS thru 3 way valve after assembly in the magnet and wash with 10 ml 2 % FCS in PBS (*see* **Note 6**).
3. Apply the parasite culture in an approximately 20 % hematocrit suspension to the column. Do not exceed a volume of 2 ml of packed RBCs.
4. Wash with 2 % FCS in PBS until wash-thru is clear (approximately 20 ml).
5. Wash with an additional 10 ml 2 % FCS in PBS.
6. Stop the flow thru at 3-way valve.
7. Apply the top adapter cap to the column.
8. Apply a 20 ml syringe with 2 % FCS in PBS in the top adapter.
9. Unscrew the column from the 3-way valve with the top adapter and 20 ml syringe still attached. Remove the column and syringe from the magnet. Gently rescue the purified parasites from the column by pressing the 20 ml syringe containing 2 % FCS in PBS.
10. Centrifuge the parasites at 800 × g for 8 min.

11. Resuspend the parasite pellet gently in 2–10 ml 2 % FCS in RPMI, depending on the pellet size.
12. Prepare a dilution of the cell suspension normally a 1:20 dilution is sufficient. Apply the diluted cells to a Neubauer chamber be able to count the number of cells per ml.
13. Prepare a cell suspension of 4×10^6 cells/ml by adding the required volume of RPMI with 2 % FCS.

3.4 Synchronization of Parasite Cultures

We routinely use MACS purification (*see* Subheading 3.3) to synchronize parasites. This is performed in a lamina flow hood with sterile columns, three way valves and RPMI. For the binding assays, very tightly synchronized cultures are not needed as parasites are purified by MACS prior to the binding assay. Other methods of synchronization such as sorbitol lysis or gelatin flotation may also be used [31, 32].

3.5 Antibody-Mediated Inhibition of Binding

1. Day 1: The synchronized parasite culture is examined by microscopy to ensure that the parasite population are at the ring stage. The parasite media is changed from normal parasite to RPMI medium with AlbuMAX II but without hypoxanthine (incubation medium) (*see* **Note 7**).
2. Add premade ^{3}H-hypoxanthine (*see* **Note 2**): 1 ml of solution per 5 ml of parasite culture.
3. The culture flask is gassed as above and incubated 20 h at 37 °C.
4. A 96 well microtiter plate (Falcon plate no 1172) is coated with CSA by adding 100 μl of 2 μg/ml decorin in PBS per well (*see* **Note 8**).
5. Cover the plate with an adherent film to reduce evaporation and incubate the plate overnight at 4 °C.
6. Day 2: The wells of the binding plate (Falcon 351172) are blocked for 2 h at RT with 1 % BSA (weight per volume) in PBS by adding 100 μl to each well.
7. Empty the plate by quick inversion and wash the plate two times with 200 μl of RPMI with 2 % FCS per well (*see* **Note 8**).
8. Add 50 μl of binding inhibitor (for example IgG, serum, CSA) to the plate at a 2× concentration of the final dilution in RPMI with 2 % FCS (*see* **Note 9**).
9. Incubate the plate at 37 °C while the parasites are MACS purified.
10. The parasites are purified 20–22 h after incubation in medium containing tritiated hypoxanthine using the MACS column as above.
11. Add 50 μl of MACS purified parasites adjusted to 4×10^6 infected RBCs/ml (*see* **Note 10**). Keep the parasites at 37 °C in RPMI 2 % FCS.

12. Incubate the plate for 1.5 h at 37 °C without shaking.
13. Wash the plates using a pipetting robot (Biomek 2000) using 37 °C RPMI with 2 % FCS at 37 °C.
14. Washing program setup (*see* **Note 11**):
    (a) Transfer RPMI with 2 % FCS from a half module container to column 1 on the plate using the 8 channel pipetting tool. Settings: 150 μl, Dispense height 15 %, Dispense rate 8.
    (b) Transfer 200 μl from row 1 to a half module waste container with "washing at sides" enabled. Use the same settings for transfer and washing. Settings: volume 200 μl suspense height 15 %, suspense rate 8.
    (c) Repeat for rows **2–12**.
    (d) Repeat **steps** (**a**)–(**c**) twice (so that the plate is washed 3 times in all).
15. The plate is harvested with 10 × 200 μl distilled water in the cell harvester onto the filter plate.
16. Dry the filter plate and cover the bottom of the wells with white adherent film.
17. Add 50 μl Microscint-20 solution per well and cover with transparent adherent film.
18. Count the plate in a scintillation counter.

3.6 Concluding Remarks

Measurements of IE binding are inherently difficult as it is highly influenced by the progression of the parasite development inside the red cell, and the homogeneity of *var* gene expression of the parasite population. We regularly examine the *var* gene expression by real time PCR and the expression of antigens on the surface of the IE by flow-cytometry of our parasite cultures. In addition, we test for mycoplasma infection and test the parasite genotype for contamination by nested PCR of the genes coding for merozoite surface protein 1 and glutamate rich protein. However, once parasites cultures have been selected to express only one variant of PfEMP1 the 96-well assay is sufficiently robust to run samples in duplicate, although we most commonly use triplicate measurements. To ensure that washing has progressed evenly throughout the plate we routinely include one row (12 wells) without inhibitor, as a positive control of binding, and one row coated with BSA, as a negative control of binding.

In terms of antibody-mediated inhibition, we include serum from non-immunized or mock immunized animals as negative controls. Importantly, we have found unspecific inhibition using plasma collected with heparin as anticoagulant. Although costly and time consuming such unspecific effects can be avoided by purifying IgG, note however that not all IgG subclasses from animal serum are evenly purified by immunoglobulin purifying kits such as

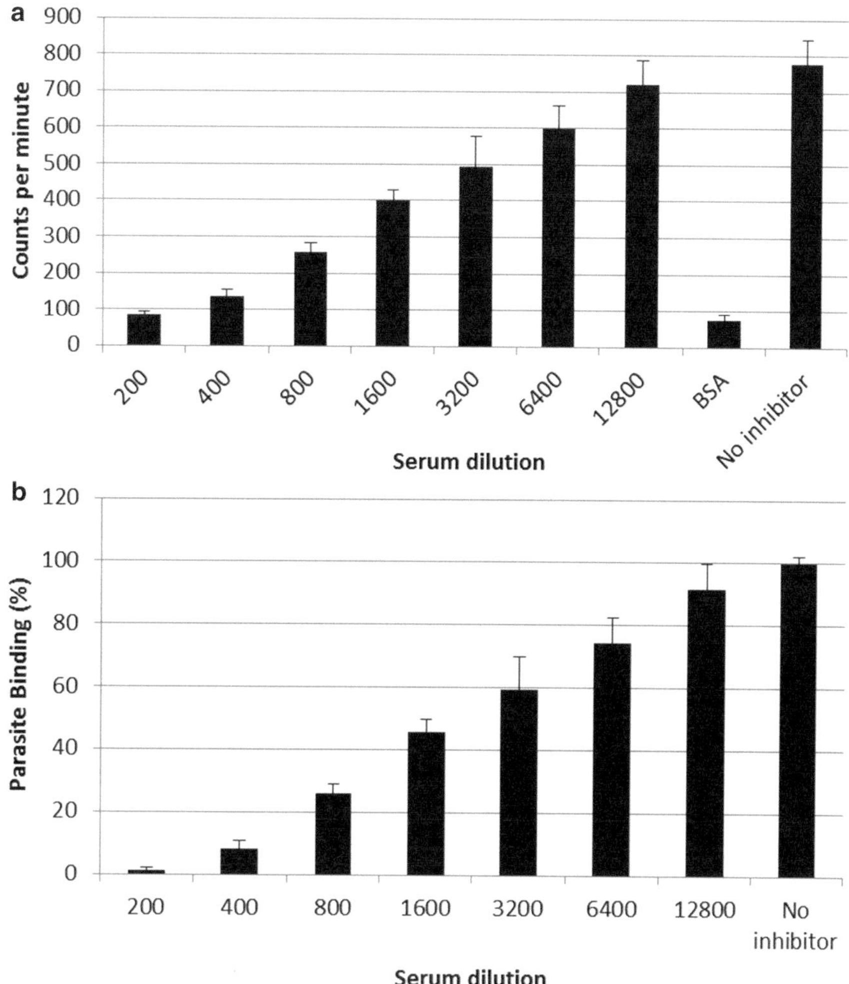

Fig. 1 Antibody-mediated inhibition of binding. Data shown are from the same assay analyzed either using the raw CPM values (**a**) or using data adjusted to percent binding by dividing with the positive control after subtracting the negative control (**b**). The inhibitor used is dilutions of pooled serum from rats immunized three times with the minimal binding epitope ID1-ID2a of VAR2CSA. Error bars represent standard deviations of triplicate measurements (**a**) or coefficients of variation (100 × (Standard deviation/mean)) of triplicate measurements (**b**)

protein G (*see* also **Note 7**). To test for specificity of binding for VAR2CSA expressing parasites soluble CSA (200 μg/ml) may be used. Assays performed on the same day may be compared to each other by recording the average counts per minutes (CPM) as shown in Fig. 1a. If assays from a series of experiments have to be compared, we record either the ratio of binding = ("CPM test sample" – "CPM negative control")/("CPM positive control" – "CPM negative control") or the percentage of binding (100 × ratio of binding) (*see* Fig. 1b). The transformation to ratios or percent binding is necessary as the efficiency of tritiated hypoxanthine incorporation varies from day to day and for different parasite genotypes.

4 Notes

1. The AlbuMAX II and hypoxanthine are made as a stock solution by dissolving 100 g of AlbuMAX II and 400 mg of hypoxanthine in 2 L of RPMI 1640 medium. The solution is sterile filtered through 0.8 μm and 0.2 μm filters. Use 50 ml of this stock solution per 500 ml bottle of culture medium.
2. A stock solution of tritiated hypoxanthine is prepared by adding 100 ml of sterile PBS to 5 mCi of tritiated hypoxanthine. This stock is diluted 1:6 with parasite incubation medium for parasite culture overnight. Furthermore ensure that you adhere to national rules when handling radioactive isotopes such as tritium.
3. Washed, uninfected RBCs for subculture should be kept in the refrigerator for 24 h before first usage (to reduce active leukocyte numbers), and can be kept in the refrigerator for up to 14 days.
4. Parasites can be obtained from different sources: (1) from peripheral blood before or at delivery collected by venipuncture in vacutainers with citrate phosphate dextrose adenine (CPDA) anticoagulant, (2) by perfusion of infected placental tissue as described by Moore et al. [33] or (3) from cryopreserved infected RBCs. It is important to keep all media preheated to 37 °C and to minimize handling time outside the 37 °C incubator. When gassing the culture flasks, fit the gas hose with a 0.2-μm filter unit, and use a sterile needle (preferably blunt to avoid accidents). Sub-cultivate parasite isolates to keep parasitemia below 5–10 % by adding appropriate volumes of infected erythrocytes to fresh uninfected RBCs. Orbital shaking and human serum instead of AlbuMAX II during culture increases parasite survival [34].
5. By cutting only the tip of the needle holster cutting accidents are avoided and needle diameter is kept intact, which is important to ensure the correct flow rate during MACS purification.
6. The column can be reused by keeping it in 96 % ethanol. If the column has been used before, wash the column with 10 ml ethanol, 10 ml ddH_2O, and 10 ml 2 % FCS in PBS. Make sure that the column is not emptied at any time during assembly and purification, since this will create air bubbles inside the column.
7. As human serum components may affect binding avidity the AlbuMAX II and FCS during culture and binding respectively may be substituted with normal human serum [35, 36], note however since human serum contains hypoxanthine this will decrease the amount of tritiated hypoxanthine uptake by the

parasites and thereby decrease the signal to noise ratio. A 50 ml flask with 5 % parasites is sufficient for one to two 96-well plates whereas a 250 ml flask is needed if 4 plates are to be processed.

8. Use gloves while handling purified receptors such as decorin to ensure minimal contamination by proteases. Likewise use pure PBS and do not vortex decorin too rigorously as this reduces the level of binding. Empty the plate and process it immediately, preferably by multichannel pipetting to avoid wells from drying, which reduces the level of binding. Alternatively add 25 or 50 μl of RPMI with 2 % FCS before addition of inhibitor for the wells not to dry (this will affect the final volume and hence concentration of inhibitors). Importantly, proteoglycans such as decorin will not bind all types of plastic surfaces therefore the coating should be investigated prior to setting up new assays.

9. We use an entire row of wells without inhibitor to verify that binding is even throughout the plates, however reserve at least triplicate wells for measurements of binding without inhibitor.

10. If inhibitor serum amounts are scarce the total volume in the well may be reduced by using 25 μl of inhibitor solution and 25 μl of 8×10^6 infected cells per ml. The most convenient way to add inhibitors is from another 96 well plate allowing the use of multichannel pipetting.

11. As variations between pipetting robots may occur, the washing rate, height and volume should be investigated. The most convenient way to do this is to test the primary settings using a BSA coated plate incubated with uninfected erythrocytes. Binding can be inspected in an inverted microscope. This way it is possible to test at which conditions uninfected erythrocytes are removed from the bottom of the wells. The fine tuning is then performed using the specific receptor–parasite pair to test at which conditions the signal to noise ratio is highest.

    It is possible to perform the assay without a pipetting robot as the plate may be washed using an electronic 8 channel pipette. Dispense the washing medium slowly at the sides of the wells (many electronic pipettes features the possibility to reduce the dispensing rate). Empty the plate by quick inversion. This is repeated three times. This method, however, increases inter- and intra-assay variation significantly. A manual pipette may also be used but this increases variation even further. Finally, instead of counting cells using tritium labelled hypoxanthine, parasites may be counted using a parasite specific lactate dehydrogenase assay [37].

References

1. Smith JD, Rowe JA, Higgins MK et al (2013) Malaria's deadly grip: cytoadhesion of Plasmodium falciparum-infected erythrocytes. Cell Microbiol 15:1976–1983
2. Bull PC, Lowe BS, Kortok M et al (1998) Parasite antigens on the infected red cell surface are targets for naturally acquired immunity to malaria. Nat Med 4:358–360
3. Chan JA, Howell KB, Reiling L et al (2012) Targets of antibodies against Plasmodium falciparum-infected erythrocytes in malaria immunity. J Clin Invest 122:3227–3238
4. Nielsen MA, Staalsoe T, Kurtzhals JA et al (2002) Plasmodium falciparum variant surface antigen expression varies between isolates causing severe and nonsevere malaria and is modified by acquired immunity. J Immunol 168:3444–3450
5. Gupta S, Snow RW, Donnelly CA et al (1999) Immunity to non-cerebral severe malaria is acquired after one or two infections. Nat Med 5:340–343
6. Cohen S, McGregor IA, Carrington S (1961) Gamma-globulin and acquired immunity to human malaria. Nature 192:733–737
7. McGregor IA, Carrington SP, Cohen S (1963) Treatment of East African *P. falciparum* malaria with West African human γ-globulin. Trans R Soc Trop Med Hyg 57:170–175
8. Jensen ATR, Magistrado P, Sharp S et al (2004) Plasmodium falciparum associated with severe childhood malaria preferentially expresses PfEMP1 encoded by group A var genes. J Exp Med 199:1179–1190
9. Salanti A, Dahlback M, Turner L et al (2004) Evidence for the Involvement of VAR2CSA in Pregnancy-associated Malaria. J Exp Med 200:1197–1203
10. Bigey P, Gnidehou S, Doritchamou J et al (2011) The NTS-DBL2X region of VAR2CSA induces cross-reactive antibodies that inhibit adhesion of several Plasmodium falciparum isolates to chondroitin sulfate A. J Infect Dis 204:1125–1133
11. Turner L, Lavstsen T, Berger SS et al (2013) Severe malaria is associated with parasite binding to endothelial protein C receptor. Nature 498:502–505
12. Salanti A, Staalsoe T, Lavstsen T et al (2003) Selective upregulation of a single distinctly structured var gene in chondroitin sulphate A-adhering Plasmodium falciparum involved in pregnancy-associated malaria. Mol Microbiol 49:179–191
13. Beeson JG, Ndungu F, Persson KE et al (2007) Antibodies among men and children to placental-binding Plasmodium falciparum-infected erythrocytes that express var2csa. Am J Trop Med Hyg 77:22–28
14. Oleinikov AV, Voronkova VV, Frye IT et al (2012) A plasma survey using 38 PfEMP1 domains reveals frequent recognition of the Plasmodium falciparum antigen VAR2CSA among young Tanzanian children. PLoS One 7, e31011
15. Fried M, Avril M, Chaturvedi R et al (2013) Multilaboratory approach to preclinical evaluation of vaccine immunogens for placental malaria. Infect Immun 81:487–495
16. Nielsen MA, Pinto VV, Resende M et al (2009) Induction of adhesion-inhibitory antibodies against placental Plasmodium falciparum parasites by using single domains of VAR2CSA. Infect Immun 77:2482–2487
17. Ghumra A, Khunrae P, Ataide R et al (2011) Immunisation with recombinant PfEMP1 domains elicits functional rosette-inhibiting and phagocytosis-inducing antibodies to Plasmodium falciparum. PLoS One 6, e16414
18. Moll K, Pettersson F, Vogt AM et al (2007) Generation of cross-protective antibodies against Plasmodium falciparum sequestration by immunization with an erythrocyte membrane protein 1-duffy binding-like 1 alpha domain. Infect Immun 75:211–219
19. Doritchamou J, Bigey P, Nielsen MA et al (2013) Differential adhesion-inhibitory patterns of antibodies raised against two major variants of the NTS-DBL2X region of VAR2CSA. Vaccine 31:4516–4522
20. Beeson JG, Mann EJ, Elliott SR et al (2004) Antibodies to variant surface antigens of Plasmodium falciparum-infected erythrocytes and adhesion inhibitory antibodies are associated with placental malaria and have overlapping and distinct targets. J Infect Dis 189:540–551
21. Boeuf P, Hasang W, Hanssen E et al (2011) Relevant assay to study the adhesion of Plasmodium falciparum-infected erythrocytes to the placental epithelium. PLoS One 6, e21126
22. Fernandez P, Kviebig N, Dechavanne S et al (2008) Var2CSA DBL6-epsilon domain expressed in HEK293 induces limited cross-reactive and blocking antibodies to CSA binding parasites. Malar J 7:170
23. Fernandez P, Petres S, Mecheri S et al (2010) Strain-transcendent immune response to recombinant Var2CSA DBL5-epsilon domain block P. falciparum adhesion to placenta-derived BeWo cells under flow conditions. PLoS One 5, e12558

24. Fried M, Duffy PE (2002) Analysis of CSA-binding parasites and antiadhesion antibodies. Methods Mol Med 72:555–560
25. Magistrado PA, Minja D, Doritchamou J et al (2011) High efficacy of anti DBL4varepsilon-VAR2CSA antibodies in inhibition of CSA-binding Plasmodium falciparum-infected erythrocytes from pregnant women. Vaccine 29:437–443
26. Obiakor H, Avril M, Macdonald NJ et al (2013) Identification of VAR2CSA domain-specific inhibitory antibodies of the Plasmodium falciparum erythrocyte membrane protein 1 using a novel flow cytometry assay. Clin Vaccine Immunol 20:433–442
27. Tuikue Ndam NG, Fievet N, Bertin G et al (2004) Variable adhesion abilities and overlapping antigenic properties in placental Plasmodium falciparum isolates. J Infect Dis 190:2001–2009
28. Lucchi NW, Koopman R, Peterson DS et al (2006) Plasmodium falciparum-infected red blood cells selected for binding to cultured syncytiotrophoblast bind to chondroitin sulfate A and induce tyrosine phosphorylation in the syncytiotrophoblast. Placenta 27:384–394
29. Viebig NK, Nunes MC, Scherf A et al (2006) The human placental derived BeWo cell line: a useful model for selecting Plasmodium falciparum CSA-binding parasites. Exp Parasitol 112:121–125
30. Haase RN, Megnekou R, Lundquist M et al (2006) Plasmodium falciparum parasites expressing pregnancy-specific variant surface antigens adhere strongly to the choriocarcinoma cell line BeWo. Infect Immun 74:3035–3038
31. Goodyer ID, Johnson J, Eisenthal R et al (1994) Purification of mature-stage Plasmodium falciparum by gelatine flotation. Ann Trop Med Parasitol 88:209–211
32. Lambros C, Vanderberg JP (1979) Synchronization of Plasmodium falciparum erythrocytic stages in culture. J Parasitol 65:418–420
33. Moore JM, Nahlen B, Ofulla AV et al (1997) A simple perfusion technique for isolation of maternal intervillous blood mononuclear cells from human placentae. J Immunol Methods 209:93–104
34. Ribacke U, Moll K, Albrecht L et al (2013) Improved in vitro culture of Plasmodium falciparum permits establishment of clinical isolates with preserved multiplication, invasion and rosetting phenotypes. PLoS One 8, e69781
35. Frankland S, Adisa A, Horrocks P et al (2006) Delivery of the malaria virulence protein PfEMP1 to the erythrocyte surface requires cholesterol-rich domains. Eukaryot Cell 5:849–860
36. Frankland S, Elliott SR, Yosaatmadja F et al (2007) Serum lipoproteins promote efficient presentation of the malaria virulence protein PfEMP1 at the erythrocyte surface. Eukaryot Cell 6:1584–1594
37. Prudhomme JG, Sherman IW (1999) A high capacity in vitro assay for measuring the cytoadherence of Plasmodium falciparum-infected erythrocytes. J Immunol Methods 229:169–176

Part IV

Parasite Manipulation

Chapter 21

Generation of Transgenic Rodent Malaria Parasites Expressing Human Malaria Parasite Proteins

Ahmed M. Salman, Catherin Marin Mogollon, Jing-wen Lin, Fiona J.A. van Pul, Chris J. Janse, and Shahid M. Khan

Abstract

We describe methods for the rapid generation of transgenic rodent *Plasmodium berghei* (*Pb*) parasites that express human malaria parasite (HMP) proteins, using the recently developed GIMO-based transfection methodology. Three different genetic modifications are described resulting in three types of transgenic parasites. (1) Additional Gene (AG) mutants. In these mutants the HMP gene is introduced as an "additional gene" into a silent/neutral locus of the *Pb* genome under the control of either a constitutive or stage-specific *Pb* promoter. This method uses the GIMO-transfection protocol and AG mutants are generated by replacing the positive–negative selection marker (SM) h*dhfr::yfcu* cassette in a neutral locus of a standard GIMO mother line with the HMP gene expression cassette, resulting in SM free transgenic parasites. (2) Double-step Replacement (DsR) mutants. In these mutants the coding sequence (CDS) of the *Pb* gene is replaced with the CDS of the HMP ortholog in a two-step GIMO-transfection procedure. This process involves first the replacement of the *Pb* CDS with the h*dhfr::yfcu* SM, followed by insertion of the HMP ortholog at the same locus thereby replacing h*dhfr::yfcu* with the HMP CDS. These steps use the GIMO-transfection protocol, which exploits both positive selection for *Pb* orthologous gene-deletion and negative selection for HMP gene-insertion, resulting in SM free transgenic parasites. (3) Double-step Insertion (DsI) mutants. When a *Pb* gene is essential for blood stage development the DsR strategy is not possible. In these mutants the HMP expression cassette is first introduced into the neutral locus in a standard GIMO mother line as described for AG mutants but under the control elements of the *Pb* orthologous gene; subsequently, the *Pb* ortholog CDS is targeted for deletion through replacement of the *Pb* CDS with the h*dhfr::yfcu* SM, resulting in transgenic parasites with a new GIMO locus permissive for additional gene-insertion modifications.

The different types of transgenic parasites can be exploited to examine interactions of drugs/inhibitors or immune factors with HMP molecules in vivo. Mice either immunized with HMP-vaccines or treated with specific drugs can be infected/challenged with these transgenic mutants to evaluate drug or vaccine efficacy in vivo.

Key words Malaria, *Plasmodium berghei*, Human parasites, Transgenic rodent parasites, GIMO-transfection, Challenge model, Vaccine-candidates, Drug-targets

Ashley M. Vaughan (ed.), *Malaria Vaccines: Methods and Protocols*, Methods in Molecular Biology, vol. 1325, DOI 10.1007/978-1-4939-2815-6_21, © Springer Science+Business Media New York 2015

1 Introduction

Rodent malaria parasites are used as models for human malaria and in particular to aid drug discovery and vaccine development. These models are used to study drug action and to identify targets for protective immune responses, in vivo. Although a high level of orthology exists between the genes of *Plasmodium* species that infect rodents and humans [1, 2], critical differences often exist in the sequence and structure between the encoded proteins. In addition, human malaria parasites (HMP; e.g., *P. falciparum* and *P. vivax*) express genes that are absent from rodent parasite genomes. These genetic differences complicate the analysis of drugs/inhibitors or immune factors in rodent models and the effective translation of findings in model systems to human malaria. "Humanizing" rodent parasites by introducing HMP genes into rodent parasite genomes can help to circumvent problems of interpreting data from different interventions, arising from structural differences that exist between functional HMP and rodent malaria parasite orthologs. In addition, it increases the possibilities of analyzing HMP-specific proteins in vivo [3].

Here we describe methods to generate "humanized" rodent malaria parasites in the *P. berghei* (*Pb*) model. Efficient methods exist for *Pb* genetic modification including a recently described method for GIMO-transfection (Gene Insertion-Marker Out; [4]) that greatly simplifies and speeds up the generation of transgenic parasites expressing heterologous proteins, free of drug-selection marker genes. Three different genetic modifications are described here resulting in three types of transgenic parasites that express HMP proteins. (1) *Additional Gene* (*AG*) mutants. In these mutants the HMP gene is introduced as an additional gene into a silent/neutral locus of the *Pb* genome under the control of a constitutive or stage-specific *Pb* promoter. This method is mainly used when a functional ortholog of the HMP gene is absent in the rodent malaria parasite genome. This method makes use of the GIMO-transfection method and AG mutants are created by replacing the positive–negative selection marker (SM) h*dhfr::yfcu* cassette in a neutral locus of a standard GIMO mother line with the HMP gene expression cassette, resulting in SM free transgenic parasites. (2) *Double-step Replacement* (*DsR*) mutants. In these mutants the coding sequence (CDS) of the *Pb* gene is replaced with the CDS of the orthologous HMP gene, in a two-step GIMO transfection. First, the *Pb* gene is deleted by double crossover homologous recombination with a construct having the h*dhfr::yfcu* SM flanked by the 5′ untranslated region (UTR; containing the gene promoter) and 3′ UTR (containing the transcriptional terminator sequences) of the *Pb* gene as gene targeting regions (TRs), thereby creating an "GIMO locus". Next, this GIMO locus is replaced by the HMP gene expression cassette with the HMP homolog flanked by the same 5′ UTR and 3′ UTR regions of the orthologous *Pb* gene. This method creates transgenic parasites expressing an HMP gene free of SM. (3) *Double-step Insertion* (*DsI*) mutants. When a *Pb* gene is essential for blood stage development the DsR approach is not suitable, as it is not possible to first create a GIMO-based deletion mutant in the first step. Therefore, in DsI mutants the HMP gene is first introduced into the neutral locus of an existing GIMO mother line under the control of 5′ UTR and 3′ UTR of the *Pb* ortholog. This step, in common with the AG method, results in a transgenic mutant expressing an additional copy of HMP but under the control elements of the *Pb* ortholog in a neutral locus, free of SM. Subsequently, the *Pb* ortholog is deleted. This method generates transgenic parasites not only expressing the HMP gene but also containing a GIMO locus (in the *Pb* gene). The absence of SM in the DsR and AG mutants and the GIMO locus created in DsI mutants facilitates rapid additional genetic modifications in these lines, for example to introduce additional HMP genes or reporter genes encoding fluorescent or luminescent proteins.

These different transgenic parasites can be exploited to examine interactions of drugs/inhibitors or induced immune factors against HMP molecules, in vitro and in vivo. Mice either immunized with candidate HMP-vaccines or treated with specific antibodies or drugs/inhibitors can be infected or challenged with these transgenic parasites to evaluate the efficacy of drugs/inhibitors or vaccines in vivo [3]. Humanized rodent parasites have been used to assess the efficacy of candidate vaccines against the *P. vivax* TRAP protein [5], the *P. falciparum* and *P. vivax* CS proteins [6, 7], the *P. falciparum* and *P. vivax* P25 proteins [8, 9] and the *P. falciparum* MSP1 gene [10, 11]. In addition, humanized *Pb* parasites expressing *P. falciparum* cyclic GMP-dependent protein kinase (PKG) and *P. falciparum* hexose transporter 1 have been generated, permitting in vivo screening of inhibitors interfering with PKG and antimalarial sugar analogs respectively [12, 13].

In this chapter we principally describe the generation of GIMO-based mutants in the rodent malaria parasite, *P. berghei*; however, similar reagents (e.g., a GIMO mother line and constructs) also exist for the rodent parasite *P. yoelii* [4].

2 Materials

2.1 Standard Parasites Lines Used for Generation Transgenic Parasites Expressing HMP Genes

1. Wild type (WT) lines of *P. berghei* ANKA or NK65; the most frequently used is the reference ANKA line, cl15cy1 [14].
2. The reporter *Pb* ANKA parasite line *Pb*GFP-Luc$_{con}$ (676m1cl1) expresses a fusion protein of GFP (mutant3) and firefly luciferase (LUC-IAV) under the constitutive *eef1a* promoter and is SM free [15]. The reporter cassette is integrated into the neutral *230p* locus (PBANKA_030600). For details of

PbGFP-Luccon, see RMgmDB entry #29 (http://www.pberghei.eu/index.php?rmgm=29) and **Note 1**.

3. The reporter *Pb* ANKA parasite line *Pb*GFP-Luc$_{ama1}$ (1037m1f1m1cl1) expresses a fusion protein of GFP (mutant3) and firefly luciferase (LUC-IAV) under the schizont-specific *ama-1* promoter and is SM free [16]. The reporter cassette is integrated into the neutral *230p* locus (PBANKA_030600). For details of *Pb* GFP-Luc$_{ama1}$, see RMgmDB entry 32 (http://www.pberghei.eu/index.php?rmgm=32) and **Note 1**.
4. The standard PbANKA-*230p* GIMO mother line (GIMO$_{PbANKA}$ 1596cl1). The line contains a positive–negative selection marker (SM) cassette, a fusion gene of h*dhfr* (human dihydrofolate reductase; positive SM) and y*fcu* (yeast cytosine deaminase and uridyl phosphoribosyl transferase; negative SM) under control of the constitutive *eef1a* promoter, stably integrated into the neutral *230p* locus (PBANKA_030600) through double crossover recombination [4]. The GIMO mother line is used for introduction of transgenes into the modified *230p* locus through transfection with constructs that target the *230p* locus. These constructs insert into the *230p* locus ("gene insertion"), thereby removing the h*dhfr::yfcu* SM ("marker out") from the genome of the mother line. Transgenic parasites that are SM free are subsequently selected by applying negative drug selection using 5-FC. This selection procedure is performed in vivo in mice. For details of the PbANKA-*230p* GIMO mother line, see RMgmDB entry #687 (http://www.pberghei.eu/index.php?rmgm=687). We have generated a comparable standard GIMO mother line for the rodent parasite *P. yoelii* XNL Py17XNL-*230p* GIMO mother line (GIMO$_{Py17X,}$ 1923cl1; *see* **Note 2**).
5. The standard PbANKA-*s1* GIMO mother line (2149cl1). The line contains a positive–negative h*dhfr::yfcu* selection marker (SM) cassette, under control of the constitutive *eef1a* promoter stably integrated into the neutral *s1* gene-locus (PBANKA_120680) through double crossover recombination. The neutral *s1* locus has also been used in *P. yoelii* to introduce reporter proteins [17]. In addition, it contains GFP under the constitutive *eef1a* promoter integrated into the neutral *230p* locus (PBANKA_030600). This line is currently unpublished but is available from the Leiden Malaria Research Group. The GIMO mother line is used for introduction of transgenes into the modified *s1* locus through transfection with constructs that target the *s1* locus. These constructs insert into the *s1* locus ("gene insertion"), thereby removing the h*dhfr::yfcu* selectable marker ("marker out") from the genome of the mother line. Transgenic parasites that are marker-free

are subsequently selected by applying negative drug selection using 5-FC. This selection procedure is performed in vivo in mice. The PbANKA-s1 GIMO mother line contains a GFP-luciferase fusion expression cassette in the *230p* locus and therefore transgenic parasites made in this line express both GFP and luciferase under the constitutive *eef1α* promoter. In contrast, transgenic parasites made in the PbANKA-*230p* GIMO do not express a reporter protein.

2.2 Laboratory Animals and Mosquitoes

2.2.1 Laboratory Animals

In our laboratory, we mainly use Swiss Webster mice (6 weeks old; 25–26 g) for generation of the transgenic parasite lines. However, other mouse strains such as C57BL/6 and BALB/c can also be used. All experiments using mice must be performed according to the appropriate National guidelines and regulations.

2.2.2 Laboratory Mosquitoes

Anopheles stephensi. For procedures of maintenance/rearing of mosquitoes and infection of mosquitoes, *see* ref. [18].

2.3 Basic DNA Constructs/Plasmids

1. Plasmid pL0043 [4]. This is a basic construct that is used to rapidly introduce transgenes into the *230p* locus (PBANKA_030600) of the PbANKA-*230p* GIMO mother line. This construct integrates by double crossover recombination and replaces the positive–negative SM (h*dhfr::yfcu*) cassette with the transgene-expression cassette (*see* **Note 3** for details of the generation of pL0043). We have generated a similar construct (pL1849) to rapidly introduce transgenes into the *230p* locus (PY17X_0306600) of the PyXNL-*230p* GIMO mother line. This construct integrates by double crossover homologous recombination and replaces the positive–negative SM with the transgene-expression cassette. The construct pL1849 was generated using a modified 2-step PCR method (*see* **Note 4**).
2. *Plasmid* pL2023. This is a basic construct that can be used to rapidly introduce transgenes into the *Pb s1* locus (PBANKA_120680) of the PbANKA-*s1* GIMO mother line. This construct integrates by double crossover recombination and replaces the positive–negative (h*dhfr::yfcu*) SM. *See* **Note 5** for details of the generation of pL2023 (pL2023 is currently unpublished but is available from the Leiden Malaria Research Group).
3. *Plasmid* pL0034. This construct contains the positive–negative (h*dhfr::yfcu*) SM cassette. It can be used to clone any specific 5′ and 3′ gene targeting region (TR) to generate a targeted gene-deletion mutant in the *Pb* genome by double crossover homologous recombination; replacing the *Pb* target gene with the h*dhfr::yfcu* SM, thereby generating a gene-specific GIMO locus (selected by positive selection using pyrimethamine).

The generated gene-specific GIMO line can then be used, in a subsequent transfection to introduce the orthologous HMP gene into this GIMO locus. Specifically, by using a modified DNA construct that contains the *Pb* gene 5′ and 3′ TRs (these TRs must include the complete *Pb* gene promoter and transcription terminator sequences), replacing the SM with a HMP CDS, thereby creating a HMP expression cassette. The GIMO protocol can then be employed to insert the HMP expression cassette (gene insertion) and replacing the introduced h*dhfr::yfcu* SM cassette (marker out), using negative selection. This results in generation of DsR mutants (Subheading 3.2) without SM.

2.4 Reagents

For reagents for in vitro cultivation of schizonts and transfection of *P. berghei see* ref. [14].

1. Glycerol. Stock solution: 30 % (vol/vol) glycerol in PBS. Store at 4 °C.
2. Phosphate-buffered saline (PBS). Stock solution: 0.01 M KH_2PO_4, 0.1 M Na_2HPO_4, 1.37 M NaCl, 0.027 M KCl; pH 7.0. For a working solution, dilute the stock solution with nine volumes of distilled water. Adjust the pH to 7.2 with 1 M HCl and sterilize by autoclaving for 20 min at 120 °C.
3. Heparin, Grade I-A, cell culture tested, 140 mUSP units/mg. Heparin stock solution: dissolve the heparin powder in distilled water to a concentration of 25,000 units/ml. Filter-sterilize (0.2 μm) and store at 4 °C. For a working solution, add 0.2 ml of the stock solution to 25 ml RPMI 1640 culture medium without FBS to create a final solution of 200 units/ml. Store at 4 °C.
4. Pyrimethamine solution (Sigma). Dissolve pyrimethamine powder (5-4-Chlorophenyl-6-ethyl 2,4-pyrimidinediamine) in DMSO to a final concentration of 7 mg/ml (stirring on a vortex) and dilute 100 times with normal tap water with an adjusted pH of 3.5–5.0 (with 1 M HCl). Store at 4 °C and use the solution for the drinking water of mice during the complete selection period.
5. 5-FC solution. Negative selection of mutants is performed by providing 5-fluorocytosine (5-FC) in the drinking water of mice, 1 day after the mice have been infected with transfected parasites. The 2 mg/ml final concentration of 5-FC diluted with drinking water is provided to mice during the complete selection period (*see* ref. 19 for details of the 5-FC drinking water protocol).
6. DNA constructs (5–10 μg) in 5–10 μL TE buffer or water used for transfection (stored at −20 °C).

2.5 Equipment

For equipment for in vitro cultivation of schizonts and transfection of *P. berghei see* ref. [14].

1. Nucleofector device (Lonza) (http://www.lonza.com/).
2. Anesthesia induction chamber: Fluovac isoflurane–halothane scavenger (Stoelting Co.). Mice are anesthetized in the "induction chamber," which is prefilled with the anesthetic vapor (a mixture of isoflurane and air) via the vaporizer unit. The injection of parasites or collecting blood by heart puncture is performed in mice that are kept under anesthesia by holding their muzzles to the small mask that is connected to the vaporizer unit.
3. Insulin syringes.

3 Methods

Three different genetic modifications are described resulting in three types of transgenic parasites that express HMP proteins: (1) Additional Gene mutants (AG; Subheading 3.1); (2) Double-step Replacement mutants (DsR; Subheading 3.2); and (3) Double-step Insertion mutants (DsI; Subheading 3.3). All mutants are generated using GIMO-transfection method [4]. For GIMO-transfection constructs are used, which contain the positive–negative drug-selection marker (SM) h*dhfr::yfcu*. This marker is a fusion of a positive SM (human h*dhfr* conferring resistance to pyrimethamine) and the negative SM (*yfcu* conferring sensitivity to 5-fluorocytosine; 5-FC). Parasites expressing h*dhfr::yfcu* are resistant to the pyrimethamine but are sensitive to 5-FC. GIMO-transfection uses positive selection for targeted gene-deletion and negative selection to rapidly generate gene-insertion transgenic parasites free of SM.

3.1 Transgenic Parasites with an HMP Gene in a Neutral Locus: Additional Gene (AG) Mutants

When a functional ortholog of an HMP gene is absent in the *Pb* genome, the HMP gene can be introduced into a neutral/silent locus of the *Pb* genome. Moreover, this approach can be used when the stage specificity and/or level of HMP expression needs to be altered. *See* Table 1 for different promoter regions used to drive transgene expression. The HMP gene is introduced into a standard GIMO mother line (Subheading 2.1) using a modified GIMO construct (Fig. 1; Subheading 2.3). The standard constructs target the *230p* or *s1* gene locus, as they contain targeting regions (TRs) to these genes as well as containing a multiple cloning site, where the HMP expression cassette can be introduced. The HMP expression cassette consists of the HMP CDS flanked upstream by the desired 5′ UTR (containing the *Pb* promoter) and downstream by the 3′ UTR (containing the transcriptional

Table 1
Different *P. berghei* regulatory regions (promoter and 3′ UTR transcription terminator sequences) used to control transgene expression

Gene name	Gene product	Reference[a] or primer[b]	Timing of expression
Promoter regions			
eef1α	PBANKA_113330	RMgm-7; [15]	Constitutive
hsp70	PBANKA_071190	RMgm-928 and [31]	Constitutive (Strong)
ama1	PBANKA_091500	RMgm-32; [16]	Schizonts (blood, liver), sporozoites
Soap	PBANKA_103780	ATAAGAAT**GCGGCCGC**GTATCTAAAAAAAGCCTAATATTTCC/ CCATG**CCATGG**TTTGATTAATATAAATACAAAAAAGG	Ookinetes
Dynein heavy chain, putative	PBANKA_041610	AA**GGATCC**TTTTTATCATTTGGATAATTAATTC/ AA**GATATC**ATATTTAAACAGATTAAGTACCG	Male gametocytes
lap4/ccp2	PBANKA_131950	AA**GATATC**TTTATAAATGAAGCAATACCAC/ TT**GGATCC**TTCTATTAATAAAAAATATAAATATATG	Female gametocytes
uis4	PBANKA_050120	TAT**CCTGCAGG**GTGATAGTGTAGATTTTTTTGTTTGAC/ ATAAGAAT**GCGGCCGC**AGACGTAATAATTATGTGCTGAAAGG	Sporozoites (early) liver stages
cs/csp	PBANKA_040320	GCTC**CTTAAG**ACATAAAAGGGAATATGGAATATACTAGC/ CG**GGATCC**AAATATATGCGTGTATATATAGATTTTG	Sporozoites, liver stage

Trap	PBANKA_134980	CAT**GGGCCC**GAAAGGAAAATGGGCAAATTATGTGTC/ ACT**GTTAAC**GGAAATTGTCTTACCCATATTATTCCTAC	Sporozoites
sequestrin/lisp2	PBANKA_100300	CAT**GGGCCC**GTCCTTATGGGCATATAACATCG/ A**AGGCCT**ATGTGTAAAAAAGTAAAATGATTATAATAGAAGTG	Middle/late liver stages
3′ UTR regions			
pbdhfr/ts	PBANKA_071930	CG**GGATTCC**GTTTTTCTTACTTATATATTTATACC/ GCTC**GGTACC**CGAAATTGAAGG	NA
Cam	PBANKA_101060	TGC**TCTAGA**ATTATTAATATATATGAATATATATACATCGTTGTATGCG/ CGG**GGTACC**GACCATATAAGAATTAACCC	NA
dhfs-fpgs	PBANKA 134000	RMgm-757; [31]	NA
dhps;ppk	PBANKA_142670	RMgm-757; [31]	NA
uis4	PBANKA_050120	CG**GATATC**TATAATTCATTATGAGTAGTGTAATTCAG/ GGCC**GGTACC**TTTCGCTTTAATGCTTGTCATC	NA
trap	PBANKA_134980	CG**GGATCC**AACTTAAGAGTATTATTTTTGTTTCG/ ATAAGAAT**GCGGCCGC**CATATATATCTAGATGATTATTCTTATGTTAC	NA
sequestrin/lisp2	PBANKA_100300	CCGG**GGTACC**ATGCATATAAGAAAAAGCCCAAACC/ ATAAGAAT**GCGGCCGC**TCGAAGAAATTCGAGTTAAGAAATTAAATGATGG	NA

[a]Reference to a line where gene regulatory sequence has been used to regulate transgene expression either as an entry in the RMgm Database (www.pberghei.eu; i.e., RMgm-#ID) or in a publication

[b]The primer sequences (i.e., Forward/Reverse) surrounding the regulatory region are shown with the restriction site used (*bold and underlined*) to introduce the region into the transfection construct

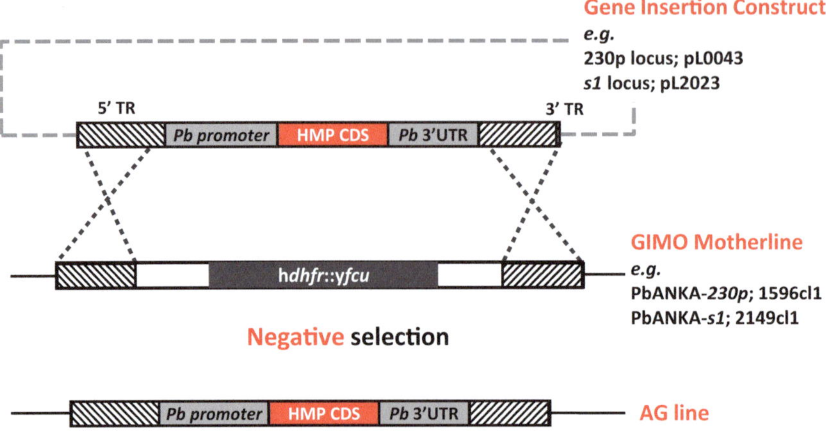

Fig. 1 Generation of AG mutants. Additional Gene (AG) mutants have a human malaria parasite (HMP) gene introduced into a neutral locus (*230p* or *s1* locus) of the *P. berghei* GIMO mother line genome by GIMO-transfection. Schematic representation of the construct to introduce the human malaria parasite (HMP) gene into the *230p* or *s1* locus of GIMO mother lines, resulting in the generation of the AG mutant after negative selection with 5-FC is shown. Two basic constructs can be used to rapidly introduce transgenes into neutral *Pb* loci by GIMO transfection; specifically pL0043 to introduce transgenes into the *230p* locus (for transfection into the *Pb*ANKA-*230p* GIMO mother line; 1596cl1) and pL2023 for the *s1* locus (for transfection into the *Pb*ANKA-*s1* GIMO mother line; 2149cl1). These basic constructs contain 5′ and 3′ TRs for these loci as well as a multiple-cloning site. The final Gene Insertion construct contains the HMP CDS is flanked upstream by the 5′ UTR (containing the gene promoter region) and downstream by 3′ UTR (containing the transcription terminator sequence) regions of the *Pb* ortholog, both of which can be PCR-amplified from *Pb* gDNA. The selection of the *Pb* promoter region is dependent on the timing and strength of HMP gene expression required (*see* Table 1). The HMP CDS can be PCR-amplified from HMP genomic DNA or cDNA. The construct is targeting the *230p* or *s1* target regions (*hatched boxes*) by double crossover homologous recombination (DXO), resulting in replacement of the h*dhfr::yfcu* selectable marker cassette that is present in the GIMO parasites with the HMP gene expression cassette (*see* **Note 6** for details)

terminator sequence) regions. *See* Fig. 1 and **Note 6** for details on the generation of these constructs.

Two different standard *Pb* GIMO lines exist containing the h*dhfr::yfcu* SM cassette either in the neutral *230p* locus (the PbANKA-*230p* GIMO mother line [4]), or the silent *s1* locus (the PbANKA-*s1* GIMO mother line) *see* Subheading 2.1. The latter line is currently unpublished but is available from the Leiden Malaria Research Group. This line exhibits normal development throughout the complete life cycle (CJJ and SMK, unpublished observations). The neutral *s1* locus has also been used in *P. yoelii* to introduce reporter proteins [17]. For introducing an HMP gene as an additional copy in *P. yoelii* XNL, a GIMO line exists (the PyXNL-*230p* GIMO mother line; [4]), which contains the h*dhfr::yfcu* SM cassette into the neutral *230p* locus (*see* **Note 2**).

3.1.1 Transfection of Parasites and Injection into Mice

1. Prepare 5–10 μg of linearized DNA construct in 5–10 μL water or TE buffer. This construct is based on a standard GIMO construct and contains the 5′ and 3′ TRs of the *230p* or *s1* targeting regions of the GIMO mother line and an HMP gene expression cassette (i.e., the HMP gene CDS flanked by 5′ UTR (promoter) and 3′ UTR of a chosen *Pb* gene; Fig. 1, **Note 6**).
2. Collect cultured (in vitro matured) *P. berghei* schizonts of the standard PbANKA-*230p* or PbANKA-*s1* GIMO mother lines (Subheading 2.1) for transfection as described in ref. [14].
3. Transfect the schizonts with the DNA construct using a Nucleofector device using the transfection protocol and conditions as described in ref. [14].
4. Inject the transfected parasites into a mouse tail vein using insulin syringes under anesthesia.

3.1.2 Negative Selection of Parasites (5-FC) and Cloning

1. Select transfected parasites by negative selection with 5-FC: provide the mouse with drinking water containing 5-FC one day after infection with transfected parasites. Provide the water for a period of 8–11 days up to the collection of infected blood.
2. Collect transfected and selected parasites between day 8 and 11 after infecting mice with transfected parasites. In successful transfection experiments, the parasitemia usually increases to 2–5 % between days 8 and 11. Collect 0.6–1 ml of blood from the mouse with a parasitemia of 2–5 % by heart puncture under anesthesia.
3. Use 0.2 ml of infected blood for storage in liquid nitrogen (these parasites are used for cloning transfected parasites): transfer 0.2 ml of the suspension to an Eppendorf tube containing 0.3 ml glycerol-PBS stock solution; distribute this suspension equally among two cryogenic vials, 0.25 ml per tube, and store these tubes within 20 min in liquid nitrogen.
4. Use the remainder of the blood (0.4–0.8 ml) to genotype the transfected parasite population by Southern analysis of separated chromosomes (*see* **Note 7a**, Fig. 2) or digested genomic DNA or by diagnostic PCR as described in ref. [14].
5. If the genotyping shows correct deletion of the h*dhfr::yfcu* SM cassette, clone the parasites by the method of limiting dilution. Infect a mouse with transfected parasites from the liquid nitrogen storage and collect blood at a parasitemia of 0.2–1 % for limiting dilution of parasites and injecting 10 mice with 0.3 parasites per mouse using insulin syringes under anesthesia as described in ref. [20].
6. Collect cloned parasite lines at day 8/9 after cloning. The parasitemia usually increases to 0.5–2 % at day 8. Collect 0.6–1 ml of blood from the mouse with a parasitemia of 1–3 %

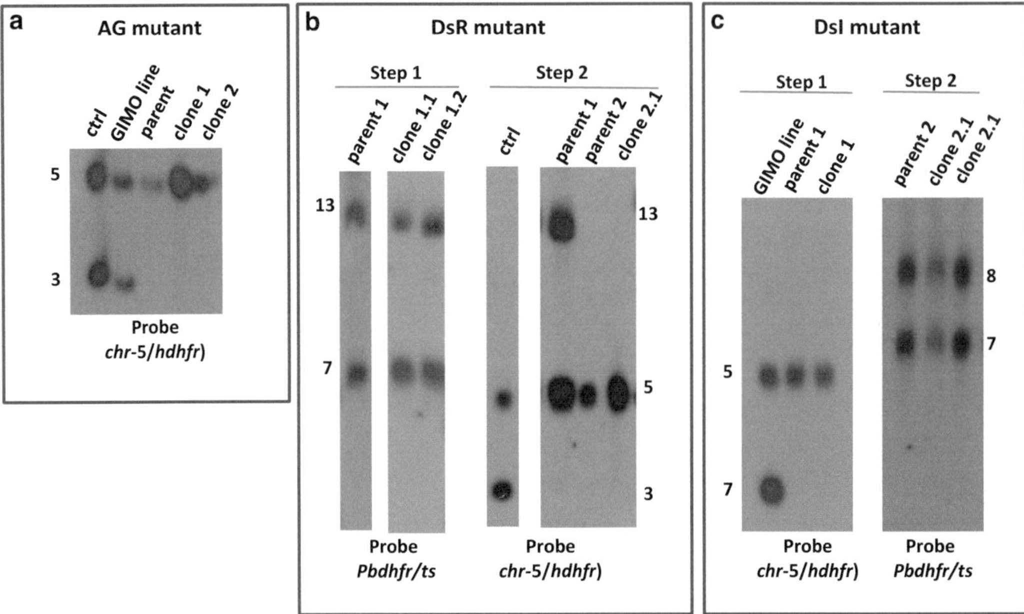

Fig. 2 Genotyping of AG, DsR, and DsI mutants. (**a**) *AG mutants*: Southern analysis of chromosomes (chrs) separated by pulsed-field gel electrophoresis (PFGE) to confirm integration of the DNA construct in the GIMO locus by showing the removal of the h*dhfr::y fcu* SM cassette both in uncloned (parent) and cloned parasites. The Southern blot is hybridized with a mixture of two probes: one recognizing h*dhfr* and a control probe recognizing chr 5. As an additional control (ctrl), parasite line 2117cl1 is used with the h*dhfr::y fcu* SM integrated into chr 3. (**b**) *DsR mutants*: Southern analysis of PFGE-separated chrs to confirm integration of the DNA construct into the target *Pb* gene both in uncloned (parent 1) and cloned parasites selected in step 1 of the DsR transfection protocol. The chrs are hybridized using a probe recognizing the 3′UTR *Pbdhfr/ts* of the SM of the integrated construct which also hybridizes to the endogenous *Pbdhfr/ts* on chr 7. For genotyping of selected parasites in step 2 of the DsR protocol (i.e., the uncloned parent 2 and cloned parasites): Southern analysis of PFGE-separated chrs to confirm integration of the orthologous HMP gene in the GIMO locus by showing the absence of the h*dhfr::y fcu* SM cassette. Separated chrs are hybridized with a mixture of two probes: one recognizing h*dhfr* and a control pb25 probe recognizing chromosome 5 as described above for the AG mutants. (**c**) *DsI mutants*: Southern analysis of PFGE-separated chrs to confirm integration of the DNA construct in the GIMO locus by showing the absence of the h*dhfr::y fcu* SM cassette both in uncloned (parent 1) and cloned parasites in step 1. Chrs are hybridized with a mixture of two probes: one recognizing h*dhfr* and a control probe recognizing pb25 on chr 5 as described above for the AG mutants. For genotyping of selected parasites in step 2 (the uncloned parent 2 and cloned parasites) we usually perform Southern analysis of PFGE-separated chromosomes to confirm integration of the DNA construct in the target *Pb* gene both in uncloned (parent 1) and cloned parasites selected with positive selection in step 1. The chrs are hybridized using a probe recognizing the 3′UTR *Pbdhfr/ts* of the SM of the integrated construct which also hybridizes to the endogenous *Pbdhfr/ts* on chr 7 as described above for step 1 of the DsR protocol

by heart puncture under anesthesia. Use 0.2 ml of infected blood for storage in liquid nitrogen: transfer 0.2 ml of the suspension to an Eppendorf tube containing 0.3 ml glycerol-PBS stock solution; distribute this suspension equally among two cryogenic vials, 0.25 ml per tube, and store these tubes within 20 min in liquid nitrogen.

7. Use the remainder of the blood (0.4–0.8 ml) to genotype the cloned parasite population by Southern analysis of separated chromosomes (*see* **Note 7a**, Fig. 2) or digested genomic DNA or by diagnostic PCR as described in ref. [14].
8. The cloned AG parasites with a correct genotype are used for phenotype analysis to (1) determine (normal) development throughout the life cycle and (2) to confirm correct HMP expression (*see* Subheading 3.4).

3.2 Transgenic Parasites Expressing HMP Proteins: Double Step Replacement (DsR) Mutants

In DsR mutants the CDS of the *Pb* gene is replaced with the CDS of the HMP ortholog in a two-step transfection procedure (Fig. 3, **Note 8**). First, parasites are transfected with a gene-deletion construct designed to replace the *Pb* CDS with the h*dhfr::yfcu* SM cassette. This results in deletion of the *Pb* gene; however, selection of gene-deletion mutants (by positive selection with pyrimethamine) is only possible if the gene is not essential for blood stages. In the transfected parasites the locus of interest will contain unaltered 5′ and 3′ sequences upstream and downstream of the CDS. Clonal lines of these gene-deletion mutants will then be transfected with a second gene-insertion constructs that leads to replacement of the h*dhfr::yfcu* SM cassette with the orthologous HMP gene. Transfected parasites will be selected with 5-FC, which will kill the non-transfected parasites that still harbor h*dhfr::yfcu*. This method creates parasites that express an HMP gene under the control of regulatory sequences of the *Pb* ortholog, which are free of SM, permitting additional genetic modifications.

3.2.1 Transfection of Parasites and Injection into Mice: Transfection Step 1

1. Prepare 5–10 μg of linear DNA construct in 5–10 μL water or TE buffer. This construct (*Construct 1*) is a gene-deletion construct containing the h*dhfr::yfcu* SM cassette flanked by the 5′ and 3′ TRs of the *Pb* gene and is based on standard construct pL0034 (Subheading 2.3; Fig. 3, *see* **Note 8**).
2. Collect cultured (in vitro matured) *P. berghei* schizonts of wild type (WT; Subheading 2.1) or reference reporter lines (e.g., *Pb*GFP-Luc$_{con}$ or *Pb*GFP-Luc$_{ama1}$; Subheading 2.1, *see* **Note 1**) for transfection as described in ref. [14].
3. Transfect the schizonts with *Construct 1* using a Nucleofector device using the transfection protocol and conditions as described in ref. [14].
4. Inject the transfected parasites into a tail vein of a mouse using insulin syringes under anesthesia.

3.2.2 Positive Selection of Parasites (Pyrimethamine) and Cloning: Transfection Step 1

1. Select transfected parasites by positive selection with pyrimethamine: provide the mouse with drinking water containing pyrimethamine 1 day after infection with transfected parasites. Provide the water for a period of 8–11 days up to the collection of infected blood.

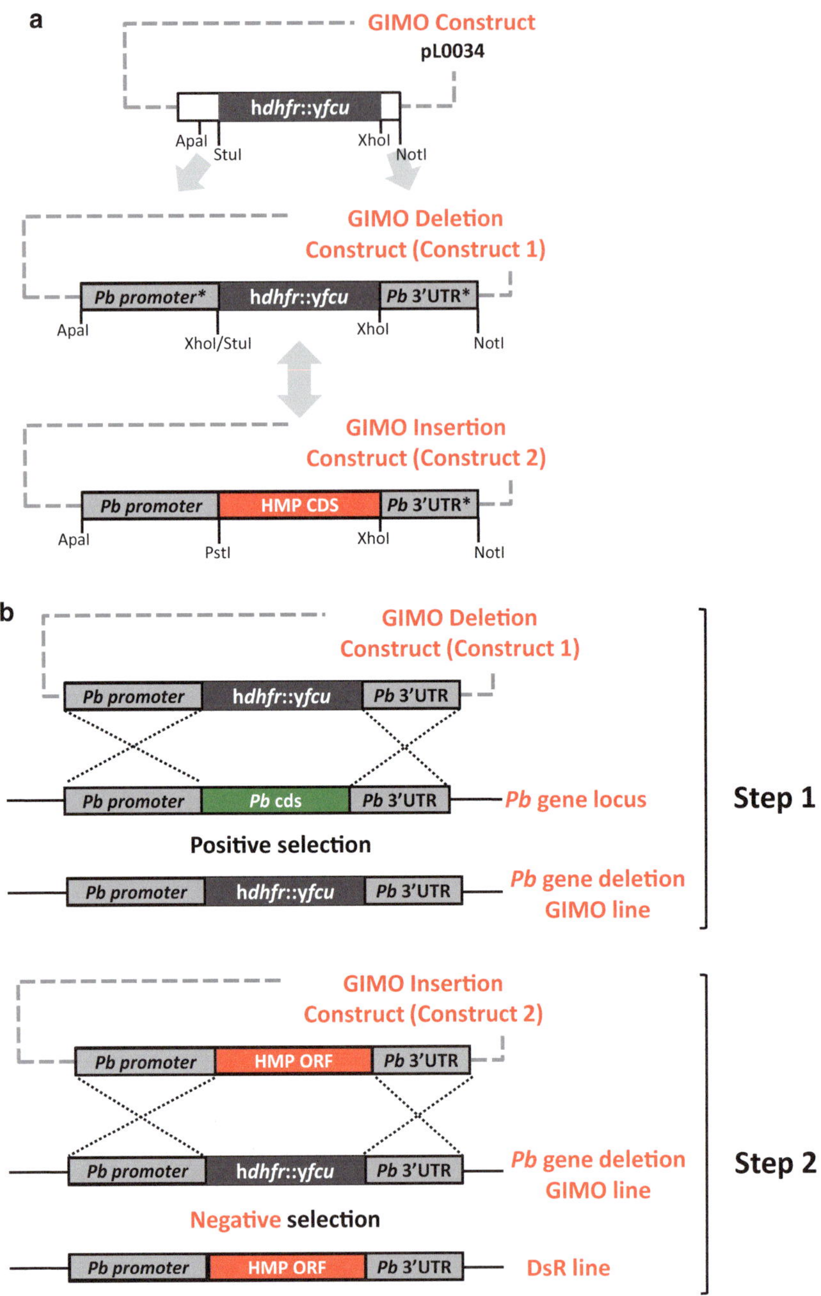

Fig. 3 Generation of DsR mutants. (**a**) Generation of the two constructs for generation of DsR mutants. Schematic representation describing the generation of *Construct 1* (*GIMO Deletion construct*) by cloning 5′- and 3′-TRs of the *Pb* gene (these regions need to include the complete *Pb* gene promoter and transcriptional terminator sequences) into the cloning sites of the basic construct pL0034, upstream and downstream of the h*dhfr*::yfcu SM, respectively. *Note: the hdhfr::yfcu SM cassette (shown in the schematic as hdhfr::yfcu) is the complete expression cassette; flanked by the constitutive Pb eef1α promoter and the Pb dhfr/ts transcription terminator sequences.* TRs can be PCR-amplified from *Pb* gDNA. Introducing additional restriction sites in the used primers for amplifying the *Pb* 5′- and 3′-TRs should be considered to facilitate the subsequent release of the SM in order to generation *Construct 2 (GIMO Insertion construct).* This schematic shows as an example the

2. Collect transfected and selected parasites between day 8 and 11 after infecting mice with transfected parasites. In successful transfection experiments, the parasitemia usually increases to 2–5 % between days 8 and 11. Collect 0.6–1 ml of blood from the mouse with a parasitemia of 2–5 % by heart puncture under anesthesia.
3. Use 0.2 ml of infected blood for storage in liquid nitrogen (these parasites are used for cloning transfected parasites): transfer 0.2 ml of the suspension to an Eppendorf tube containing 0.3 ml glycerol-PBS stock solution; distribute this suspension equally among two cryogenic vials, 0.25 ml per tube, and store these tubes within 20 min in liquid nitrogen.
4. Use the remainder of the blood (0.4–0.8 ml) to genotype the transfected parasite population by Southern analysis of separated chromosomes (*see* **Note 7b**, Fig. 2) or digested genomic DNA or by diagnostic PCR as described in ref. [14].
5. If genotyping shows correct deletion of the *Pb* CDS, the parasites are cloned by the method of limiting dilution. Infect a mouse with transfected parasites from the liquid nitrogen storage and collect blood at a parasitemia of 0.2–1 % for limiting dilution of parasites and injecting 10 mice with 0.3 parasites per mouse using insulin syringes under anesthesia as described in ref. [20]. Genotyping and cloning of the transfected parasites is an essential step before proceeding with transfection step 2 (*see* **Note 9**).

Fig. 3 (continued) 5′-TR created with an *XhoI* restriction site at the 5′ end and a *PstI*/*XhoI* double restriction sites at the 3′ end. Similarly the 3′-TR has been generated with an *XhoI* restriction site at the 5′ end and *NotI* restriction sites at the 3′ end. Therefore *Construct 1* has been constructed with a specific restriction site (*XhoI*) both just before and after the h*dhfr*::y*fcu* SM cassette, and digestion with this enzyme releases the h*dhfr*::y*fcu* SM cassette from the plasmid resulting in a linear DNA construct containing both 5′ and 3′ TRs with complementary ends. Self-ligation can then be performed to generate a "marker-free" construct with only the 5′- and 3′-TRs and a multiple-cloning site in between these TR which can in turn be used to insert the orthologous HMP gene and thereby create *Construct 2* (GIMO Insertion construct). The HMP CDS being flanked upstream by the orthologous *Pb* 5′ UTR (containing the gene promoter region) and downstream by Pb 3′ UTR (containing the transcription terminator sequence), *see* **Note 8** for details. (**b**) *Generation of DsR mutants* where the *Pb* target gene (TG) is replaced with the orthologous gene of a human malaria parasite (HMP). *1st step*: The *GIMO Deletion construct* (*Construct 1*) is used to replace the *P. berghei* gene with the positive/negative selectable maker (h*dhfr*::y*fcu*) cassette, resulting in the generation of the TG GIMO line after positive selection with pyrimethamine. *Construct 1* targets the TG at the target regions (*hatched boxes*) by double crossover homologous recombination. After genotyping and confirming the correct construct integration, this line is cloned. *2nd step*: The *GIMO insertion construct* (*Construct 2*) is used to replace the SM in the GIMO line with the HMP CDS, under negative (5-FC) selection, resulting in DsR mutants. *Construct 2* integrates by double crossover homologous recombination using the same TRs employed in *Construct 1*, resulting in the introduction of the HMP gene under the control of the *Pb* target gene promoter and transcriptional terminator sequences.

6. Collect cloned parasite lines at day 8/9 after cloning. The parasitemia usually increases to 0.5–2 % at day 8. Collect 0.6–1 ml of blood from the mouse with a parasitemia of 1–3 % by heart puncture under anesthesia. Use 0.2 ml of infected blood for storage in liquid nitrogen (these parasites are used for "transfection step 2" (see below)): transfer 0.2 ml of the suspension to an Eppendorf tube containing 0.3 ml glycerol-PBS stock solution; distribute this suspension equally among two cryogenic vials, 0.25 ml per tube, and store these tubes within 20 min in liquid nitrogen.
7. Use the remainder of the blood (0.4–0.8 ml) to genotype the cloned parasite population by Southern analysis of separated chromosomes (*see* **Note 7b**, Fig. 2) or digested genomic DNA or by diagnostic PCR as described in ref. [14].

3.2.3 Transfection of Parasites and Injection into Mice: Transfection Step 2

1. Prepare 5–10 μg of linear DNA construct in 5–10 μL water or TE buffer. This construct (*Construct 2*) contains the HMP-CDS flanked by the same *Pb* 5′ UTR and 3′ UTR sequences present in *Construct 1* (*see* Fig. 3, **Note 8**).
2. Collect cultured (in vitro matured) schizonts of cloned gene-deletion parasites (as generated in transfection step 1) for transfection as described in ref. [14].
3. Transfect the schizonts with *Construct 2* using an Nucleofector device using the transfection protocol and conditions as described in ref. [14].
4. Inject the transfected parasites into a tail vein of a mouse using insulin syringes under anesthesia.

3.2.4 Negative Selection of Parasites (5-FC) and Cloning: Transfection Step 2

1. Select transfected parasites by negative selection with 5-FC: provide the mouse with drinking water containing 5-FC one day after infection with transfected parasites. Provide the water for a period of 8–11 days up to the collection of infected blood.
2. Collect transfected and selected parasites between day 8 and 11 after infecting mice with transfected parasites. In successful transfection experiments, the parasitemia usually increases to 2–5 % between days 8 and 11. Collect 0.6–1 ml of blood from the mouse with a parasitemia of 2–5 % by heart puncture under anesthesia.
3. Use 0.2 ml of infected blood for storage in liquid nitrogen (these parasites are used for cloning transfected parasites): transfer 0.2 ml of the suspension to an Eppendorf tube containing 0.3 ml glycerol-PBS stock solution; distribute this suspension equally among two cryogenic vials, 0.25 ml per tube, and store these tubes within 20 min in liquid nitrogen.

4. Use the remainder of the blood (0.4–0.8 ml) to genotype the transfected parasite population by Southern analysis of separated chromosomes (*see* **Note 7**, Fig. 2) or digested genomic DNA or by diagnostic PCR as described in ref. [14].
5. If the genotyping shows correct deletion of the h*dhfr::yfcu* SM cassette clone the parasites by the method of limiting dilution. Infect a mouse with transfected parasites from the liquid nitrogen storage and collect blood at a parasitemia of 0.2–1 % for limiting dilution of parasites and injecting 10 mice with 0.3 parasites per mouse using insulin syringes under anesthesia as described in ref. [20].
6. Collect cloned parasite lines at day 8/9 after cloning. The parasitemia usually increases to 0.5–2 % at day 8. Collect 0.6–1 ml of blood from the mouse with a parasitemia of 1–3 %. Use 0.2 ml of infected blood for storage in liquid nitrogen (these parasites are used for "transfected step 2" (see below)): transfer 0.2 ml of the suspension to an Eppendorf tube containing 0.3 ml glycerol-PBS stock solution; distribute this suspension equally among two cryogenic vials, 0.25 ml per tube, and store these tubes within 20 min in liquid nitrogen.
7. Use the remainder of the blood (0.4–0.8 ml) to genotype the cloned parasite population by Southern analysis of separated chromosomes (*see* **Note 7**, Fig. 2) or digested genomic DNA or by diagnostic PCR as described [14].
8. The cloned DsR parasites with a correct genotype are used for phenotype analysis to (1) determine (normal) development throughout the life cycle and (2) to confirm correct HMP expression (*see* Subheading 3.4).

3.3 Transgenic Parasites Expressing HMP Proteins: Double-Step Insertion (DsI) Mutants

When a gene is essential for blood stages it is not possible to use the DsR approach as described in Subheading 3.2, since the initial gene deletion step will yield no deletion mutants. In DsI mutants the HMP CDS is therefore first introduced into the neutral locus of an existing GIMO mother line (Subheading 2.1) as was described for AG mutants using a construct (*Construct 1*) copy of HMP but under the control elements of the *Pb* ortholog in a neutral locus, free of SM (*see* Fig. 4, **Note 10**). Subsequently, the *Pb* ortholog is targeted for deletion through replacement of the *Pb* gene with the h*dhfr::yfcu* SM, resulting in transgenic parasites with a new GIMO locus permissive for rapid additional gene-insertion modifications (*see* Fig. 4, **Note 10**).

3.3.1 Transfection of Parasites and Injection into Mice: Transfection Step 1

1. Prepare 5–10 μg of linear DNA construct in 5–10 μL water or TE buffer. This construct (*Construct 1*) is based on a standard GIMO construct and contains an HMP flanked by the 5′ UTR and 3′ UTR regulatory sequences of the orthologous *Pb* gene (*see* Fig. 4, **Note 10**).

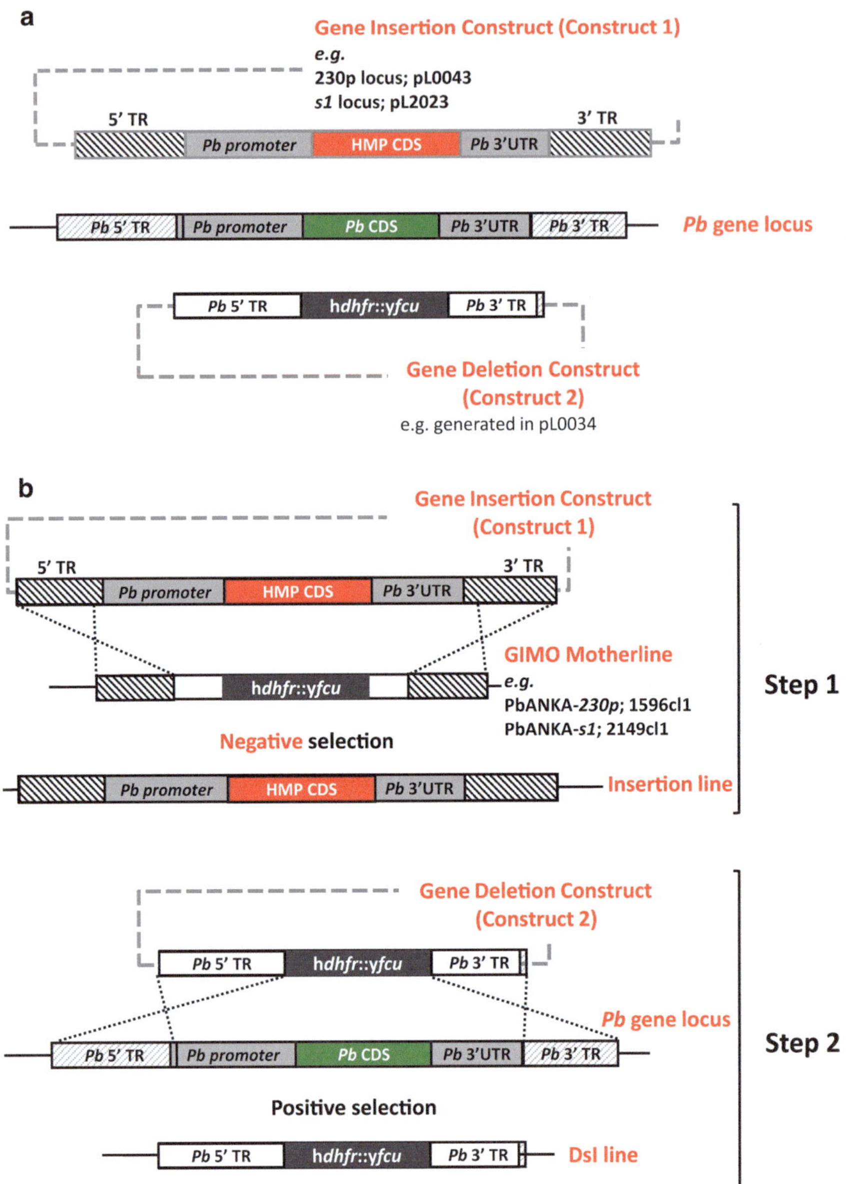

Fig. 4 Generation of DsI mutants. (**a**) Generation of the two constructs for generation of DsI mutants. Schematic representation describing the generation of *Construct 1* (*Gene Insertion construct*). Two basic constructs can be used to rapidly introduce transgenes by GIMO transfection into neutral *Pb loci*; specifically pL0043 to introduce transgenes into the *230p* locus (for transfection into the PbANKA-230p GIMO mother line; 1596cl1) and pL2023 for the *s1* locus (for transfection into the PbANKA-s1 GIMO mother line; 2149cl1). *See* Fig. 1 for details on the generation of constructs using these plasmids and the 5′ and 3′ Targeting regions (5′ and 3′ TR). The HMP CDS is flanked upstream by the gene promoter region and transcription terminator sequence of the *Pb* ortholog, both of which can be PCR-amplified from *Pb* gDNA. *Construct 1* is linearized using appropriate restriction enzymes outside of these 5′ and 3′ TRs before transfection. *Construct 2 (Deletion construct)*. This construct can be generated by cloning 5′ and 3′ TRs of the *Pb* gene into the cloning sites of basic construct pL0034, upstream and downstream of the SM, respectively. Both TRs can be PCR-amplified from *Pb* gDNA.

2. Collect cultured (in vitro matured) *P. berghei* schizonts of a standard GIMO line (Subheading 2.1) for transfection as described in ref. [14].
3. Transfect the schizonts with the DNA construct using an Nucleofector device using the transfection protocol and conditions as described in ref. [14].
4. Inject the transfected parasites into a tail vein of a mouse using insulin syringes under anesthesia.

3.3.2 Negative Selection of Parasites (5-FC) and Cloning: Transfection Step 1

1. Select transfected parasites by negative selection with 5-FC: provide the mouse with drinking water containing 5-FC one day after infection with transfected parasites. Provide the water for a period of 8–11 days up to the collection of infected blood.
2. Collect transfected and selected parasites between day 8 and 11 after infecting mice with transfected parasites. In successful transfection experiments, the parasitemia usually increases to 2–5 % between days 8 and 11. Collect 0.6–1 ml of blood from the mouse with a parasitemia of 2–5 % by heart puncture under anesthesia.
3. Use 0.2 ml of infected blood for storage in liquid nitrogen (these parasites are used for cloning transfected parasites): transfer 0.2 ml of the suspension to an Eppendorf tube containing 0.3 ml glycerol-PBS stock solution; distribute this suspension equally among two cryogenic vials, 0.25 ml per tube, and store these tubes within 20 min in liquid nitrogen.
4. Use the remainder of the blood (0.4–0.8 ml) to genotype the transfected parasite population by Southern analysis of separated chromosomes (*see* **Note 7c**, Fig. 2) or digested genomic DNA or by diagnostic PCR as described [14].

Fig. 4 (continued) *Note: It is important to choose at least one (ideally both) Pb TR (here shown as hatched boxes) that are different from the promoter/terminator regions used in Construct 1 to avoid targeting the HMP gene when it has been introduced into the neutral locus.* The generated construct is linearized using appropriate restriction enzymes outside of the 5′ and 3′ TRs. *See* **Note 10** for details. (**b**) *Generation of DsI mutants,* the HMP is introduced into a neutral locus and the *Pb* ortholog is subsequently deleted; *1st step*: the HMP expression cassette is introduced into a neutral locus (the *230p* or *s1* locus) in a standard GIMO mother line as described for AG mutants but under the control elements of *Pb* orthologous gene using the *Construct 1 (Gene Insertion construct).* The construct targets the *230p* or *s1* target regions by double crossover homologous recombination, under negative (5-FC) selection, resulting in replacement of the h*dhfr*/y*fcu* selectable marker cassette present in the GIMO Mother line. After genotyping and confirming the correct construct integration this line is cloned. *2nd step*: The essential *Pb* ortholog gene CDS is targeted for deletion through replacement of the *Pb* CDS with the h*dhfr*::y*fcu* SM using *Construct 2* (*Deletion construct*), by homologous double crossover recombination performed under positive selection with pyrimethamine resulting in the generation of the *DsI mutant*

5. If the genotyping shows correct deletion of the h*dhfr::yfcu* SM cassette clone the parasites by the method of limiting dilution. Infect a mouse with transfected parasites from the liquid nitrogen storage and collect blood at a parasitemia of 0.2–1 % for limiting dilution of parasites and injecting 10 mice with 0.3 parasites per mouse using insulin syringes under anesthesia as described in ref. [20]. Genotyping and cloning of the transfected parasites is an essential step before proceeding with transfection step 2 (*see* **Note 9**).
6. Collect cloned parasite lines at day 8/9 after cloning. The parasitemia usually increases to 0.5–2 % at day 8. Collect 0.6–1 ml of blood from the mouse with a parasitemia of 1–3 % by heart puncture under anesthesia. Use 0.2 ml of infected blood for storage in liquid nitrogen (these parasites are used for "transfected step 2" (see below)): transfer 0.2 ml of the suspension to an Eppendorf tube containing 0.3 ml glycerol-PBS stock solution; distribute this suspension equally among two cryogenic vials, 0.25 ml per tube, and store these tubes within 20 min in liquid nitrogen.
7. Use the remainder of the blood (0.4–0.8 ml) to genotype the cloned parasite population by Southern analysis of separated chromosomes or digested genomic DNA (*see* **Note 7c**, Fig. 2) or by diagnostic PCR as described in ref. [14].

3.3.3 Transfection of Parasites and Injection into Mice: Transfection Step 2

1. Prepare 5–10 μg of linear DNA construct in 5–10 μL water or TE buffer. This construct (*Construct 2*) contains h*dhfr::yfcu* SM cassette flanked by 5′ and 3′ UTR regions outside of the *Pb* gene regulatory sequences (*see* Fig. 4, **Note 10**).
2. Collect cultured (in vitro matured) schizonts of cloned transgenic HMP-expressing parasites (as generated in transfection step 1) for transfection as described in ref. [14].
3. Transfect the schizonts with *Construct 2* using an Nucleofector device using the transfection protocol and conditions as described in ref. [14].
4. Inject the transfected parasites into a tail vein of a mouse using insulin syringes under anesthesia.

3.3.4 Positive Selection of Parasites (Pyrimethamine) and Cloning: Transfection Step 2

1. Select transfected parasites by positive selection with pyrimethamine: provide the mouse with drinking water containing pyrimethamine 1 day after infection with transfected parasites. Provide the water for a period of 8–11 days up to the collection of infected blood.
2. Collect transfected and selected parasites between day 8 and 11 after infecting mice with transfected parasites. In successful transfection experiments, the parasitemia usually increases to 2–5 % between days 8 and 11. Collect 0.6–1 ml of blood from the mouse with a parasitemia of 2–5 % by heart puncture under anesthesia.

3. Use 0.2 ml of infected blood for storage in liquid nitrogen (these parasites are used for cloning transfected parasites): transfer 0.2 ml of the suspension to an Eppendorf tube containing 0.3 ml glycerol-PBS stock solution; distribute this suspension equally among two cryogenic vials, 0.25 ml per tube, and store these tubes within 20 min in liquid nitrogen.
4. Use the remainder of the blood (0.4–0.8 ml) to genotype the transfected parasite population by Southern analysis of separated chromosomes (*see* **Note** 7, Fig. 2) or digested genomic DNA or by diagnostic PCR as described in ref. [14].
5. If genotyping shows correct deletion of the *Pb* CDS clone the parasites by the method of limiting dilution. Infect a mouse with transfected parasites from the liquid nitrogen storage and collect blood at a parasitemia of 0.2–1 % for limiting dilution of parasites and injecting 10 mice with 0.3 parasites per mouse using insulin syringes under anesthesia as described in ref. [20].
6. Collect cloned parasite lines at day 8/9 after cloning. The parasitemia usually increases to 0.5–2 % at day 8. Collect 0.6–1 ml of blood from the mouse with a parasitemia of 1–3 % by heart puncture under anesthesia. Use 0.2 ml of infected blood for storage in liquid nitrogen (these parasites are used for "transfection step 2" (see below)): transfer 0.2 ml of the suspension to an Eppendorf tube containing 0.3 ml glycerol-PBS stock solution; distribute this suspension equally among two cryogenic vials, 0.25 ml per tube, and store these tubes within 20 min in liquid nitrogen.
7. Use the remainder of the blood (0.4–0.8 ml) to genotype the cloned parasite population by Southern analysis of separated chromosomes (*see* **Note** 7, Fig. 2) or digested genomic DNA or by diagnostic PCR as described in ref. [14].
8. The cloned DsI parasites with a correct genotype are used for phenotype analysis to (1) determine (normal) development throughout the life cycle and (2) to confirm correct HMP expression (*see* Subheading 3.4).

3.4 Phenotype Analysis of Transgenic Parasites Expressing HMP Genes

Before using transgenic *Pb* parasites expressing HMP genes in assays for drug- or vaccine evaluation, the phenotype is analyzed to (1) determine whether HMP gene expression affects normal development and (2) to confirm correct timing and level of HMP gene expression. Below we briefly mention several assays that are used for such analyses and refer to published methods.

3.4.1 Transgenic Parasites Expressing HMP Genes in Asexual Blood Stages

1. Determination of blood stage growth. A standard method to analyze growth is determined from the multiplication rate of asexual blood stages in vivo during the cloning procedure of mutants [16] and is calculated as follows: the percentage of infected erythrocytes in Swiss OF1 mice injected with a single parasite is quantified at days 8–11 by examination of

Giemsa-stained blood films. The mean asexual multiplication rate per 24 h is then calculated assuming a total of 1.2×10^{10} erythrocytes per mouse (2 ml of blood). The percentage of infected erythrocytes in mice infected with a single parasite of a *Pb* ANKA reference lines ranges between 0.5 and 2 % at day 8 after infection, resulting in a mean multiplication rate of 10 per 24 h [16].

A second frequently used method to determine asexual growth rate is by examining the course of parasitemia after infecting mice with a standard dose of infected red blood cells (irbc, i.e., 10^3–10^4 irbc). The course of parasitemia can be determined by counting irbc in Giemsa stained blood films of tail blood samples or, when parasites express GFP or Luciferase, by standard FACS [21] or simple bioluminescence assays [22] respectively.

2. Determination of HMP expression. This is performed using standard Northern analysis of transcription, Western and or immunofluorescence analysis of protein expression methods.

3.4.2 Transgenic Parasites Expressing HMP Genes in Transmission Stages (Gametocytes, Zygotes, Oocysts, and Sporozoites)

1. Gametocyte production is usually determined by counting mature gametocytes in tail blood of mice that have either synchronized or non-synchronized blood stage infections [23]. Ookinete production is usually determined in standard in vitro cultures of ookinetes [24] and is usually defined as the percentage of female gametocytes/gametes that develop into mature ookinetes. The ratio of unfertilized female gametocytes/gametes to ookinetes is determined in Giemsa stained slides of samples taken from the ookinete cultures at 16–24 h [25]. Oocysts and sporozoites production is determined in *A. stephensi* mosquitoes that are infected on gametocytemic mice. This is usually performed by microscopic analysis of dissected midguts and salivary glands [26].
2. Determination of HMP expression. This is performed using standard Northern analysis of transcription, Western and or immunofluorescence analysis of protein expression methods.

3.4.3 Transgenic Parasites Expressing HMP Genes in Liver Stages

1. Sporozoite infectivity and liver stage development can be determined in cultures of hepatocytes (e.g., HepG2, Huh7) or in mice infected with sporozoites, either by mosquito bite or by intravenous injection of sporozoites [27]. Sporozoites are obtained by standard methods of dissection of salivary glands of infected mosquitoes [27]. Sporozoite infectivity and liver parasite loads can be quantified by qPCR [28] or, when parasites express Luciferase, by bioluminescence assays (both in vitro and in vivo imaging; [27]) or by measuring the prepatent period (time taken, in days, to achieve a parasitemia in the blood of 0.5–2 % after infection of mice with defined numbers of sporozoites; [29]).

2. Determination of HMP expression. This is performed using standard Northern analysis of transcription, Western and or immunofluorescence analysis of protein expression methods.

4 Notes

1. *Pb*GFP-Luc$_{ama1}$ (1037m1f1m1cl1) and the *Pb*GFP-Luc$_{con}$ (676m1cl) are reporter parasites expressing a fusion protein of GFP (mutant3) and firefly luciferase (LUC-IAV). These lines are suitable reporter lines for use in simple and sensitive in vitro and in vivo screening assays to test inhibitors and chemicals for antimalarial activity against blood stages [22]. These assays are based on the determination of luciferase activity (luminescence) in small blood samples containing transgenic blood-stage parasites that express luciferase under the control of a promoter that is either schizont-specific (*ama-1*) or constitutive (*eef1*α). The reading of luminescence assays is rapid, requires a minimal number of handling steps and no experience with parasite morphology or handling fluorescence-activated cell sorters, produces no radioactive waste and test plates can be stored for prolonged times before processing. In addition, the *Pb*GFP-Luc$_{con}$ (676m1cl) line can be used to determine the number of parasites in the liver (i.e., liver loads) in live animals over time, using in vivo imaging methodologies [27, 30].
2. The standard PyXNL-*230p* GIMO mother line (GIMO$_{Py17X}$, 1923cl1). The line contains a positive–negative selectable marker (SM) cassette, a fusion gene of h*dhfr* (*human dihydrofolate reductase*; positive SM) and y*fcu* (*yeast cytosine deaminase and uridyl phosphoribosyl transferase*; negative SM) under control of the constitutive *eef1a* promoter stably integrated into the neutral *230p* locus (PY17X_0306600) through double crossover recombination [4]. The GIMO mother line is used for introduction of transgenes into the modified *230p* locus through transfection with constructs that target the *230p* locus. These constructs insert into the *230p* locus ("gene insertion"), thereby removing the h*dhfr::yfcu* selectable marker ("marker out") from the genome of the mother lines. Transgenic parasites that are SM free are subsequently selected by applying negative drug selection using 5-FC. This selection procedure is performed in vivo in mice. For details of the PyXNL-*230p* GIMO mother line, see RMgmDB entry #688 (http://www.pberghei.eu/index.php?rmgm=688).
3. To generate pL0043, the *230p* TRs as well as the ampicillin resistance gene were amplified from plasmid pL1063 (MRA-852, www.mr4.org) using primers 5116/5117 (GGGGTACCGAGCTCGAATTCTCTTGAGC;

GGGGTACCGAGCTCGAATTCTCTTGAGC). A multiple cloning site (MCS) was amplified from pCRII-Blunt-TOPO vector (Zero Blunt TOPO PCR Cloning Kit, Invitrogen, Groningen, The Netherlands) using M13 forward and reverse primers. The two PCR products were digested with *Asp*718I and *Not*I restriction enzymes and ligated together creating the targeting construct pL0043.

4. pL1849 was generated using a modified 2-step PCR method (*see* **Note 5**). In the first PCR reaction, 5′- and 3′-TRs (both 1 kb) of *230p* were amplified from *P. yoelii* 17XNL genomic DNA with the primer set 6523/6524 (GAACTCGTACT CCTTGGTGACGGGTACCGTGATGGAATGGCAACA TCTG; *CATCTACAAGCATCGTCGACCTC*GGTTGGAC AATGTAATGCTAC) and 6525/6526 (*CCTTCAATTTC GGATCCACTAG*AAGTAAAAGGGGTAAGACAGC; *CCTTCAATTTCGGATCCACTAG*AAGTAAAA GGGGTAAGACAGC). These primers contain 59-extensions homologues to the h*dhfr::yfcu* selection marker cassette and 59-terminal extensions with an anchor-tag suitable for the second PCR reaction. A 55 nt oligo (oligo 6598; GAGGTCGACGATGCTTGTAGATGCCCGGGCCTT CAATTTCGGATCCACTAG) containing a *Xma*I restriction site flanked by 2 sequences homologues to the h*dhfr::yfcu* selection cassette was used to join the two *230p* TR regions. In the second PCR reaction an fragment containing both *230p* TRs interrupted by the *Xma*I site was amplified, using the external anchor-tag primers 4661/4662 (GAACTCGTACT CCTTGGTGACG; GAACTCGTACTCCTTGGTGACG), resulting in the PCR product of 2 kb. The PCR product was cloned into TOPO TA vector (TOPO TA Cloning Kit, Invitrogen, Groningen, The Netherlands) resulting in construct pL1849.

5. To generate plasmid pL2023, the 5′- and 3′-TRs (each about 0.8 kb) of the *s1* locus were PCR-amplified *Pb* genomic DNA using primer pairs 1003/1004 (5′TR; CATGGGCCC ACCATGCTTTGTCTGAGAGTG and AAGGCCTGGTA CCATACTGTTCTTCCCAATGGATC) flanked by *Apa*I restriction site at the 5′ end and both *StuI/KpnI* restriction sites at its 3′ end of the PCR fragment and the primers 1005/1006 (3′UTR; ATAAGAATGCGGCCGCCTGCAG CATTCAAATGCTTGAAGGCGATG and ACATGGCGCC AAGCTTATGGCACATGGATCGAACAG), flanked by *NotI/PstI* restriction sites at the 5′ end and *Kas*I/*Hind*III restriction sites at its 3′ end of the PCR fragment. The 5′ and 3′ TRs were subsequently cloned into the sites of *Apa*I/*Stu*I and *Not*I/*Kas*I of pL0034, upstream and downstream of the h*dhfr::yfcu* SM cassette, respectively, resulting construct

pL1928, which has been used to generate PbANKA-*s1* GIMO mother line, 2149cl1, using positive selection (Subheading 2.1).

Currently pL1928 is unpublished but is available from the Leiden Malaria Research Group. Plasmid pL1928 has been constructed with a specific restriction site (*Kpn*I) both just before and after the h*dhfr::yfcu* SM cassette, therefore digestion with this enzyme releases the h*dhfr::yfcu* SM cassette from the plasmid resulting in a linear DNA construct containing both 5′ and 3′ TRs of the *s1* locus with complementary ends. Self-ligation was performed to generate a "marker-free" *s1* targeting construct (pL2023) with only the 5′- and 3′-s1 TRs flanking a multiple-cloning site. Therefore, pL2023 is a basic construct that can be used to rapidly clone HMP genes into the neutral *s1 Pb* locus and introduced into a PbANKA-s1 mother line that also expresses a florescent-bioluminescent reporter (i.e., GFP-luciferase; PbANKA-*s1* GIMO mother line, 2149cl1).

6. Constructs to generate AG mutants (Subheading 3.1):
   Two basic constructs (Subheading 2.3) can be used to rapidly introduce transgenes into neutral *Pb* loci by GIMO transfection; specifically pL0043 to introduce transgenes into the *230p* locus (for transfection into the PbANKA-230p GIMO mother line; 1596cl1) and pL2023 for the *s1* locus (for transfection into the PbANKA-s1 GIMO mother line; 2149cl1). These basic constructs contain 5′ and 3′ TRs for these loci as well as a multiple-cloning site. This multi-cloning site is used to introduce the HMP CDS, which can be PCR-amplified from HMP genomic DNA (gDNA) or cDNA. The HMP CDS is flanked upstream by the 5′ UTR (containing the gene promoter region) and downstream by 3′ UTR (containing the transcription terminator sequence) regions of a chosen *Pb* gene, both of which can be PCR-amplified from *Pb* gDNA (Fig. 3a). The selection of the *Pb* promoter region is dependent on the timing and strength of HMP gene expression required, and a variety of standard *Pb* promoter regions have been characterized and are available (*see* Table 1 for details). The regions critical for HMP gene expression (i.e., the promoter and HMP CDS) of the final construct must be sequenced to ensure that the HMP gene will be correctly expressed in the AG mutant. In addition, an expression cassette containing a reporter gene can also be introduced into this construct if required. For example the GFP::luciferase expression cassette can be PCR-amplified from construct pL1063 [15]. In case of using PbANKA-s1 (2149cl1) GIMO mother line there is no need to include the GFP-Luciferase cassette into the *s1* targeting construct, since this line already contains the GFP-Luciferase cassette integrated into the neutral *230p* locus. The final *Construct 1* is linearized using appropriate restriction enzymes outside of the 5′ and 3′ TRs.

7. Genotyping of AG, DsR, and DsI mutants (*see* Fig. 2)

   (a) AG mutants: We usually perform Southern analysis of chromosomes separated by pulsed-field gel electrophoresis (PFGE) to confirm integration of the DNA construct in the GIMO locus by showing the absence of the h*dhfr::yfcu* SM cassette both in uncloned (parent) and cloned parasites. Separated chromosomes are hybridized with a mixture of two probes: one recognizing h*dhfr* (recognizing the SM in chr 3 and chr 12 for the *230p* and *s1* mother lines respectively) and a control probe (we frequently use *pb25* gene probe that recognizes *Pb* chromosome 5). As an additional control (ctrl), parasite line is used with the h*dhfr::yfcu* SM integrated into a known Pb chromosome (we frequently use line 2117cl1 that has the SM in chr 3).

   (b) DsR mutants: We usually perform Southern analysis of PFGE-separated chromosomes to confirm integration of the DNA construct in the target *Pb* gene both in uncloned (parent 1) and cloned parasites selected with positive selection in step 1. The chromosomes are hybridized using a probe recognizing the *Pbdhfr/ts* 3′UTR of the SM of the integrated construct which also hybridizes to the endogenous *Pbdhfr/ts* gene on chromosome 7. The ratio between the hybridization signal of the target chromosome and of chromosome 7 is informative for both the success of vector integration, the contamination with wild-type parasites and the possible presence of plasmids that usually migrate at the height of chromosome 9–11. For genotyping of selected parasites in step 2 (uncloned/parent 2 and cloned) we usually perform Southern analysis of PFGE-separated chromosomes to confirm integration of the orthologous HMP gene in the GIMO locus by showing the absence of the h*dhfr::yfcu* SM cassette. Separated chromosomes are hybridized with a mixture of two probes: one recognizing h*dhfr* and a control probe (for example recognizing chr 5; *pb25*) as described under (a) for the AG mutants.

   (c) DsI mutants: We usually perform Southern analysis of PFGE-separated chromosomes to confirm integration of the DNA construct in the GIMO locus by showing the absence of the h*dhfr::yfcu* SM cassette both in uncloned (parent 1) and cloned parasites in step 1. Separated chromosomes are hybridized with a mixture of two probes: one recognizing h*dhfr* and a control (*pb25*) probe recognizing chromosome 5 as described under (**a**) for the AG mutants. For genotyping of selected parasites in step 2 (uncloned/parent 2 and cloned) we usually perform

Southern analysis of PFGE-separated chromosomes to confirm integration of the DNA construct in the target *Pb* gene both in uncloned (parent 1) and cloned parasites selected with positive selection in step 1. The chromosomes are hybridized using a probe recognizing the 3′UTR *Pbdhfr/ts* of the SM of the integrated construct which also hybridizes to the endogenous *Pbdhfr/ts* on chromosome 7 as described under (**b**) for step 1.

8. Generation of the two constructs for generation of DsR mutants (Subheading 3.2).

   Construct 1 (GIMO Deletion construct): This construct can be generated by cloning 5′ and 3′ TRs of the *Pb* gene (these regions need to include the complete *Pb* gene promoter and transcriptional terminator sequences) into the cloning sites of the basic construct pL0034 (Subheading 3.2), upstream and downstream of the h*dhfr::yfcu* SM, respectively. Both TRs can be PCR-amplified from *Pb* gDNA. The targeting regions need to be chosen outside of the *Pb* CDS sequence and preferably > 0.6 kb in size (Fig. 2). The generated construct is linearized using appropriate restriction enzymes outside of the 5′ and 3′ TRs. The first transfection with *Construct 1* is aiming to replace the *Pb* CDS with the h*dhfr::yfcu* SM cassette. *Construct 1* can be transfected into a standard reporter parasite line *Pb*GFP-Luc$_{con}$ (676m1cl1; Subheading 2.1, **item 1**) to generate a *Pb* gene deletion GIMO mother line that also encodes the GFP-Luciferase expression cassette.

   Construct 2 (GIMO Insertion construct): This construct is generated based on *Construct 1*, replacing the h*dhfr::yfcu* SM cassette in *Construct 1* with HMP gene CDS sequence, which can be PCR-amplified from HMP gDNA or cDNA, resulting a HMP gene expression construct under the control of the 5′ and 3′ regulatory elements of the *Pb* ortholog. *Construct 1* can be constructed with specific restriction sites just before and after the h*dhfr::yfcu* SM cassette; therefore digestion with these enzymes will release the h*dhfr::yfcu* SM cassette from the plasmid resulting in a linear DNA construct containing only both 5′ and 3′ TRs of the target *Pb gene*. This linear construct can be used as a vector to clone/insert the orthologous HMP into it to generate *Construct 2* which contains the HMP CDS flanked upstream by the orthologous *Pb* 5′ UTR (containing the gene promoter region) and downstream by Pb 3′ UTR (containing the transcription terminator sequence) (Fig. 2).

   The generated *Construct 2* is linearized using appropriate restriction enzymes outside of the 5′ and 3′ TRs. A second transfection is performed in the gene-deletion GIMO mother line with *Construct 2* resulting in a replacement of the h*dhfr::yfcu* SM cassette with the orthologous HMP gene.

This method creates parasites that express an HMP gene under the control of the *Pb* ortholog regulatory sequences, these mutants are also SM free, facilitating easier additional genetic modifications.

9. Both for the generation of the DsR and DsI mutants, genotyping and cloning of the transfected parasites in step 1 is an essential step before proceeding with transfection step 2. In our experience, the use of parasites from uncloned populations (selected in step 1) for transfection in step 2 increases the chance to select for incorrect mutants in step 2.

10. Generation of the two constructs for generation of DsI mutants (Subheading 3.3).

    Construct 1 (Gene Insertion construct): Two basic constructs can be used to rapidly introduce transgenes by GIMO transfection into neutral *Pb* loci (Subheading 2.3); specifically pL0043 to introduce transgenes into the *230p* locus (for transfection into the PbANKA-230p GIMO mother line; 1596cl1) and pL2023 for the *s1* locus (for transfection into the PbANKA-s1 GIMO mother line; 2149cl1). These basic constructs contain 5′ and 3′ TRs for these loci as well as a multiple-cloning site. This multi-cloning site is used to introduce the HMP CDS, which can be PCR-amplified from HMP genomic DNA or cDNA. The HMP CDS is flanked upstream by the 5′ UTR (containing the full gene promoter region) and downstream by 3′ UTR (containing the transcription terminator sequence) regions of the *Pb* ortholog, both of which can be PCR-amplified from *Pb* gDNA (Fig. 3a). The regions critical for HMP gene expression (i.e., the promoter and HMP CDS) of the final construct must be sequenced to ensure that the HMP gene will be correctly expressed in the DsI mutant. For stage-specific expression or overexpression, other control elements of *Pb* genes could also be used (*see* Table 1). In addition, an expression cassette containing a reporter gene can also be introduced into this construct if required. For example GFP::luciferase expression cassette, which can be PCR-amplified from construct pL1063 [15]. However, when using construct pL2023 there is no need to include the GFP-Luciferase cassette into this construct, since PbANKA-s1 (2149cl1) GIMO mother line already contains the GFP-Luciferase cassette integrated into the neutral *230p* locus. The final *Construct 1* is linearized using appropriate restriction enzymes outside of the 5′ and 3′ TRs.

    Construct 2 (Deletion construct): This construct can be generated by cloning 5′ and 3′ TRs of the *Pb* gene into the cloning sites of basic construct pL0034 (Subheading 3.2), upstream and downstream of the h*dhfr::yfcu* SM, respectively. Both TRs can be PCR-amplified from *Pb* gDNA. It is important to choose at least one (ideally both) *Pb* TR that is different from the promoter/terminator regions used for HMP gene expression, to avoid removing the HMP gene introduced into the neutral locus. For small or medium sized genes (<3 kb), the targeting regions could be chosen outside of the *Pb* gene (*see* Fig. 3). For genes >3 kb in size, or where the regions between the neighboring genes are small (i.e., <1 kb), the 5′ and/or 3′ TR could also be designed within the *Pb* CDS. The generated construct is linearized using appropriate restriction enzymes outside of the 5′ and 3′ TRs.

Acknowledgements

Ahmed M. Salman was supported by EVIMalaR's (FP7) PhD Programme, Catherin Marin Mogollon by Colciencias Ph.D. fellowship (Call 568 from 2012 Resolution 01218 Bogotá, Colombia), and Jing-wen Lin by a MRC (UK) career development fellowship.

References

1. Carlton JM et al (2002) Genome sequence and comparative analysis of the model rodent malaria parasite Plasmodium yoelii yoelii. Nature 419(6906):512–519
2. Kooij TW, Janse CJ, Waters AP (2006) Plasmodium post-genomics: better the bug you know? Nat Rev Microbiol 4(5):344–357
3. Cockburn IA et al (2013) In vivo imaging of CD8+ T cell-mediated elimination of malaria liver stages. Proc Natl Acad Sci U S A 110(22):9090–9095
4. Lin JW et al (2011) A novel 'gene insertion/marker out' (GIMO) method for transgene expression and gene complementation in rodent malaria parasites. PLoS One 6(12), e29289
5. Bauza K et al (2014) Efficacy of a Plasmodium vivax malaria vaccine using ChAd63 and modified vaccinia Ankara expressing thrombospondin-related anonymous protein as assessed with transgenic Plasmodium berghei parasites. Infect Immun 82(3):1277–1286
6. Espinosa DA et al (2013) Development of a chimeric Plasmodium berghei strain expressing the repeat region of the P. vivax circumsporozoite protein for in vivo evaluation of vaccine efficacy. Infect Immun 81(8):2882–2887
7. Persson C et al (2002) Cutting edge: a new tool to evaluate human pre-erythrocytic malaria vaccines: rodent parasites bearing a hybrid Plasmodium falciparum circumsporozoite protein. J Immunol 169(12):6681–6685
8. Goodman AL et al (2011) A viral vectored prime-boost immunization regime targeting the malaria Pfs25 antigen induces transmission-blocking activity. PLoS One 6(12), e29428
9. Ramjanee S et al (2007) The use of transgenic Plasmodium berghei expressing the Plasmodium vivax antigen P25 to determine the transmission-blocking activity of sera from malaria vaccine trials. Vaccine 25(5):886–894
10. Cao Y, Zhang D, Pan W (2009) Construction of transgenic Plasmodium berghei as a model for evaluation of blood-stage vaccine candidate of Plasmodium falciparum chimeric protein 2.9. PLoS One 4(9), e6894
11. de Koning-Ward TF et al (2003) A new rodent model to assess blood stage immunity to the Plasmodium falciparum antigen merozoite surface protein 119 reveals a protective role for invasion inhibitory antibodies. J Exp Med 198(6):869–875
12. Tewari R, Patzewitz EM, Poulin B, Stewart L, Baker DA (2014) Development of a transgenic

Plasmodium berghei line (Pbpfpkg) expressing the P. falciparum cGMP-dependent protein kinase, a novel antimalarial drug target. PLoS One 9(5), e96923

13. Blume M et al (2011) A constitutive pan-hexose permease for the Plasmodium life cycle and transgenic models for screening of antimalarial sugar analogs. FASEB J 25(4): 1218–1229
14. Janse CJ, Ramesar J, Waters AP (2006) High-efficiency transfection and drug selection of genetically transformed blood stages of the rodent malaria parasite Plasmodium berghei. Nat Protoc 1(1):346–356
15. Janse CJ et al (2006) High efficiency transfection of Plasmodium berghei facilitates novel selection procedures. Mol Biochem Parasitol 145(1):60–70
16. Spaccapelo R et al (2010) Plasmepsin 4-deficient Plasmodium berghei are virulence attenuated and induce protective immunity against experimental malaria. Am J Pathol 176(1):205–217
17. Jacobs-Lorena VY, Mikolajczak SA, Labaied M, Vaughan AM, Kappe SH (2010) A dispensable Plasmodium locus for stable transgene expression. Mol Biochem Parasitol 171(1):40–44
18. Sinden R (1997) Infection of mosquitoes with rodent malaria. In: Crampton J, Beard CB, Louis C (eds) The molecular biology of insect disease vectors. Springer, Netherlands, pp 67–91
19. Orr RY, Philip N, Waters AP (2012) Improved negative selection protocol for Plasmodium berghei in the rodent malarial model. Malar J 11:103
20. Menard R, Janse C (1997) Gene targeting in malaria parasites. Methods 13(2):148–157
21. Janse CJ, Franke-Fayard B, Waters AP (2006) Selection by flow-sorting of genetically transformed, GFP-expressing blood stages of the rodent malaria parasite, Plasmodium berghei. Nat Protoc 1(2):614–623
22. Lin JW et al (2013) Screening inhibitors of P. berghei blood stages using bioluminescent reporter parasites. Methods Mol Biol 923: 507–522
23. Janse CJ, Waters AP (1995) Plasmodium berghei: the application of cultivation and purification techniques to molecular studies of malaria parasites. Parasitol Today 11(4): 138–143
24. Janse CJ et al (1985) In vitro formation of ookinetes and functional maturity of Plasmodium berghei gametocytes. Parasitology 91(Pt 1):19–29
25. van Dijk MR et al (2001) A central role for P48/45 in malaria parasite male gamete fertility. Cell 104(1):153–164
26. Ramakrishnan C et al (2013) Laboratory maintenance of rodent malaria parasites. Methods Mol Biol 923:51–72
27. Annoura T, Chevalley S, Janse CJ, Franke-Fayard B, Khan SM (2013) Quantitative analysis of Plasmodium berghei liver stages by bioluminescence imaging. Methods Mol Biol 923:429–443
28. Bruna-Romero O et al (2001) Detection of malaria liver-stages in mice infected through the bite of a single Anopheles mosquito using a highly sensitive real-time PCR. Int J Parasitol 31(13):1499–1502
29. Annoura T et al (2012) Assessing the adequacy of attenuation of genetically modified malaria parasite vaccine candidates. Vaccine 30(16): 2662–2670
30. Ploemen IH et al (2009) Visualisation and quantitative analysis of the rodent malaria liver stage by real time imaging. PLoS One 4(11), e7881
31. Kooij TW, Rauch MM, Matuschewski K (2012) Expansion of experimental genetics approaches for Plasmodium berghei with versatile transfection vectors. Mol Biochem Parasitol 185(1):19–26

Part V

Vaccination

Chapter 22

Vaccination Using Gene-Gun Technology

Elke S. Bergmann-Leitner and Wolfgang W. Leitner

Abstract

DNA vaccines against infection with *Plasmodium* have been highly successful in rodent models of malaria and have shown promise in the very limited number of clinical trials conducted so far. The vaccine platform is highly attractive for numerous reasons, such as low cost and a very favorable safety profile. Gene gun delivery of DNA plasmids drastically reduces the vaccine dose and does not only have the potential to make vaccines more accessible and affordable, but also simplifies (a) the testing of novel antigens as vaccine candidates, (b) the testing of antigen combinations, and (c) the co-delivery of antigens with molecular adjuvants such as cytokines or costimulatory molecules. Described in this chapter are the preparation of the inoculum (i.e., DNA plasmids attached to gold particles, coating to the inside of plastic tubing also referred to as gene gun "bullets" or cartridges), the gene gun vaccination procedure, and the challenge of mice with *Plasmodium berghei* parasites to test the efficacy of the experimental vaccine.

Key words DNA vaccines, Immunization, Gene gun, Particle-mediated epidermal delivery, Biolistic vaccine

1 Introduction

The use of plasmid DNA as a vaccine for vertebrates was first described in the late 1980s (reviewed in ref. 1). The technology rapidly gained popularity due to: (1) the low cost and simplicity of producing the vaccine, (2) the ease of its use, and (3) the induction of humoral as well as cellular immunity in a variety of animal models as well as the protective efficacy of the vaccine in numerous disease models. While the efficacy and immunogenicity of the vaccines initially appeared to be confined to small mammals, due to the presence of a perceived "primate barrier", several modifications to the plasmids used for vaccination as well as improvements in the delivery methods (such as in vivo electroporation following intramuscular injection [2]) have made DNA vaccines a useful platform for human vaccination [3]. Although in some clinical trials DNA vaccination by itself (e.g., against influenza [4] or HIV [5]) has shown to induce satisfactory immune responses, most clinical trials of DNA vaccines involve heterologous prime-boost regimens with

Ashley M. Vaughan (ed.), *Malaria Vaccines: Methods and Protocols*, Methods in Molecular Biology, vol. 1325, DOI 10.1007/978-1-4939-2815-6_22, © Springer Science+Business Media New York 2015

DNA plasmids being used to prime the immune response and a recombinant vector being used for the final boost, for example for HIV [6] or cancer [7].

DNA vaccination as a strategy to prevent malaria infection was first explored in the *P. berghei* [8] and in the *P. yoelii* [9] models of rodent malaria. In both models, as well as additionally studied malaria models, even the first generation of DNA plasmids yielded impressive efficacy, which has since been improved further. Malaria DNA vaccines were subsequently explored in nonhuman primates, delivering the plasmids by injection and in vivo electroporation [10, 11] as well as by gene gun immunization [12]. The protective efficacy of DNA plasmids encoding malaria antigens has only been tested in a very small number of clinical trials so far, with one showing immunogenicity but no protection against parasite challenge when immunizing with DNA vectors encoding several pre-erythrocytic antigens [13]. On the other hand, boosting a DNA vaccine-induced response against pre-erythrocytic antigens with an adenovirus vector encoding the same antigens, did induce protective immunity, albeit at lower levels than the current lead malaria vaccine, RTS,S [14]. Unfortunately, no efficacy studies of human malaria DNA vaccines delivered by gene gun are available to date, although the benefits of this approach are undeniable [15].

While DNA vaccine trials in malaria models, as well as clinical trials, have established the potential usefulness of this platform for the prevention of malaria infection, they have also exposed a lack of understanding of various details and parameters. These include: (1) Any successful malaria vaccine will likely require multiple immunizations; however, although the effect that the vaccination regimen and interval between immunizations has on the immunogenicity and efficacy of vaccines [16] and specifically DNA vaccines against malaria [8], has been recognized, these parameters have not been optimized yet; (2) numerous plasmid vectors are available for DNA vaccination, but which plasmids are most suitable for a malaria DNA vaccine remains to be determined; (3) the efficacy of DNA vaccines can be enhanced with conventional or DNA-encoded "molecular" adjuvants, such as cytokines. Unexpectedly, however, the co-delivery of granulocyte macrophage colony-stimulating factor (GM-CSF) with a malaria DNA vaccine did not yield protective immunity in humans thus highlighting the need to explore additional antigen-adjuvant combinations; (4) while a variety of parasite derived antigens, representing each developmental stage, have been explored as DNA-encoded vaccine-candidates, the large genome of the protozoan parasite still harbors many antigens, which have not yet been tested. These and many other parameters can easily be studied using gene gun delivery of DNA plasmids. Gene gun-based immunization has already been used for vaccinating nonhuman primates and humans with malaria DNA vaccines, and in a rigorous side-by-side comparison with injected plasmid in a preclinical model of *P. berghei*, gene gun-based vaccination was superior. The gene gun delivers a fraction of the inoculum required when using other vaccination methods. Vaccine delivery is noninvasive and well tolerated, and would thus be an attractive approach for large-scale immunization campaigns in developing countries [17]. A major advantage of the approach is the ability to co-deliver multiple molecules encoded on different plasmids to the same host cell, thus ensuring co-expression without the need for bi/multi-cistronic vectors. This facilitates the testing of immunomodulatory molecules ("mix-and-match") and allows the adjustment of differential expression levels by simply changing the ratio of plasmids used. This turned out to be crucial when using plasmid-encoded helper antigens or the co-delivery of pro-apoptotic molecules [18].

2 Materials

The methods described here for preparing the vaccine and gene gun-based vaccination are not specific for malaria DNA vaccines. Gene-gun technology (aka "biolistic plasmid delivery") has been used for the delivery of plasmids encoding various types of antigens such as influenza [19] or tumor antigens [18, 20]. Thus, the following protocols are appropriate for any preclinical gene gun-based immunization approach. Note that several types of gene guns are available for non-clinical use. The described protocol has been shown to work well for the Helios® gun system (Bio-Rad) and may have to be tweaked for other devices. Prepare all solutions with ultrapure water (prepared by purifying deionized water, 18 MW-cm resistivity at 25 °C). The use of high-quality (e.g., molecular-grade) reagents is crucial since contaminants can act as adjuvants and thus introduce variability as well as unacceptable artifacts by altering the immunogenicity of the vaccine. The main contaminant in inadequately purified plasmid preparations is endotoxin (lipopolysaccharide, LPS), a potent innate immune stimulator even at very small concentrations. LPS contamination is particularly a concern when delivering larger amounts of DNA through injection. The effect of LPS, when only minute amounts of DNA (and LPS) are delivered by gene gun, has not been sufficiently studied yet. Nevertheless, it represents an undesirable variable, which can easily be avoided by routinely removing all LPS from plasmids used for vaccination.

2.1 Materials for Preparing Gene Gun "Cartridges"

1. Gold particles: Micron-sized gold particles can be obtained from Bio-Rad or directly from the manufacturer (DeGussa Corporation Metal Group, Ferro Electronic Material Systems). Particles have an average diameter of approximately 1.4–1.6 μm (*see* **Note 1**).
2. Microcentrifuge tubes: 1.5 ml.

3. Microcentrifuge.
4. Spermidine: (1,8-Diamino-4-azaoctane, *N*-(3-Aminopropyl) 1,4-diaminobutane). Prepare stock solutions (0.05 M) with tissue-culture grade deionized water (*see* **Note 2**).
5. Calcium chloride ($CaCl_2$): Prepare 1 M stock solution of $CaCl_2$ with deionized water (*see* **Note 3**).
6. Anhydrous (200 proof) ethanol (*see* **Note 4**).
7. ETFE (Tefzel®) tubing: pretreated Ethylene tetrafluoroethylene tubing (Bio-Rad) (*see* **Note 5**).
8. Compressed nitrogen (*see* **Note 6**).
9. Plasmids: highly purified plasmids suitable for immunizations (*see* **Note 7**).
10. Compressed helium: Purity grade >4.5 (i.e., 99.995 %) with a maximum pressure of 2,600 psi.
11. Parafilm.
12. Airtight containers (such as 20 ml Wheaton scintillation vials).
13. 3 ml syringes and short (~0.5 in.) piece of silicone tubing that can be attached to the Tefzel® tubing as an adaptor (to load tubing and to remove ethanol from tubing).
14. Desiccant pack (desiccation pellets); to be added to the storage container for the cartridges.
15. Desiccant (e.g., silica gel) with color indicator (showing saturation of desiccant), and Desiccator.
16. Razor blades, one sided for cutting tubing to size.
17. Sonicating water bath.
18. Electric clipper (e.g., Oster) with clipper blade size 40.
19. Tris–EDTA (optional, for diluting plasmid preparations). When using commercially obtained Tris–EDTA, make sure it is explicitly endotoxin-free.
20. Tubing preparation station ("Bullet maker"; Bio-Rad), set up on an even, stable surface.
21. Siliconized microfuge tubes (e.g., from Costar Inc.): 0.5 and 1.5 ml.

2.2 Materials for Preparing Sporozoites for Malaria Challenge (Vaccine Testing)

1. Mosquito dissection medium: RPMI-1640 with 5 % mouse serum (*see* **Note 8**).
2. Glass wool.
3. Small glass plate or petri dish for dissection.
4. 20-gauge hypodermic needle.
5. 27-gauge needles (for injection).
6. 1 ml syringes with 0.1 ml increments.

7. Hemocytometer.
8. Phase-contrast microscope (minimum 200× magnification).
9. Microscopic (glass) slides.
10. Microscopic slide carrier and glass trough for slide staining.
11. Giemsa staining solution (stock solution from Sigma or equivalent).
12. Methanol.
13. Scalpel.
14. Surgical scissors.
15. Bunsen burner or cigarette lighter.

3 Methods

The overall workflow is summarized in Fig. 1.

3.1 Preparing the Gold Slurry

1. Weigh 30 mg gold particles into a microcentrifuge tube, and add 100 μl of 0.05 M spermidine (*see* **Note 1**).
2. Vortex *vigorously*, then briefly (~20–30 s) incubate in a sonicating water bath to break up any remaining clumps.
3. Add 60 μg of plasmid DNA to tube (*see* **Note 7**), and vortex briefly. DNA concentration should be ~1 mg/ml or higher. If the plasmid concentration is much lower than 1 mg/ml, precipitate the plasmid and resuspend in a smaller volume of Tris–EDTA buffer. Avoid adding more than 100 μl of plasmid per batch of gold slurry. When co-delivering multiple plasmids, keep the total plasmid loading rate below approximately 5 μg DNA/mg gold to avoid aggregation of gold particles, which interferes with the coating of the Teflon tubing (*see* **Note 9**).
4. While vortexing (low speed to avoid spilling), add 200 μl $CaCl_2$ to the tube to precipitate the DNA onto the gold particles. Add the $CaCl_2$ dropwise to avoid high local concentrations of $CaCl_2$ in the tube, but add the entire volume of $CaCl_2$ within a few seconds.
5. Wait until the gold particles have settled (~30 s) and spin the tube for 20 s at maximum speed in a microcentrifuge.
6. *Carefully* remove (by pipetting, not decanting) the supernatant without disturbing the pellet.
7. Close tube, break up the gold pellet (e.g., by running the tube over a rough surface such as a tube rack) and add 0.5 ml ethanol (*see* **Note 10**).
8. Spin tube for 30 s and repeat washing procedure two more times.

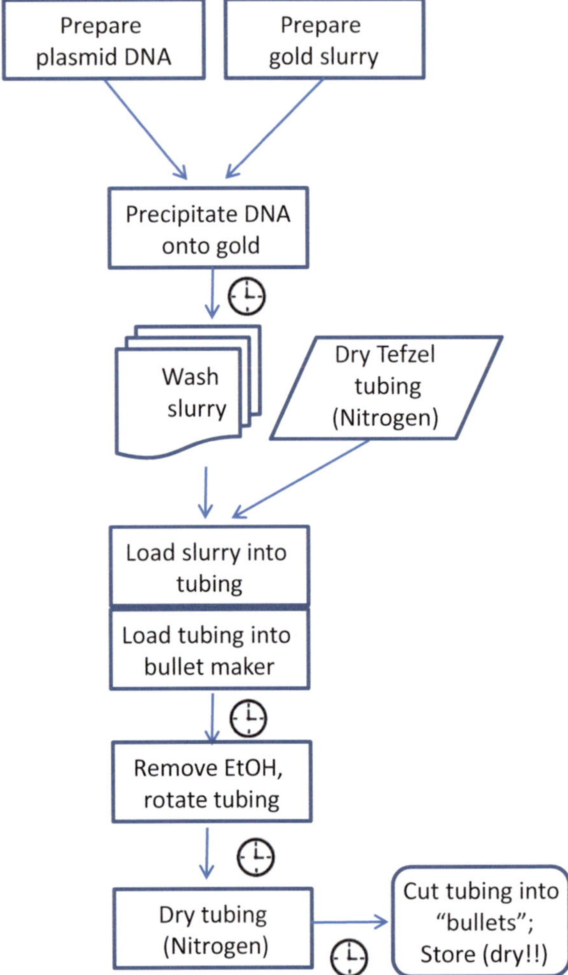

Fig. 1 Flowchart of the major steps involved in preparing the cartridges for immunization by gene gun. The *clock symbol* indicates incubation periods

9. Resuspend gold in a total of 3 ml of 200 proof ethanol in a 15 ml polypropylene tube after the third wash. This slurry can be stored at −20 °C for extended periods of time. When using such banked (i.e., frozen) slurry, allow it to warm to room temperature before opening the tube to avoid condensation. Any dilution of the ethanol with water interferes with the process of coating the gold beads in the Tefzel® cartridges. For extended storage, tubes should be capped tightly, and caps should be sealed with Parafilm.

3.2 Preparing the Gene Gun Cartridges

1. Purge the empty Tefzel® tubing with nitrogen gas for at least 15 min (to remove moisture) at a pressure of 1–2 psi and a flow rate 0.4–0.5 L/min before loading the gold slurry into the Tefzel® tubing.

2. Turn off the flow of nitrogen gas.
3. Cut a section of the N_2-purged Tefzel® tube (~30 in./76 cm) and attach to a 3 ml-syringe through a piece of silicone tubing (used as an adaptor).
4. *Quickly* draw the freshly resuspended slurry into the tubing and *immediately* insert into the tubing station. Note that the gold particles settle very quickly, resulting in an uneven distribution of gold in the tubing if not loaded quickly.
5. Allow the gold to settle for several minutes with the syringe still attached to the tubing.
6. Remove the ethanol with the syringe or peristaltic pump at a rate of 0.5–1 in (~1.3–2.5 cm)/s. Make sure to remove the ethanol at a constant speed, since any fluctuations in the speed will disturb the settled gold particles. Then, remove the syringe or peristaltic pump from the tubing.
7. *Immediately* turn the tubing 90° inside the tubing prep station, wait for a few seconds, and then turn again 90° and wait for a few seconds before starting the motor on the tubing station. This manual rotation initiates the breaking up of the thick gold slurry, which may not be accomplished efficiently by the rotation of the tubing station alone.
8. Turn on the tubing station and rotate the tubing for ~15 s without nitrogen; then initiate the flow of nitrogen (~0.4 L/min) and continue to rotate for another 3–4 min to *completely* evaporate the remaining ethanol.
9. Examine the Tefzel® tubing and remove any sections that are not evenly coated with gold.
10. Cut the tubing into 0.5 in. (1.27 cm) sections (also referred to as cartridges) with a razor blade or, optionally, with a tube cutter (Bio-Rad). Frequently change razor blades used for cutting the Tefzel® tubing. Dull blades result in the tubing being squeezed, which damages the gold coating inside the tubing.
11. Store the cartridges in airtight containers (e.g., glass scintillation vials) with a desiccant pack, and seal the cap with Parafilm. Ideally, the vials are stored at 4 °C in a desiccator.

3.3 Immunization

Note: Anesthesia of small animals (rodents) for gene gun immunization is neither necessary nor recommended.

1. Remove abdominal hair with an electric clipper. Chemical depilation (e.g., with Nair®) should be avoided because of the unknown and poorly studied effect which depilation agents may have on the immune status of the skin.
2. Apply three *non-overlapping* shots on the abdomen of each mouse for each immunization using a helium pressure of 300 psi (*see* **Notes 11** and **12**).

3.4 Malaria Challenge and Testing of Vaccine Efficacy

Note: The recommended challenge protocol is the subcutaneous injection of purified sporozoites. It combines the advantages of the needle-based challenge (simplicity) with the relevance of the mosquito-bite challenge (delivery of sporozoites into the skin). Although the challenge by an infectious mosquito bite is the most relevant method to test the efficacy of a malaria vaccine candidate, it is laborious and logistically challenging. The intravenous injection of sporozoites is not recommended since the route of delivery is highly artificial, carrying the risk of misjudging the efficacy of pre-erythrocytic vaccines as humoral immune mechanisms are bypassed.

1. Prepare Ozaki tubes [21] as follows:
   (a) Puncture the bottom of a siliconized 0.5 ml microfuge tube with a hot 20-gauge hypodermic needle;
   (b) Plug the hole with balled-up glass wool the size of a pin head (used as a filter to capture mosquito debris);
   (c) Place the Ozaki tube into a 1.5 ml siliconized tube.
2. Obtain mosquitoes 18–20 days after they have fed on *P. berghei*-infected mice or hamsters. The rating of the mosquitoes is ideally done based on the oocyst count, which is an indication of the mosquitoes' infectivity rate and the sporozoite burden in the salivary gland.
3. Kill mosquitoes by quickly submersing them in 70 % Ethanol (*see* **Note 13**), then transfer mosquitoes to dissection medium.
4. Remove mosquitoes from the liquid by pouring them onto a glass plate or petri dish. Pull head from thorax using a scalpel. Collect mosquito heads and thoraces in Ozaki tubes (*see* **Notes 14** and **15**).
5. Spin Ozaki tubes at 8,000 × *g* for 1 min at RT.
6. Remove Ozaki tube from receptacle tube. Resuspend the pellet (i.e., isolated sporozoites) with the liquid in the receptacle tube and transfer the suspension into a fresh siliconized microfuge tube (collection tube).
7. Return Ozaki tube to receptacle tube, add 100 ml dissection medium, and repeat **steps 5** and **6** two more times.
8. Pool the suspensions from all three centrifugation (wash-) steps, and mix gently. Remove aliquot for cell counting.
9. Load hemocytometer with an aliquot of sporozoite suspension, and wait 5 min until the parasites have settled before counting.
10. Count sporozoites at 200–400× magnification using a phase-contrast objective.
11. Adjust the concentration of sporozoites so that 100 μl of RPMI-1640 with 10 % mouse serum contain the sporozoites required to challenge one mouse (*see* **Note 16**).

12. Inject sporozoites subcutaneously with a 27-gauge needle into the left and right inguinal region of the mouse dispensing 50 μl per side. Raise a skin-flap when injecting to assure subcutaneous (not intramuscular or intraperitoneal) delivery.
13. Seven and fourteen days after challenge, prepare blood smears by cutting the very tip of the mouse's tail with surgical scissors. Only mice without blood parasitemia on day 14 are scored as sterilely protected.
14. Spot blood onto microscopic slide and prepare a thin blood smear.
15. Air-dry slides, then fix smears by submerging the slides in methanol.
16. Transfer slides into a 10 % Giemsa solution and stain for 15 min at RT.
17. Remove slides from the glass trough, and differentiate the staining by immersing the slides in water.
18. Air-dry slides, then evaluate blood smears microscopically at 1,000× magnification (*see* **Note 17**).
19. Calculate vaccine efficacy (*see* **Note 18**).

4 Notes

1. Gold aliquots (30 mg/microcentrifuge tube) can be stored alone (at RT) or frozen together with spermidine (100 μl/tube).
2. Spermidine deaminates over time. Therefore, it is important to store aliquots in the freezer and to avoid repeated thawing (i.e., store small aliquots in microcentrifuge tubes).
3. $CaCl_2$ is used to precipitate plasmid onto gold particles. Aliquots of stock solution (1 M) can be stored at room temperature or frozen. Calcium chloride is an irritant and eye protection should be worn when handling.
4. Anhydrous (100 %; 200 proof) ethanol is used to wash the plasmid-coated gold particles. Contaminating water interferes with plasmid binding and coating of the Tefzel® tubing with the gold particles. It is essential to keep the ethanol water-free; it should not be cooled for use. Although this enhances its ability to precipitate DNA it leads to condensation. Ethanol bottles should only be opened for brief periods of time and ethanol from bottles, which had previously been used multiple times, should not be used to prepare the final gold slurry, but only for washing of the formulated gold (protocol Subheading 3.1, **step 8**).

5. ETFE (Tefzel®) tubing is specifically pre-treated Ethylene Tetrafluoroethylene tubing and can be purchased from Bio-Rad. Untreated tubing may not allow proper coating of the tubing with the gold slurry.
6. Compressed nitrogen should have a purity grade of >4.5 (i.e., 99.995 %) and a maximum pressure of 2,600 psi, using a single-stage, low-pressure nitrogen tank regulator (final pressure between 30 and 50 psi).
7. High-quality plasmid is isolated most effectively using the EndoFree plasmid kit from Qiagen (Plasmid Maxi Kit). This will assure efficient removal of endotoxin derived from the recombinant bacteria used for plasmid production. If cesium chloride gradient centrifugation is used for plasmid purification, an additional (potential) contaminant is $CsCl_2$, which needs to be removed from the final plasmid preparation. Various commercially available mammalian expression vectors have successfully been used to deliver malaria antigens such as pCI (Promega) and pcDNA3 (Invitrogen). More recent plasmids designed for use in humans lack antibiotic resistance genes. For the proper choice and purification of plasmids used for immunization, *see* [22]. Prior to using newly generated constructs for immunizations it is essential to perform in vitro transfections e.g., cells that are easy to transfectable such as BHK cells are recommended [23, 24] to determine (a) the quality of the resulting protein product (i.e., appropriate length and absence of truncated protein; recognition by specific antibodies) and (b) the effect of the protein on the viability of the transfected cells. For example, the circumsporozoite protein antigen contains a ribosome-binding motif and, therefore, interferes with protein biosynthesis in experimentally transfected or naturally infected cells, which results in host cell-apoptosis. Analyzing both transfected cells and culture supernatant of transfected cells (by Western Blotting) reveals whether the plasmid-encoded protein is secreted or retained in the transfected cell. Cytoplasmic accumulation of protein could be due to the lack of appropriate secretion sequences or unique properties of the protein such as the presence of protozoan GPI-anchor sequences, which result in cytoplasmic retention thus altering the immunogenicity of the protein [25, 26].
8. The quality of the mouse serum used for the parasite resuspension-medium is crucial when performing subcutaneous (s.c.) or intradermal (i.d.) challenges. We have noticed that using medium with freshly (i.e., same day) obtained serum (harvested through cardiac puncture of designated donor mice, ideally litter mates of immunized mice) yielded sporozoites that had the highest functional activity as measured by sporozoite motility assays as well as the number of successful challenges.

Avoid using previously frozen mouse serum or serum that had been stored in the refrigerator for extended periods of time.

9. Reported bead loading rates range from 0.1 to 5 μg DNA per mg of gold beads. The "standard" bead loading rate, routinely used for malaria studies, is 2 μg plasmid DNA/mg gold resulting in Tefzel® cartridges, which deliver a calculated amounts of 0.5 mg gold coated with 1 μg DNA per "shot". At this bead loading rate, the surface of the gold particles is only partially coated with DNA and, therefore, the bead loading rate can be increased up to tenfold. However, increasing the bead loading rate also increases clumping of the gold, which results in poor coating of the Tefzel® cartridges and thus variable and inadequate delivery of gold particles during immunization. Increasing the amount of plasmid encoding the vaccine (i.e., antigen of interest) is not advisable since it does not appear to increase vaccine efficacy. The proposed bead loading rate for the plasmid encoding the (primary) malaria antigen leaves sufficient capacity for co-delivered plasmids (i.e., plasmids encoding additional pathogen-derived antigens or molecular adjuvants). Co-delivered plasmids should not exclusively be tested at a 1:1 ratio, but titration experiments should be conducted to determine the most effective ratio. Higher doses of co-delivered pro-apoptotic molecules to increase immunogenicity result in premature host cell death and thereby reduce the immunogenicity of the vaccine [27, 28]. The co-delivery of large amounts of helper-antigens (designed to trigger a "bystander" CD4 helper response) can lead to immunodominance of the helper antigen thus not providing the desired adjuvant effect [18]. However, gene gun vaccination permits the rapid and straight-forward comparison of multiple ratios of antigen–molecular adjuvant without the need for cloning different plasmids. The same is true for the co-delivery of multiple plasmids encoding different malaria antigens.

10. Adding polyvinylpyrrolidone (PVP) to the gold slurry as described in other gene gun protocols is not recommended. PVP is an adhesive used to facilitate the binding of gold particles to the Tefzel® tubing, but particularly at lower (i.e., 300 psi) helium pressure used for vaccine delivery, it can cause retention of some gold in the tubing and therefore, inadequate immunization.

11. Note that *Plasmodium* parasites are highly sensitive to innate immune responses [29]. The duration of the innate immune responses following vaccination is determined by the type of vaccine, the delivery method, as well as adjuvant used. Factors such as the amount of plasmid delivered or the type of plasmid used further contribute to the adjuvanticity of DNA vaccines. Therefore, it is imperative to include relevant vector controls

in the immunization experiment to control for innate protection against infection. If animals immunized with vector controls cannot be infected reliably with *Plasmodium*, the interval between the last immunization and the challenge has to be extended. For some malaria antigens, the interval between the last immunization and challenge also determines the durability of the protective immune response with short intervals resulting in only transient protection. Therefore, when testing the protective efficacy of any malaria vaccine, it is advisable to (a) explore different intervals between the last immunization and the parasite challenge and (b) rechallenge protected animals to determine the durability of the immune protection since the first exposure to the parasites may have resulted in the editing of the protective response and thus loss of protection [24, 30].

12. Before discarding spent cartridges, check for residual gold in the tubing. Retention of gold in the spent cartridge is rare when no PVP had been used (*see* **Note 10**). If excessive amounts of gold are left in the cartridge after a shot, the helium pressure used to deliver the gold particles may be too low. However, before simply increasing the pressure, consider that this will alter the depth of tissue penetration of the gold particles, which is determined by both gas pressure and size of gold particles. If using gold particles of different sizes than recommended, it is advisable to determine the location of the gene gun-delivered gold (using several pressure settings) by conventional histology of the targeted skin to assure their presence in the epidermis. Before using the gene gun for the first time consult the manufacturer's manual to assure that the helium pressure used does not exceed the maximum pressure for the specific type of gun.
13. The time the infectious mosquitoes spend in 70 % ethanol before harvesting sporozoites should be minimized. Diffusion of the alcohol into the tissue ultimately kills the parasites, so it is imperative to work quickly at this stage.
14. Assure that the mosquito parts do not dry up since this will greatly affect the viability of the sporozoites. One Ozaki tube can be filled with material derived from as many as 100 mosquitoes.
15. Alternatively, sporozoites can be obtained by carefully removing the heads from the mosquitoes and slowly pulling out the attached salivary glands. These salivary glands are spun down in siliconized microfuge tubes. This method will yield the highest purity of sporozoites, but requires a significant amount of practice and skill. The Ozaki method is more popular because of its ease of use and high yields.

16. The dose of sporozoites required for a reliable infection of 90 % of control animals depends on the mouse strain [31]. BALB/c exhibit inherent resistance to *P. berghei* and, therefore, require 3,000–4,000 sporozoites to become infected while C57BL6 mice can be reliably challenged with as few as 300 sporozoites. Outbred mice such as the CD-1 or AJ-mice require very high doses (12,000 sporozoites/mouse).
17. To reliably determine the absence of blood-stage parasites (i.e., to be able to conclude that a mouse is sterilely protected); at least 20 microscopic fields have to be evaluated.
18. Formula to calculate vaccine efficacy:

$$1-(I_v / I_c)$$

where I_v and I_c are the % infected animals in vaccinated and control plasmid groups, respectively.

For the statistical analysis of the results, the Fisher's Exact Test is appropriate.

Disclaimer

The opinions or assertions contained herein are the private views of the authors, and are not to be construed as official, or as reflecting true views of the Department of the Army, the Department of Defense, or the Department of Health and Human Services.

References

1. Donnelly JJ et al (1997) DNA vaccines. Annu Rev Immunol 15:617–648
2. Kopycinski J et al (2012) A DNA-based candidate HIV vaccine delivered via in vivo electroporation induces CD4 responses toward the alpha4beta7-binding V2 loop of HIV gp120 in healthy volunteers. Clin Vaccine Immunol 19(9):1557–1559
3. Ferraro B et al (2011) Clinical applications of DNA vaccines: current progress. Clin Infect Dis 53(3):296–302
4. Ledgerwood JE et al (2012) Influenza virus h5 DNA vaccination is immunogenic by intramuscular and intradermal routes in humans. Clin Vaccine Immunol 19(11):1792–1797
5. Vardas E et al (2012) Indicators of therapeutic effect in FIT-06, a Phase II trial of a DNA vaccine, GTU((R))-Multi-HIVB, in untreated HIV-1 infected subjects. Vaccine 30(27):4046–4054
6. Koup RA et al (2010) Priming immunization with DNA augments immunogenicity of recombinant adenoviral vectors for both HIV-1 specific antibody and T-cell responses. PLoS One 5(2), e9015
7. Diaz CM et al (2013) Phase 1 studies of the safety and immunogenicity of electroporated HER2/CEA DNA vaccine followed by adenoviral boost immunization in patients with solid tumors. J Transl Med 11:62
8. Leitner WW et al (1997) Immune responses induced by intramuscular or gene gun injection of protective deoxyribonucleic acid vaccines that express the circumsporozoite protein from Plasmodium berghei malaria parasites. J Immunol 159(12):6112–6119
9. Sedegah M et al (1994) Protection against malaria by immunization with plasmid DNA encoding circumsporozoite protein. Proc Natl Acad Sci U S A 91(21):9866–9870
10. Kumar R et al (2013) Functional evaluation of malaria Pfs25 DNA vaccine by in vivo electroporation in olive baboons. Vaccine 31(31): 3140–3147
11. Ferraro B et al (2013) Inducing humoral and cellular responses to multiple sporozoite and liver-stage malaria antigens using exogenous plasmid DNA. Infect Immun 81(10): 3709–3720

12. Walsh DS et al (2006) Heterologous prime-boost immunization in rhesus macaques by two, optimally spaced particle-mediated epidermal deliveries of Plasmodium falciparum circumsporozoite protein-encoding DNA, followed by intramuscular RTS,S/AS02A. Vaccine 24(19):4167–4178
13. Richie TL et al (2012) Clinical trial in healthy malaria-naive adults to evaluate the safety, tolerability, immunogenicity and efficacy of MuStDO5, a five-gene, sporozoite/hepatic stage Plasmodium falciparum DNA vaccine combined with escalating dose human GM-CSF DNA. Hum Vaccin Immunother 8(11):1564–1584
14. Chuang I et al (2013) DNA prime/Adenovirus boost malaria vaccine encoding P. falciparum CSP and AMA1 induces sterile protection associated with cell-mediated immunity. PLoS One 8(2), e55571
15. Bergmann-Leitner ES, Leitner WW (2013) Improving DNA vaccines against malaria: could immunization by gene gun be the answer? Ther Deliv 4(7):767–770
16. Ledgerwood JE et al (2013) Prime-boost interval matters: a randomized phase 1 study to identify the minimum interval necessary to observe the H5 DNA influenza vaccine priming effect. J Infect Dis 208(3): 418–422
17. Bergmann-Leitner ES, Leitner WW (2013) Gene gun immunization to combat malaria. Methods Mol Biol 940:269–284
18. Leitner WW et al (2009) Enhancement of DNA tumor vaccine efficacy by gene gun-mediated codelivery of threshold amounts of plasmid-encoded helper antigen. Blood 113(1):37–45
19. Loudon PT et al (2010) GM-CSF increases mucosal and systemic immunogenicity of an H1N1 influenza DNA vaccine administered into the epidermis of non-human primates. PLoS One 5(6), e11021
20. Leitner WW et al (2003) Alphavirus-based DNA vaccine breaks immunological tolerance by activating innate antiviral pathways. Nat Med 9(1):33–39
21. Ozaki LS, Gwadz RW, Godson GN (1984) Simple centrifugation method for rapid separation of sporozoites from mosquitoes. J Parasitol 70(5):831–833
22. Mairhofer J, Lara AR (2014) Advances in host and vector development for the production of plasmid DNA vaccines. Methods Mol Biol 1139:505–541
23. Leitner WW et al (2000) Enhancement of tumor-specific immune response with plasmid DNA replicon vectors. Cancer Res 60(1):51–55
24. Bergmann-Leitner ES et al (2005) C3d binding to the circumsporozoite protein carboxy-terminus deviates immunity against malaria. Int Immunol 17(3):245–255
25. Bergmann-Leitner ES et al (2011) Cellular and humoral immune effector mechanisms required for sterile protection against sporozoite challenge induced with the novel malaria vaccine candidate CelTOS. Vaccine 29(35):5940–5949
26. Scheiblhofer S et al (2001) Removal of the circumsporozoite protein (CSP) glycosylphosphatidylinositol signal sequence from a CSP DNA vaccine enhances induction of CSP-specific Th2 type immune responses and improves protection against malaria infection. Eur J Immunol 31(3):692–698
27. Bergmann-Leitner ES et al (2009) Molecular adjuvants for malaria DNA vaccines based on the modulation of host-cell apoptosis. Vaccine 27(41):5700–5708
28. Leitner WW, Restifo NP (2003) DNA vaccines and apoptosis: to kill or not to kill? J Clin Invest 112(1):22–24
29. Smith TG et al (2002) Innate immunity to malaria caused by Plasmodium falciparum. Clin Invest Med 25(6):262–272
30. Bergmann-Leitner ES et al (2007) C3d-defined complement receptor-binding peptide p28 conjugated to circumsporozoite protein provides protection against Plasmodium berghei. Vaccine 25(45):7732–7736
31. Leitner WW, Bergmann-Leitner ES, Angov E (2010) Comparison of Plasmodium berghei challenge models for the evaluation of pre-erythrocytic malaria vaccines and their effect on perceived vaccine efficacy. Malar J 9:145

Index

Ashley M. Vaughan (ed.), *Malaria Vaccines: Methods and Protocols*, Methods in Molecular Biology, vol. 1325, DOI 10.1007/978-1-4939-2815-6, © Springer Science+Business Media New York 2015

I

K

L

M

N

O

P

Q

R

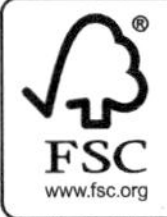

MIX
Papier aus verantwortungsvollen Quellen
Paper from responsible sources
FSC® C105338

If you have any concerns about our products,
you can contact us on
ProductSafety@springernature.com

In case Publisher is established outside the EU,
the EU authorized representative is:
Springer Nature Customer Service Center GmbH
Europaplatz 3, 69115 Heidelberg, Germany

Printed by Libri Plureos GmbH
in Hamburg, Germany